CLINICAL SKILLS FOR OSCEs

Life is short, the art long, opportunity fleeting,

experiment treacherous, judgement difficult.

Hippocrates (c. 460–370 BC). Aphorisms, Aph. 1.

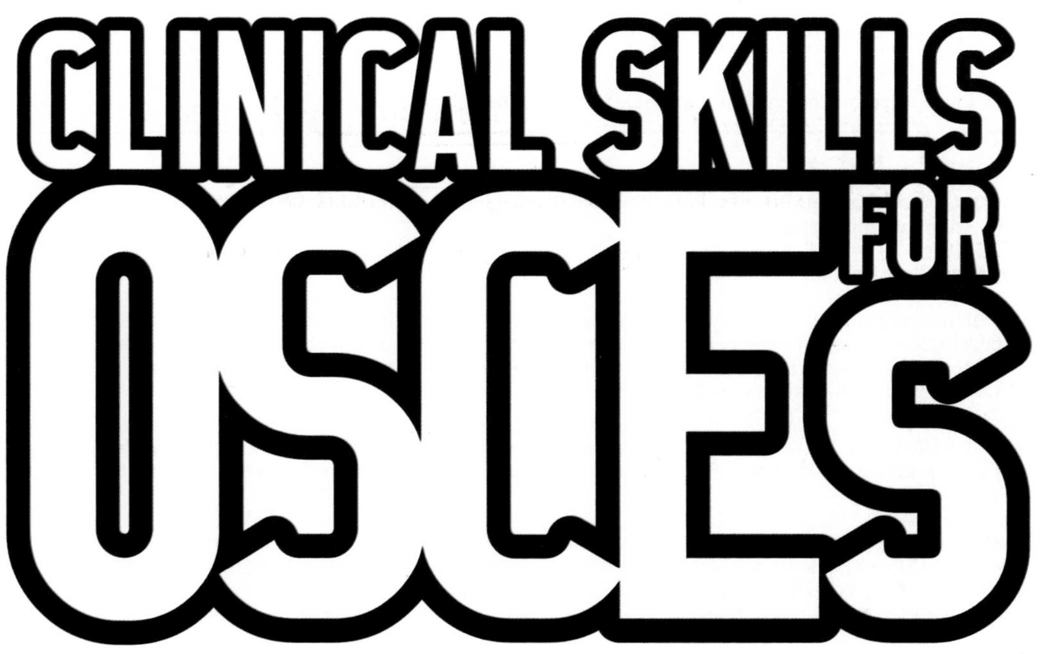

Fourth Edition

Neel Burton
Green Templeton College, University of Oxford

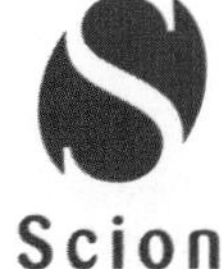
Scion

Fourth edition published in 2011 by Scion Publishing Ltd

ISBN 978 1 904842 82 8

First edition published in 2003 by BIOS Scientific Publishers
Second edition published in 2006 by Informa Healthcare
Third edition published in 2009 by Scion Publishing Ltd

A CIP catalogue record for this book is available from the British Library.

Scion Publishing Limited
The Old Hayloft, Vantage Business Park, Bloxham Road, Banbury, Oxfordshire OX16 9UX
www.scionpublishing.com

Important Note from the Publisher

The information contained within this book was obtained by Scion Publishing Limited from sources believed by us to be reliable. However, while every effort has been made to ensure its accuracy, no responsibility for loss or injury whatsoever occasioned to any person acting or refraining from action as a result of information contained herein can be accepted by the authors or publishers.

Although every effort has been made to ensure that all owners of copyright material have been acknowledged in this publication, we would be pleased to acknowledge in subsequent reprints or editions any omissions brought to our attention.

Readers should remember that medicine is a constantly evolving science and while the authors and publishers have ensured that all dosages, applications and practices are based on current indications, there may be specific practices which differ between communities. You should always follow the guidelines laid down by the manufacturers of specific products and the relevant authorities in the country in which you are practising.

Typeset by Phoenix Photosetting, Chatham, Kent, UK
Printed by Nuffield Press, Abingdon, UK

Contents

IV. NEUROLOGY

V. PSYCHIATRY

VI. ENT, OPHTHALMOLOGY, AND DERMATOLOGY

VII. PAEDIATRICS AND GERIATRICS

VIII. OBSTETRICS, GYNAECOLOGY, AND SEXUAL HEALTH

IX. ORTHOPAEDICS AND RHEUMATOLOGY

X. EMERGENCY MEDICINE AND ANAESTHESIOLOGY

XI. DATA INTERPRETATION

XII. PRESCRIBING AND ADMINISTRATIVE SKILLS

XIII. COMMUNICATION SKILLS

Preface to the Fourth Edition

This fourth edition of CSFO is largely the product of the many comments and suggestions received from students and lecturers over the years, principally from the United Kingdom but also from as far afield as Australia, Japan, and the USA.

For this fourth edition, the text has been rewritten to bring it up to date with current practice and to clear up any remaining grey areas. Detailed descriptions of differentials have been added, and there are more photographs, figures, and boxes and tables than ever before.

More conspicuously, the fourth edition includes a free clinical skills DVD. There is much about clinical skills that cannot be conveyed through the written word and that students find difficult to visualise in their mind's eye. The clinical skills DVD aims to expose you to a range of different clinicians, all performing near the level of the gold standard, and to a range of different patients. For each clinical skill, you should be able to get a feel not only for the steps involved, but also for their orchestration, and for the type of doctor–patient interaction that they call upon. Of course, the DVD cannot feature each and every clinical skill, and priority has been given to those clinical skills that are used most regularly by most junior doctors, and that are most commonly examined in the course of undergraduate medical training. The DVD also includes 100 mock marking schemes for you to practise with in pairs or in small groups.

I hope that CSFO 4e contributes to making you a better doctor and that you invest the time and efforts that it saves you on your outside interests. In the long run, being a good doctor is about being a real person, and only you can teach yourself that.

Neel Burton, Oxford, April 2011

Post-scriptum:
Comments about this book and suggestions for improving it can be made to neelburton@yahoo.com.

Preface to the First Edition

Clinical skills exams, such as Objective Structured Clinical Examinations (OSCEs), are a daunting but essential component of medical undergraduate education.

To prepare for these exams, our generation of medical students had to pull together vast amounts of information from maladapted resources. This tedious and time-consuming process can now be avoided, as all this information has been compiled into this one, handy book.

Indeed, this book covers all the clinical skills that are likely to be tested during the clinical years of a medical course. Although it aims to be comprehensive and detailed, its primary purpose is to be easy to read and to the point. *Clinical Skills for OSCEs* does not attempt to teach its reader medicine or surgery, but rather gathers and organises a large amount of information and presents it in a structured and memorable fashion.

We hope you find *Clinical Skills for OSCEs* useful both for your revision and for the consolidation of skills learnt at the patient's bedside.

Neel L Burton
Akbar H de' Medici
Nicholas C Stacey
London, August 2002

- **Don't panic.** Be philosophical about your exams. Put them into perspective. And remember that as long as you do your bit, you are statistically very unlikely to fail. Book a holiday to a sunny Greek island starting on the day after your exams to help focus your attention.

- **Read the instructions carefully and stick to them.** Sometimes it's just possible to have revised so much that you no longer 'see' the instructions and just fire out the bullet points like an automatic gun. If you forget the instructions or the actor looks at you like Caliban in the mirror, ask to read the instructions again. A related point is this: pay careful attention to the facial expression of the actor or examiner. Just as an ECG monitor provides live indirect feedback on the heart's performance, so the actor or examiner's facial expression provides live indirect feedback on your performance, the only difference being – I'm sure you'll agree – that facial expressions are far easier to read than ECG monitors.

- **Quickly survey the cubicle for the equipment and materials provided.** You can be sure that items such as hand disinfectant, a tendon hammer, a sharps bin, or a box of tissues are not just random objects that the examiner later plans to take home.

- **First impressions count.** You never get a second chance to make a good first impression. As much of your future career depends on it, make sure that you get off to an early start. And who knows? You might even fool yourself.

- **Prefer breadth to depth.** Marks are normally distributed across a number of relevant domains, such that you score more marks for touching upon a large number of domains than for exploring any one domain in great depth. Do this only if you have time, if it seems particularly relevant, or if you are specifically asked. Perhaps ironically, touching upon a large number of domains makes you look more focussed, and thereby safer and more competent.

- **Don't let the examiners put you off or hold you back.** If they are being difficult, that's their problem, not yours. Or at least, it's everyone's problem, not yours. And remember that all that is gold does not glitter; a difficult examiner may be a hidden gem.

- **Be genuine.** This is easier said than done, but then even actors are people. By convincing yourself that the OSCE stations are real situations, you are much more likely to score highly with the actors, if only by 'remembering' to treat them like real patients. This may hand you a merit over a pass and, in borderline situations, a pass over a fail. Although they never seem to think so, students usually fail OSCEs through poor communications skills and lack of empathy, not through lack of studying and poor memory.

- **Enjoy yourself.** After all, you did choose to be there, and you probably chose wisely. If you do badly in one station, try to put it behind you. It's not for nothing that psychiatrists refer to 'repression' as a 'defence mechanism', and a selectively bad memory will do you no end of good.

- **Keep to time but do not appear rushed.** If you don't finish by the first bell, simply tell the examiner what else needs to be said or done, or tell him indirectly by telling the patient, for example, "Can we make another appointment to give us more time to go through your treatment options?" Then summarise and conclude. Students often think that tight protocols impress examiners, but looking slick and natural and handing over some control to the patient is often far more impressive. And probably easier.

- **Be nice to the patient.** Have I already said this? Introduce yourself, shake hands, smile, even joke if it seems appropriate – it makes life easier for everyone, including yourself. Remember to explain everything to the patient as you go along, to ask him about pain before you touch him, and to thank him on the second bell. The patient holds the key to the station, and he may hand it to you on a silver platter if you seem deserving enough. That having been said, if you reach the end of the station and feel that something is amiss, there's no harm in gently reminding him, for example, "Is there anything else that you feel is important but that we haven't had time to talk about?" Nudge-nudge.

- **Take a step back to jump further.** Last minute cramming is not going to magically turn you into a good doctor, so spend the day before the exam relaxing and sharpening your mind. Go to the country, play some sports, rent out a DVD. And make sure that you are tired enough to fall asleep by a reasonable hour.

- **Finally, remember to practise, practise, and practise.** Look at the bright side of things: at least you're not going to be alone, and there are going to be plenty of opportunities for good conversations, good laughs, and good meals. You might even make lifelong friends in the process. And then go off to that Greek island.

Station 1

Hand washing

Hands must be washed before every episode of care that involves direct contact with a patient's skin, their food or medication, invasive devices, or dressings, and after any activity or contact that potentially contaminates the hands.

The procedure

- Remove your watch and any jewellery that you may be wearing, or indicate that you would do so.
- Roll up your sleeves.
- Turn on the hot and cold taps with your elbows and wait until the water is warm.
- Thoroughly wet your hands.
- Apply liquid soap or disinfectant from the dispenser. Liquid soap is used in most hospital situations. Disinfectants include aqueous chlorhexidine ('Hibiscrub') and povidone iodine ('Betadine'). Alcohol hand rubs offer a practical alternative to liquid soaps and disinfectants, but simple soap bars should be avoided.
- Wash your hands using the Ayliffe hand washing technique (see *Figure 1* overleaf):
  ① palm to palm
  ② right palm over left dorsum and left palm over right dorsum
  ③ palm to palm with fingers interlaced
  ④ back of fingers to opposing palms with fingers interlocked
  ⑤ rotational rubbing of right thumb clasped in left palm and left thumb clasped in right palm
  ⑥ rotational rubbing, backwards and forwards, with clasped fingers of right hand in left palm and clasped fingers of left hand in right palm.
- Rinse your hands thoroughly.
- Turn the taps off with your elbows.
- Dry your hands with a paper towel and discard it in the foot-operated bin, remembering to use the pedal rather than your clean hands!
- Consider applying an emollient.

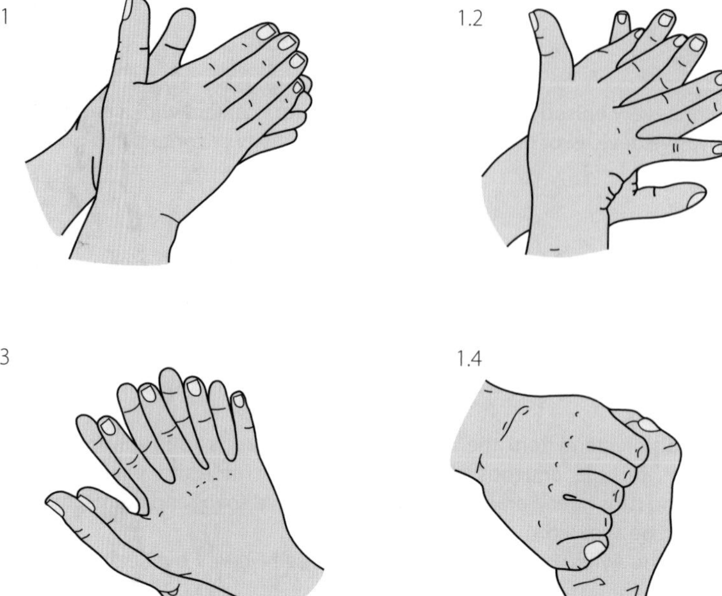

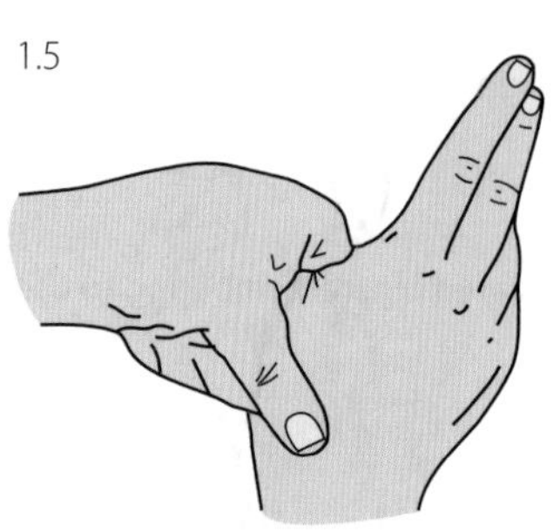

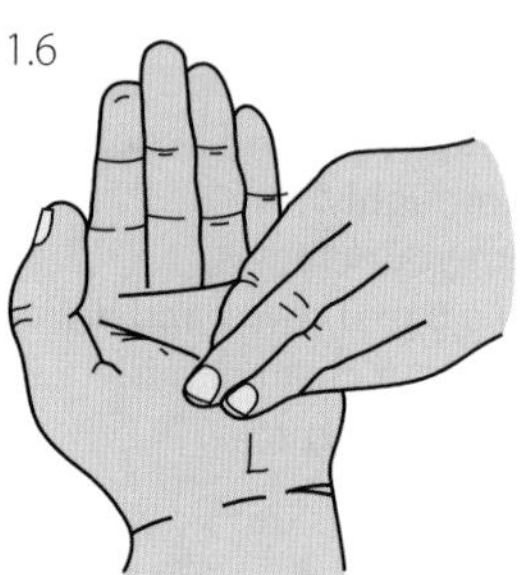

1.5

1.6

Figure 1. Ayliffe hand washing technique:

1.1 Palm to palm
1.2 Right palm over left dorsum and left palm over right dorsum
1.3 Palm to palm fingers interlaced
1.4 Backs of fingers to opposing palms with fingers interlocked
1.5 Rotational rubbing of right thumb clasped in left palm and vice versa
1.6 Rotational rubbing, backwards and forwards with clasped fingers of right hand in left palm and vice versa

Scrubbing up for theatre

The equipment	
• Scrubs. • Clogs or plastic overshoes. • Theatre cap. • Face mask.	• Sterile gown pack. • Sterile gloves. • Brush packet containing a nail brush and nail pick.

Before handwashing

State that you would:

- Change into scrubs.
- Put on clogs or plastic overshoes.
- Don a theatre cap, tucking all your hair underneath it.
- Remove all items of jewellery, including your watch.
- Enter the scrubbing room.
- Put on a face mask, and ensure that it covers both your nose and mouth.
- Open a sterile gown pack *without touching the gown*.
- Lay out a pair of sterile gloves *without touching the gloves*.

Handwashing

- Open a brush packet containing a nail brush and nail pick.
- Turn on the hot and cold taps and wait until the water is warm.

From here on, keep your hands above your elbows at all times.

The social wash

- Wash your hands with liquid disinfectant, either chlorhexidine ('Hibiscrub') or povidone iodine ('Betadine'), lathering up your arms to 2 cm above the elbows.

The second wash

- Use the nail pick from the brush packet to clean under your fingernails.
- Dispense soap on to the sponge side of the brush and use the sponge to scrub from your fingertips to 2 cm above your elbows (30 seconds per arm).

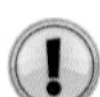

Dispense soap using your elbow or a foot pedal, not your hands.

- To rinse, start from your hands and move down to your elbows so that the rinse water does not re-contaminate your hands.

The third wash

- Using the brush side of the brush, scrub your fingernails (30 seconds per arm).
- Using the sponge side of the brush, scrub:
  - each finger and interdigital space in turn (30 seconds per arm)

- the palm and back of your hands (30 seconds per arm)
- your forearms, moving up circumferentially to 2 cm above your elbows (30 seconds per arm)

Remember to keep the brush well-soaped at all times.

- To rinse, start from your hands and move down to your elbows.
- Turn the taps off with your elbows.

After handwashing

- Use the towels in the gown pack to dry your arms from the fingertips down.
- Pick up the gown from the inside and shake it open, ensuring that it does not touch anything.
- Put your arms through the sleeves, but do not put your hands through the cuffs.
- Put on the gloves without touching the outside of the gloves. Practise this – it's not easy!
- Ask an assistant to tie up the gown for you.

After scrubbing up, keep your hands in front of your chest and do not touch any non-sterile areas, including your mask and hat.

Station 3 DVD

Venepuncture/phlebotomy

Specifications: The station consists of an anatomical arm and all the equipment that might be required. Assume that the anatomical arm is a patient and take blood from it.

Before starting

- Introduce yourself to the patient.
- Explain the procedure and ask for his consent to carry it out. For example, *"I would like to take a blood sample from you to check how your kidneys are working. This is a quick, simple, and routine procedure which involves inserting a small needle into one of the veins on your arm. You will feel a sharp scratch when the needle is inserted, and there may be a little bit of bleeding afterwards. Do you have any questions?"*.
- Ask him which arm he prefers to have blood taken from.
- Ask him to expose this arm.
- Gather the equipment in a tray.

The equipment

In a tray, gather:

- A pair of non-sterile gloves.
- A tourniquet.
- Alcohol wipes.
- A 21G (green) needle and Vacutainer holder.
- The bottles appropriate for the tests that you are sending for (these vary from hospital to hospital, but are generally yellow for biochemistry, purple for haematology, pink for group and save and crossmatch, blue for clotting, grey for glucose, and black for ESR).
- Cotton wool.

Make sure you have a sharps box close at hand. The key to passing this station is to be seen to be safe.

The procedure

- Wash your hands (see *Station 1*).
- Position the patient so that his arm is fully extended. Ensure that he is comfortable.
- Apply the tourniquet.
- Select a vein by palpation: the bigger and straighter the better. The vein selected is most commonly the median cubital vein in the antecubital fossa.
- Don a pair of non-sterile gloves.
- Clean the venepuncture site using the alcohol sterets. Explain that the alcohol sterets may feel a little cold.
- Once the alcohol has dried off, attach the needle to the Vacutainer holder.
- Tell the patient to expect a 'sharp scratch'.
- Retract the skin to stabilise the vein and insert the needle into the vein.
- Keeping the needle still, place a Vacutainer tube on the needle-holder and let it fill.
- Once all the necessary tubes are filled, release the tourniquet. Remember that the tubes need to be filled in a certain order. See the guide to Vacutainer tubes in *Station 105*.

- Release the tourniquet.
- Remove the needle from the vein and apply pressure on the puncture site.
- Dispose of the needle in the sharps box.
- Remove and dispose of the gloves in the clinical waste bin.

After the procedure

- Ensure that the patient is comfortable.
- Thank the patient.
- Label the tubes (at least: patient's name, date of birth, and hospital number; date and time of blood collection).
- Fill in the blood request form (at least: patient's name, date of birth, and hospital number; date of blood collection; tests required).
- Document the blood tests that have been ordered in the patient's notes.

Examiner's questions

If the veins are not apparent

- Lower the arm over the bedside.
- Ask the patient to exercise his arm by repeatedly clenching his fist.
- Gently tap the venepuncture site with two fingers.
- Apply a warm compress to the venepuncture site.
- Do not cause undue pain to the patient by trying over and over again – call a more experienced colleague instead.
- Use femoral stab as a last resort.

In the event of a needlestick injury

- Encourage bleeding, wash with soap and running water.
- Immediately report the injury to the local Public Health Consultant.
- If there is a significant risk of HIV, post-exposure prophylaxis should be started as soon as possible.
- Fill out an incident form.

For more information on the management of needlestick injury, refer to local or national protocols.

Cannulation and setting up a drip

Specifications: The station is likely to require you either to cannulate an anatomical arm and to put up a drip, or simply to cannulate the anatomical arm. This chapter covers both scenarios.

Before starting

- Introduce yourself to the patient.
- Explain the procedure and ask for his consent to carry it out. For example, *"I would like to insert a thin plastic tube into one of the veins on your arm. The tube will enable you to receive intravenous fluids and prevent you from becoming dehydrated. You may feel a sharp scratch when the tube is inserted. Do you have any questions?"*
- Ask him which arm he would prefer to have the cannula on.
- Ask him to expose this arm.
- Gather the equipment in a tray.

It is important to read the instructions for the station carefully. If, for example, the instructions specify that the patient is under general anaesthesia, you are probably not going to gain any marks for explaining the procedure.

Cannulation only

The equipment

In a tray, gather:

- A pair of non-sterile gloves.
- A tourniquet.
- Alcohol sterets.
- An IV cannula of appropriate size (*Table 1*). Size is primarily determined by the viscosity of the fluid to be infused and the required rate of infusion.
- A pre-filled 5 ml syringe containing saline flush.
- An adhesive plaster.
- A sharps box.

The procedure

- Wash your hands (see *Station 1*).
- Position the patient so that his arm is fully extended. Ensure that he is comfortable.
- Apply the tourniquet.
- Select a vein by palpation: the bigger and straighter the better. Try to avoid the dorsum of the hand and the antecubital fossa.
- Don a pair of non-sterile gloves.
- Clean the skin with an alcohol steret and let it dry.
- Remove the cannula from its packaging and remove its cap.
- Tell the patient to expect a 'sharp scratch'.
- Anchor the vein by stretching the skin and insert the cannula at an angle of approximately 30 degrees.
- Once a flashback is seen, advance the cannula and needle by about 2 mm.
- Pull back slightly on the needle and advance the cannula into the vein.

- Release the tourniquet.
- Press on the vein over the tip of the cannula, remove the needle completely, and immediately put it into the sharps box.
- Cap the cannula.
- Apply the adhesive plaster to fix the cannula.
- Flush the cannula with 5 ml normal saline.

Table 1. IV cannulae

Colour	Size	Water flow (ml/min)*
Blue	22G	33
Pink	20G	54
Green	18G	80
White	17G	125
Grey	16G	180
Orange	14G	270

* Approximate values. According to Poiseuille's Law, the velocity of a Newtonian fluid through a cylindrical tube is directly proportional to the fourth power of its radius.

After the procedure

- Discard any rubbish.
- Ensure that the patient is comfortable.
- Thank the patient.

Cannulation and setting up a drip

The equipment

In a tray, gather:

- A pair of gloves.
- A tourniquet.
- Alcohol sterets.
- An IV cannula of appropriate size.
- An adhesive plaster.
- A sharps box.
- An appropriate fluid bag.
- A giving set.

The procedure

- Check the fluid prescription chart (if appropriate).
- Check the fluid in the bag (solution type and concentration) and its expiry date.
- Remove the fluid bag from its packaging and hang it up on a drip stand.
- Remove the giving set from its packaging. The regulating clamp for the IV line should be closed.
- Remove the protective covering from the exit port at the bottom end of the fluid bag.
- Remove the plastic cover from the large, pointed end of the giving set.
- Drive the large, pointed end of the giving set into the exit port at the bottom end of the fluid bag.
- Remove the protective cap from the other end of the giving set.
- Squeeze and release the collecting chamber of the giving set until it is about half full.
- Open the regulating clamp and run fluid through the giving set to expel any air/bubbles.

- Close the regulating clamp.
- Wash your hands (see *Station 1*).
- Position the patient so that his arm is fully extended. Ensure that he is comfortable.
- Apply the tourniquet.
- Select a vein by palpation: the bigger and straighter the better. Try to avoid the dorsum of the hand and the antecubital fossa.
- Don a pair of non-sterile gloves.
- Clean the skin with an alcohol steret and let it dry.
- Remove the cannula from its packaging and remove its cap.
- Tell the patient to expect a 'sharp scratch'.
- Anchor the vein by stretching the skin and insert the cannula at an angle of approximately 30 degrees.
- Once a flashback is seen, advance the cannula and needle by about 2 mm.
- Pull back slightly on the needle and advance the cannula into the vein.
- Release the tourniquet.
- Press on the vein over the tip of the cannula, remove the needle and immediately put it into the sharps box.
- Cap the cannula.

Indicate that you would:

- Apply the adhesive plaster to fix the cannula.
- Attach the giving set.
- Adjust the drip-rate (1 drop per second is equivalent to about 1 litre per 6 hours).
- Check that there is no swelling of the subcutaneous tissue.
- Tape the tubing to the arm.

After the procedure

- Ensure that the patient is comfortable.
- Thank the patient.
- Discard any rubbish.
- Sign the fluid chart and record the date and time (if appropriate).

Examiner's questions: complications of cannula insertion

- Infiltration of the subcutaneous tissue
- Nerve damage
- Haematoma
- Embolism
- Phlebitis
- Thrombophlebitis
- Septic thrombophlebitis
- Local infection

Blood transfusion

Specifications: This station requires you either to cannulate an anatomical arm and set up a blood transfusion, or, more likely, simply to set up a blood transfusion. You may be instructed to talk through parts of the procedure.

Before starting

- Introduce yourself to the patient.
- Explain the requirement for a blood transfusion and ensure that he is consenting.
- Ensure that baseline observations have been recorded (pulse rate, blood pressure, and temperature).

Cannulation

See *Station 4.*

Blood transfusion

1. Sample collection

- Confirm the patient's name and date of birth and check his identity bracelet.
- Extract 10 ml of blood into a pink tube.
- Immediately label the tube and request form with the patient's identifying data: name, date of birth, and hospital number.
- Fill out a blood transfusion form, specifying the total number of units required.
- Ensure that the tube reaches the laboratory promptly.

2. Blood transfusion prescription

- Prescribe the number of units of blood required in the intravenous infusion section of the patient's prescription chart. Each unit of blood should be prescribed separately and be administered over a period of 4 hours.
- If the patient is elderly or has a history of heart failure, consider prescribing 20 mg of oral frusemide with the second and fourth units of blood.
- Arrange for the blood bag to be delivered. The blood transfusion must start within 30 minutes of the blood leaving the blood refrigerator.

3. Checking procedures

Ask a registered nurse or another doctor to go through the following checking procedures with you:

A. Positively identify the patient by asking him for his name, date of birth, and address.
B. Confirm the patient's identifying data and ensure that they match those on his identity bracelet, case notes, prescription chart, and blood compatibility report.
C. Record the blood group and serial number on the unit of blood and make sure that they match the blood group and serial number on the blood compatibility report and the blood compatibility label attached to the blood unit.
D. Check the expiry date on the unit of blood.
E. Inspect the blood bag for leaks or blood clots or discoloration.

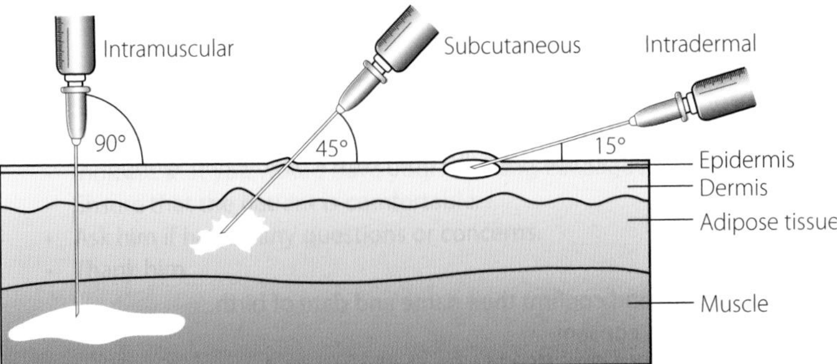

Figure 2. Intramuscular, subcutaneous, and intradermal injection techniques.

the general embarrassment of the thing. In infants and toddlers, the vastus lateralis muscle in the anterolateral aspect of the middle or upper thigh is the preferred IM injection site.

- With your free hand, slightly stretch the skin at the site of injection.
- Introduce the needle at an 80–90 degree angle to the patient's skin in a quick, firm motion.
- Pull on the syringe's plunger to ensure that you have not entered a blood vessel. If you aspirate blood, you need to start again with a new needle, and at a different site.
- Slowly inject the drug and quickly remove the needle.
- Immediately dispose of the needle in the sharps box.
- Apply gentle pressure over the injection site with some cotton wool.
- Remove the gloves.

Subcutaneous injection technique

- Bunch the skin between thumb and forefinger, thereby lifting the adipose tissue from the underlying muscle.
- Insert the needle at a 45 degree angle in a quick, firm motion.
- Release the skin.
- Pull on the syringe's plunger to ensure that you have not entered a blood vessel.
- Slowly inject the drug.
- Dispose of the needle in the sharps box.
- Apply gentle pressure over the injection site with some cotton wool.
- Remove the gloves.

Intradermal injection technique

- Stretch the skin taut between thumb and forefinger.
- Hold the needle so that the bevel is uppermost.
- Insert the needle at a 15 degree angle, almost parallel to the skin.
- Ensure that the needle is visible beneath the surface of the epidermis.
- Slowly inject the drug.
- A visible bleb should form. If not, immediately withdraw the needle and start again.
- Dispose of the needle in the sharps box.
- Remove the gloves.

After the procedure

- Ensure that the patient is comfortable.
- Sign the prescription chart and record the date, time, drug, dose, and injection site of the injection in the medical records.
- Ensure that the patient is comfortable.
- Ask him if he has any questions or concerns.
- Thank him.

Examination of a superficial mass and of lymph nodes

Before starting

- Introduce yourself to the patient.
- If allowed, take a brief history from him, for example, onset, course, effect on everyday life.
- Explain the examination and ask for his consent.
- Ask him to expose the lump completely.
- Position him appropriately and ensure that he is comfortable.

The examination

- Inspect the patient from the end of the bed, looking for other lumps and any other signs.
- Inspect the lump and note its site, colour, and any changes to the overlying skin such as inflammation or tethering. Note also the presence or absence of a punctum.
- Ask the patient if the lump is painful before you palpate it. Is the pain only brought on by palpation or is it a more constant pain?
- Warm your hands.
- Assess the temperature of the lump with the back of your hand.
- Palpate the lump in a rotary motion with the pads of your fingers. Now consider:
  - number: solitary or multiple
  - size: estimate length, width, and height, or use a ruler or measuring tape
  - shape: spherical, ovoid, irregular, other
  - edge: well or poorly defined
  - surface: smooth or irregular
  - consistency: soft, firm, hard, rubbery
  - fluctuance: rest two fingers of your left hand on either side of the lump and press on the lump with the index finger of your right hand: if your left hand fingers are displaced, the lump is fluctuant
  - pulsatility: rest a finger of each hand on either side of the lump: if your fingers are displaced, the lump is pulsatile
  - mobility or fixation both of the overlying skin to the lump, and of the lump to the underlying muscle
  - compressibility and reducibility: press firmly on the lump to see if it disappears; if it immediately reappears, it is compressible; if it only reappears upon standing or coughing, it is reducible
- Percuss the lump for dullness or resonance.
- Auscultate the lump for bruits or bowel sounds.
- Transilluminate the lump by holding it between the fingers of one hand and shining a pen torch to it with the other. A bright red glow indicates fluid whereas a dull or absent glow suggests a solid mass.
- Examine the draining lymph nodes (see further down), or indicate that you would do so.

After examining the lump

- Ask the patient if he has any questions or concerns.
- Thank the patient.
- Summarise your findings and offer a differential diagnosis.
- If appropriate, suggest further investigations, e.g. aspirate, biopsy, ultrasound, CT.

Lymph node examination

Head and neck

The patient should be sitting up and examined from behind. With the fingers of both hands, palpate the submental, submandibular, parotid, and pre- and post-auricular nodes. Next palpate the anterior and posterior cervical nodes and the occipital nodes.

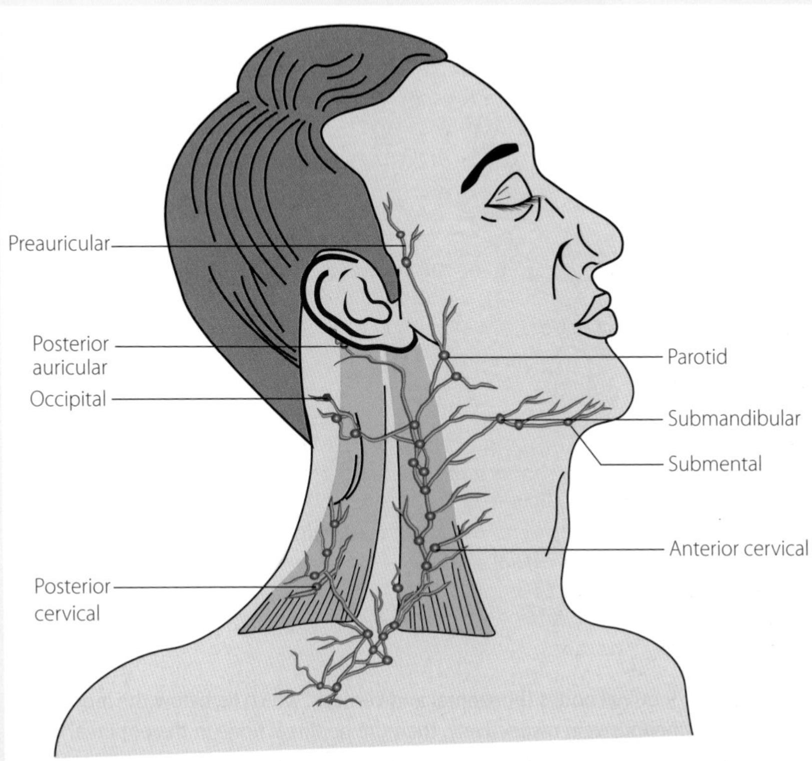

Figure 3. Lymph nodes in the head and neck.

Upper body

- Palpate the supraclavicular and infraclavicular nodes on either side of the clavicle.
- Expose the right axilla by lifting and abducting the arm and supporting it at the wrist with your right hand.
- With your left hand, palpate the following lymph node groups:
  - the apical
  - the anterior
  - the posterior
  - the nodes of the medial aspect of the humerus
- Now expose the left axilla by lifting and abducting the left arm and supporting at the wrist with your left hand.
- With your right hand, palpate the lymph node groups, as listed above.

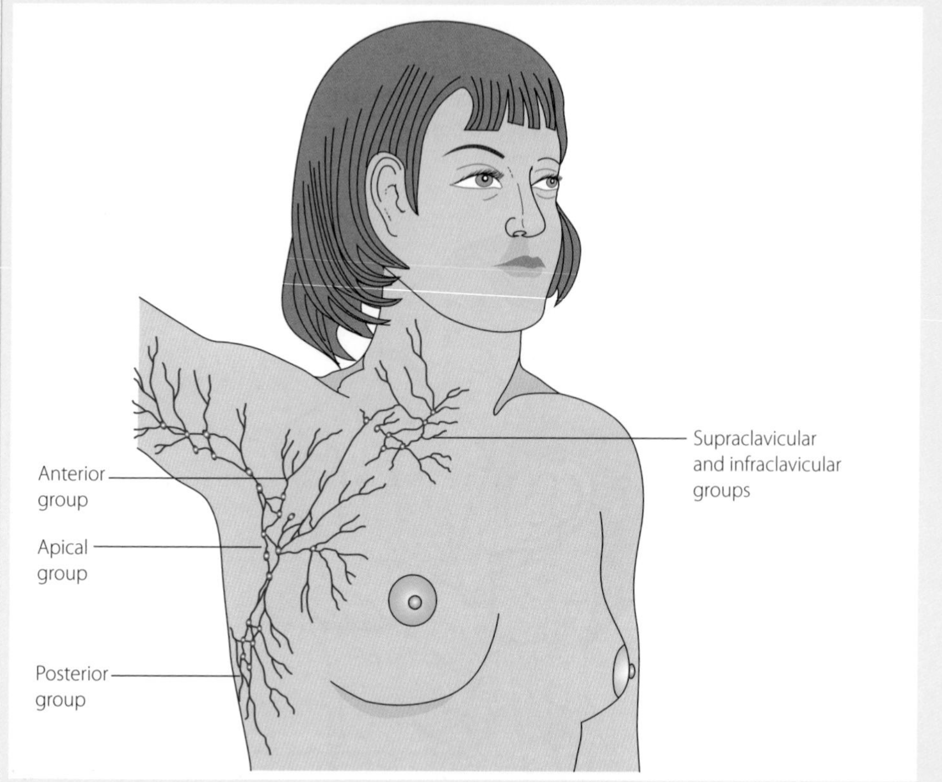

Figure 4. Lymph nodes of the upper body.

Lower body

Palpate the superficial inguinal nodes (horizontal and vertical), which lie below the inguinal ligament and near the great saphenous vein respectively, then the popliteal node in the popliteal fossa.

Common conditions most likely to come up in a lump examination station	
Epidermoid (sebaceous) cyst: • results from obstruction of sebaceous gland • may be red, hot, and tender • spherical, smooth • attached to the skin but not to the underlying muscle • may have a punctum which may exude a cottage cheese discharge	**Fibroma:** • common and benign fibrous tissue tumour • skin-coloured and painless • can be sessile or pedunculated, 'hard' or 'soft' • situated in the skin and so unattached to underlying structures
Lipoma: • common and benign soft tissue tumour • skin-coloured and painless • spherical, soft and sometimes fluctuant • not attached to the skin and therefore mobile and 'slippery'	**Skin abscess:** • collection of pus in the skin • very likely to be red, hot, and tender • may be indurated

Chest pain history

Before starting

- Introduce yourself to the patient.
- Explain that you are going to ask him some questions to uncover the nature of his chest pain, and ask for his consent to do this.
- Ensure that he is comfortable; if not, make sure that he is.

The history

- Name, age, occupation, and ethnic origin.

Presenting complaint and history of presenting complaint

- Ask about the nature of the chest pain. Use open questions and give the patient the time to tell his story. Also remember to be empathetic: chest pain can be a very frightening experience.
- Elicit the patient's ideas and concerns.
- For any pain, determine its:
  - site and radiation (into the jaw, arm, or back)
  - character
  - severity, for example, *"How would you rate the pain on a scale of 1 to 10, with 1 being no pain at all and 10 being the worst pain you have ever experienced?"*
  - onset and progression
  - timing and duration
  - aggravating and alleviating factors (exercise, movement, deep breathing, coughing, cold air, large or spicy meals, alcohol, rest, GTN, sitting up in bed)
  - associated symptoms and signs; ask specifically about sweating, nausea and vomiting, shortness of breath, dizziness, cough, haemoptysis and palpitations
  - effect on everyday life, including exercise tolerance and sleep
- Ask about any previous episodes of chest pain.

Past medical history

- Current, past, and childhood illnesses.
- In particular, ask about coronary heart disease, myocardial infarction, stroke, pneumonia, pulmonary embolism, deep vein thrombosis, hypertension, hyperlipidaemia, diabetes, smoking, alcohol use, and recent long-haul travel.
- Recent trauma or injury.
- Surgery.

Drug history

- Prescribed medication, including the oral contraceptive pill if female.
- Over-the-counter medication.
- Illicit drugs.
- Allergies.

Family history

- Parents, siblings, and children. Ask specifically about heart disease, hypertension, and other heritable cardiovascular risk factors.

Social history

- Employment.
- Housing.
- Hobbies.

After taking the history

- Ask the patient if there is anything else that he might add that you have forgotten to ask. This is an excellent question to ask in clinical practice, and an even better one to ask in exams.
- Thank the patient.
- Summarise your findings and offer a differential diagnosis.
- State that you would like to examine the patient and order some investigations, for example, ECG and chest X-ray, to confirm your diagnosis.

Common conditions most likely to come up in a chest pain history station
Angina: • heavy retrosternal pain which may radiate into the neck or left arm • brought on by effort and relieved by rest and nitrates • risk factors for ischaemic heart disease are likely • a family history of ischaemic heart disease is likely
MI: • pain typically comes on over a few minutes • pain is similar to that of angina but is typically severe, long-lasting (> 20 minutes), and unresponsive to nitrates • often associated with sweating, nausea, and breathlessness • risk factors for ischaemic heart disease are likely • a family history of ischaemic heart disease is likely
Pleuritic pain: • sharp, stabbing, 'catching' pain • may radiate to the back or shoulder • typically aggravated by deep breathing and coughing • can be caused by pleurisy which can occur with pneumonia, pulmonary embolus, and pneumothorax, or by pericarditis which can occur post-MI, in viral infections, and in autoimmune diseases • pleural pain is localised to one side of the chest and is not position dependent • pericardial pain is central and positional, aggravated by lying down and alleviated by sitting up or leaning forward
Pulmonary embolus: • sharp, stabbing pain that is of sudden onset • may be associated with shortness of breath, haemoptysis, and/or pleurisy • typically aggravated by deep breathing and coughing • risk factors such as recent surgery or prolonged bed rest may be present

Gastro-oesophageal reflux disease: • retrosternal burning • clear relationship with food and alcohol, but no relationship with effort • may be associated with odynophagia and nocturnal asthma • aggravated by lying down and alleviated by sitting up and by antacids such as Gaviscon or milk
Musculoskeletal complaint: • may be associated with a history of physical injury or unusual exertion • pain is aggravated by movement, but is not reliably alleviated by rest • the site of the pain is tender to touch
Panic attack: • rapid onset of severe anxiety lasting for about 20–30 minutes • associated with chest tightness and hyperventilation

If you cannot differentiate angina from gastro-oesophageal reflux disease, advise a therapeutic trial of an antacid or a nitrate and/or record an ECG.

Station 10

Cardiovascular risk assessment

Cardiovascular risk factors can usefully be divided into fixed (non-modifiable) and modifiable risk factors. Fixed risk factors include older age, male gender, family history, and a South Asian background. Modifiable risk factors include hypertension, hyperlipidaemia, diabetes, smoking, alcohol, exercise, and stress. Having one or more of these risk factors does not mean that a person is going to develop cardiovascular disease, but merely that he is at increased probability of developing it. Conversely, having no risk factors is not a guarantee that a person is not going to develop cardiovascular disease.

Before starting

- Introduce yourself to the patient.
- Explain that you are going to ask him some questions to assess his risk of cardiovascular disease (coronary heart disease, cerebrovascular disease, vascular disease) and ask for his consent to do this.

Remember to be tactful in your questioning, and to respond sensitively to the patient's ideas and concerns.

The risk assessment

If this information has not already been provided or disclosed, find out the patient's reason for attending. Then note or enquire about:

Fixed risk factors

1. Age.
2. Sex.
3. Ethnic background. People from a South Asian background are at a notably higher risk of cardiovascular disease.
4. Family history. Ask about a family history of cardiovascular disease and risk factors for cardiovascular disease such as hypertension, hyperlipidaemia and diabetes mellitus.

Modifiable risk factors

5. Hypertension. If hypertensive, ask about latest blood pressure measurement, time since first diagnosis, and any medication being taken.
6. Hyperlipidaemia. If hyperlipidaemic, ask about latest serum cholesterol level, time since first diagnosis, and any medication being taken.
7. Diabetes mellitus. If diabetic, ask about medication being taken, level of diabetes control being achieved, time since first diagnosis, and presence of complications.
8. Cigarette smoking. If a smoker or ex-smoker, ask about number of years spent smoking and average number of cigarettes smoked per day. Does the patient also smoke roll-ups and cannabis?
9. Alcohol. Ask about the number of units of alcohol drunk in a day. Note that depending on the amount and type that is drunk, alcohol can be either a protective factor or a risk factor.
10. Lack of exercise. Ask about amount of exercise taken in a day or week. Does the patient walk to work or walk to the shops?
11. Stress. Ask about occupational history and home life.

Table 2. Desirable lipid levels	
Total cholesterol	$\leqslant$ 5.0 mmol/l
LDL cholesterol (fasting)	$<$ 3.0 mmol/l
HDL cholesterol	$\geqslant$ 1.2 mmol/l
Total cholesterol/HDL cholesterol	$\leqslant$ 4.5
Tryglycerides (fasting)	$\leqslant$ 1.5 mmol/l
NB. Patients at high risk of cardiovascular disease should aim for even better than these figures.	

After the assessment

- If you have time, assess the extent of any cardiovascular disease.
- Ask the patient if there is anything he would like to add that you may have forgotten to ask about.
- Give him feedback on his cardiovascular risk (e.g. low, medium, high), and indicate a further course of action if appropriate (e.g. further investigations or further appointment to discuss reducing modifiable risk factors).
- Address any remaining concerns.

Station 11

Blood pressure measurement

Before starting

- Introduce yourself to the patient.
- Explain the procedure and ask for his consent to carry it out.
- Tell him that he might feel some discomfort as the cuff is inflated, and that the blood pressure measurement may have to be repeated.

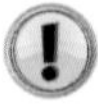

Avoid white coat hypertension by putting the patient at ease. Briefly discuss a non-threatening subject, such as the patient's journey to the clinic, or the weather.

The procedure

- Select an appropriately sized cuff and attach it to the BP machine. This is usually a standard cuff in all but children and the obese.
- Position the BP machine so that it is roughly at the level of the patient's heart.
- Position the vertical column so that it is at the level of your eyes.
- Position the patient's right arm so that it is horizontal at the level of the mid-sternum.
- Locate the brachial artery at about 2 cm above the antecubital fossa.
- Apply the cuff to the arm, ensuring that the arterial point is over the brachial artery.
- Inflate the cuff to 20–30 mmHg higher than the estimated systolic blood pressure. You can estimate the systolic blood pressure by palpating the brachial or radial artery pulse and inflating the cuff until you can no longer feel it.
- Place the stethoscope over the brachial artery pulse, ensuring that it does not touch the cuff.
- Reduce the pressure in the cuff at a rate of 2–3 mmHg.
  - The first consistent Korotkov sounds indicate the systolic blood pressure.
  - The muffling and disappearance of the Korotkov sounds indicate the diastolic blood pressure.
- Record the blood pressure as the systolic reading over the diastolic reading. Do not attempt to 'round off' your readings; to an examiner's ear, 143/88 usually rings more true than 140/90.
- If the blood pressure is higher than 140/90, indicate that you might take a second reading after giving the patient a one minute rest.
- In some situations, it may be appropriate to record the blood pressure in both arms, and also with the patient lying and standing.

After the procedure

- Ensure that the patient is comfortable.
- Tell the patient his blood pressure and explain its significance. Hypertension can only be confirmed by several blood pressure measurements taken over time.
- Thank the patient.
- Document the blood pressure recording in the patient's notes.

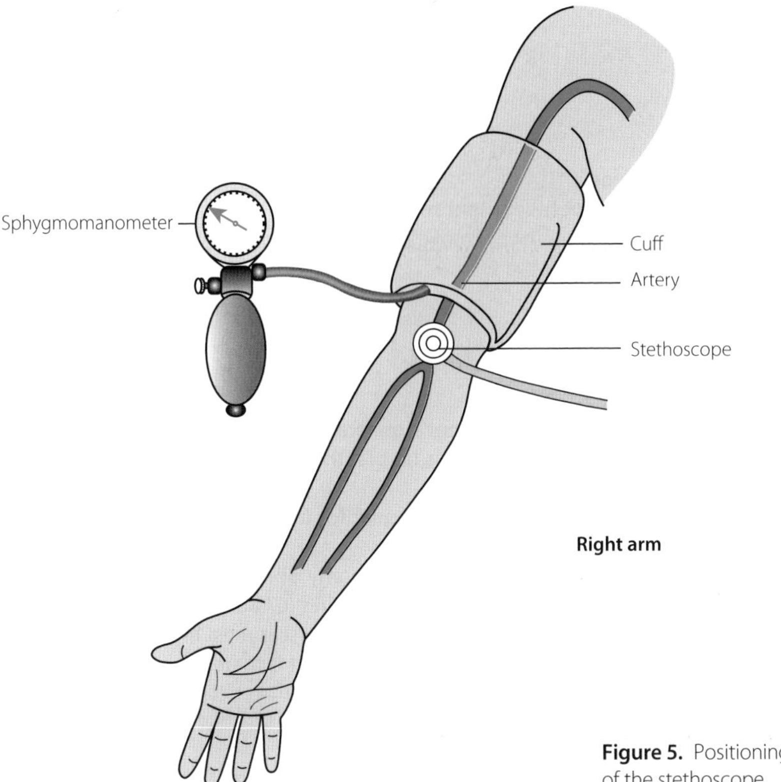

Figure 5. Positioning of the cuff and head of the stethoscope.

Examiner's questions

Causes of secondary hypertension:

- high catecholamines as in phaeochromocytoma
- high glucocorticoids as in Cushing's syndrome
- high mineralocorticoids as in Conn's syndrome
- renal disease
- renal artery stenosis
- coarctation of the aorta
- hyper- or hypo-thyroidism
- parahyperthyroidism
- pre-eclampsia
- illicit drugs

Complications of hypertension:

- cerebrovascular accident (haemorrhage or infarct)
- retinopathy
- ischaemic heart disease
- left ventricular failure
- renal failure

Investigations in hypertension:

- this involves confirming hypertension, assessing for a possible secondary cause, and assessing for end-organ damage (see above)

Cardiovascular examination

Before starting

- Introduce yourself to the patient.
- Explain the examination and ask for his consent to carry it out.
- Position him at 45 degrees, and ask him to remove his top(s).
- Ensure that he is comfortable.

The examination

General inspection

- From the end of the couch, observe the patient's general appearance (age, state of health, nutritional status, and any other obvious signs). Is he breathless or cyanosed? Is he coughing? Does he have the malar flush of mitral stenosis?
- Observe the patient's surroundings, looking in particular for items such as a nitrate spray, an oxygen mask, and IV lines and infusions.
- Inspect the chest for any scars and the precordium for any abnormal pulsation. A median sternotomy scar could indicate coronary artery bypass grafting (CABG), valve repair or replacement, or the repair of a congenital defect. A left submammary scar most likely indicates repair or replacement of the mitral valve. Do not miss a pacemaker if it is there!

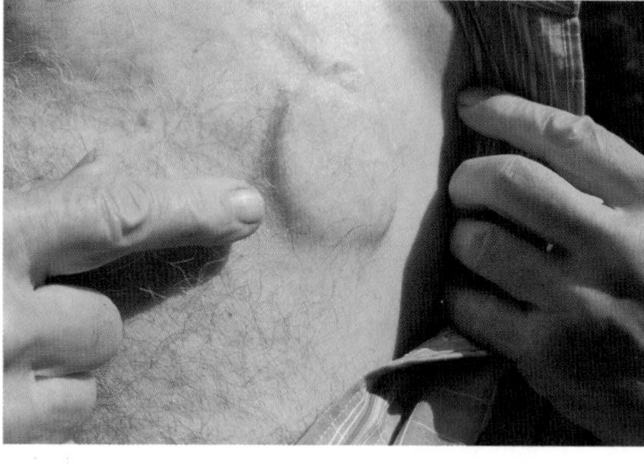

Figure 6. Pacemakers can be visible from outside the body.

Reproduced with permission from Julia Freeman-Woolpert (www.sxc.hu/profile/juliaf).

Inspection and examination of the hands

- Take both hands noting:
  - temperature
  - colour (the blue of peripheral cyanosis and the orange of nicotine stains)
  - nail bed capillary refill time
  - the presence of clubbing (endocarditis, cyanotic congenital heart disease)
  - the presence of Osler nodes and Janeway lesions (subacute infective endocarditis (see *Figure 7*))

  - the presence of splinter haemorrhages (subacute infective endocarditis)
  - the presence of koilonychia or 'spoon nails' (iron deficiency)
- Determine the rate, rhythm, volume, and character of the radial pulse.
- Raise the patient's arm above his head to assess for a collapsing or water hammer pulse (aortic regurgitation). Ask the patient whether he has any shoulder pain first.
- Simultaneously take the pulse in both arms to exclude radio-radial delay (aortic arch aneurysm). Indicate that you would also exclude radio-femoral delay (coarctation of the aorta).
- As you move up the arm, look for bruising, which may indicate that the patient is on an anti-coagulant, and for evidence of intravenous drug use, which is a risk factor for subacute infective endocarditis.
- Indicate that you would like to record the blood pressure (see *Station 11*).

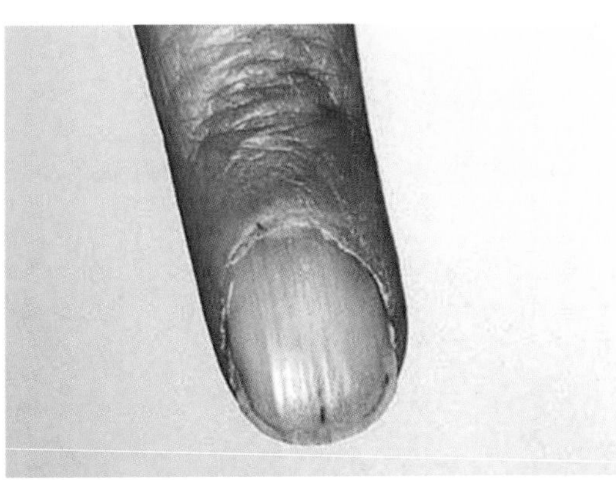

Figure 7. Splinter haemorrhage.

Inspection and examination of the head and neck

- Inspect the eyes, looking for peri-orbital xanthelasma and corneal arcus, both of which indicate hyperlipidaemia
- Gently retract an eyelid and ask the patient to look up. Inspect the conjunctivus for pallor, which is indicative of anaemia.
- Ask the patient to open his mouth, and look for signs of central cyanosis, dehydration, poor dental hygiene (subacute bacterial endocarditis), and a high arched palate (Marfan's syndrome).
- Palpate the carotid artery and assess its volume and character. Never palpate both carotid arteries simultaneously.
- Assess the jugular venous pressure (see *Figure 8*) and, if possible, the jugular venous pulse form: ask the patient to turn his head slightly to one side, and look at the internal vein medial to the clavicular head of sternocleidomastoid. Assuming that the patient is reclining at 45 degrees, the vertical height of the jugular distension from the angle of Louis (sternal angle) should be no greater than 4 cm.

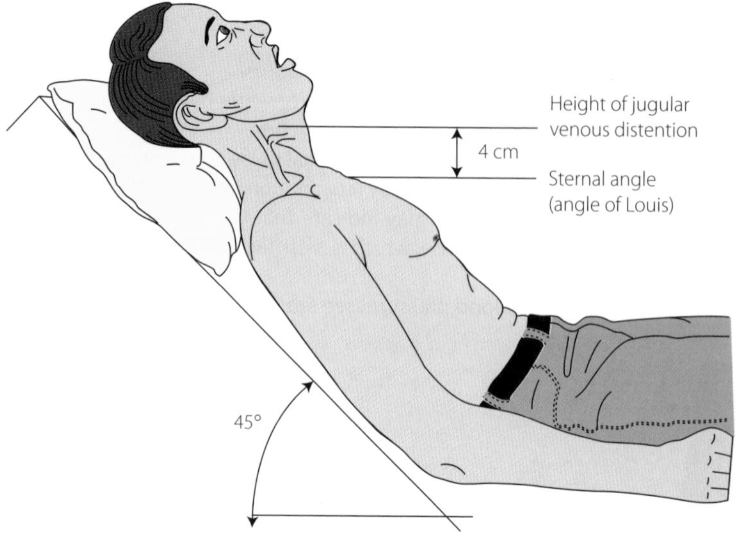

Figure 8. Assessing the jugular venous pressure.

Palpation of the heart

 *Ask the patient if he has any chest pain.*

- Determine the location and character of the apex beat. It is normally located in the fifth intercostal space at the midclavicular line. The apex may be displaced, and it may be 'heaving', suggesting left ventricular hypertrophy, or 'tapping', suggesting mitral stenosis.
- Place the flat of your hands over either side of the sternum and feel for any heaves and thrills. Heaves result from right ventricular hypertrophy (*cor pulmonale*) and thrills result from transmitted murmurs.

Auscultation of the heart

- Listen for heart sounds, additional sounds, murmurs, and pericardial rub. Using the stethoscope's diaphragm, listen in the:
  - *aortic area*
    right second intercostal space near the sternum
  - *pulmonary area*
    left second intercostal space near the sternum
  - *tricuspid area*
    left third, fourth, and fifth intercostal spaces near the sternum
  - *mitral area*
    left fifth intercostal space, in the mid-clavicular line

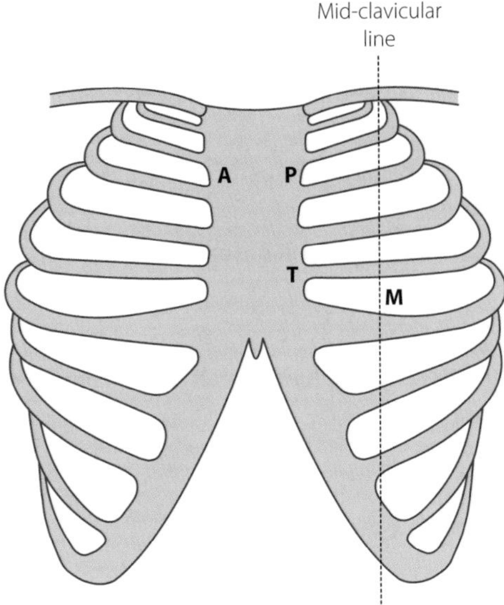

Figure 9. Auscultation points.

- In addition:
  - ask the patient to bend forward and to hold his breath at end-expiration. Using the stethoscope's diaphragm, listen at the left sternal edge in the fourth intercostal space for the mid-diastolic murmur of aortic regurgitation.
  - ask the patient to turn onto his left side and to hold his breath at end-expiration. Using the stethoscope's *bell*, listen in the mitral area for the mid-diastolic murmur of mitral stenosis.
  - listen over the carotid arteries for any bruits and the radiation of the murmur of aortic stenosis.
  - listen in the left axilla for the radiation of the murmur of mitral regurgitation.

For any murmur, determine its location and radiation, and its duration and timing in relation to the cardiac cycle. This is best done by palpating the carotid artery to determine the start of systole. Grade the murmur on a scale of I to VI according to its intensity (see *Table 3*). Common conditions associated with murmurs are listed in *Table 4*.

Table 3. Grading murmurs	
I	Barely audible murmur
II	Soft and localised murmur
III	Murmur of moderate intensity that is immediately audible
IV	Murmur of loud intensity
V	Murmur of loud intensity with a palpable precordial thrill
VI	As above, except that the murmur is audible even as the stethoscope is lifted from the chest wall

Table 4. Common conditions associated with murmurs

Aortic stenosis	Slow-rising pulse, heaving cardiac apex, mid-systolic murmur best heard in the aortic area and radiating to the carotids and cardiac apex
Mitral regurgitation	Displaced, thrusting cardiac apex, pan-systolic murmur best heard in the mitral area and radiating to the axilla
Aortic regurgitation	Collapsing pulse, thrusting cardiac apex, diastolic murmur best heard at the left sternal edge
Mitral valve prolapse	Mid-systolic click, late-systolic murmur best heard in the mitral area

Chest examination

- Percuss and auscultate the chest, especially at the bases of the lungs. Heart failure can cause pulmonary oedema and pleural effusions.

Abdominal examination

- Palpate the abdomen to exclude ascites and/or hepatomegaly.
- Check for the presence of an aortic aneurysm.
- Ballot the kidneys and listen for any renal artery bruits.

Examination of the ankles and legs

- Inspect the legs for scars that might be indicative of vein harvesting for a CABG.
- Palpate for the 'pitting' oedema of cardiac failure, which in some cases may extend all the way up to the sacrum or even the torso ('anasarca').
- Assess the temperature of the feet, and check the posterior tibial and dorsalis pedis pulses in both feet.

After the examination

- Indicate that you would look at the observation chart, dipstick the urine, examine the retina with an ophthalmoscope and, if appropriate, order some key investigations, e.g. FBC, ECG, CXR, echocardiogram.
- Cover the patient up and ensure that he is comfortable.
- Thank the patient.
- Summarise your findings and offer a differential diagnosis.

Common conditions most likely to come up in a cardiovascular examination station

- Murmurs (see *Table 4*)
- Heart failure
- Median sternotomy scar
- Pacemaker

Peripheral vascular system examination

In this station you may be asked to restrict your examination to the arterial or venous system only. You must therefore be able to separate out the signs for either (see *Table 5*).

Before starting

- Introduce yourself to the patient.
- Explain the examination and ask for his consent to carry it out.
- Ask him to expose his feet and legs and to lie down on the couch.

The examination

Inspection

- Skin changes: pallor, shininess, loss of body hair, *atrophie blanche* (ivory-white areas), haemosiderin pigmentation, inflammation, eczema, lipodermatosclerosis.
- Thickened dystrophic nails.
- Scars.
- Signs of gangrene: blackened skin, nail infection, amputated toes.
- Venous and arterial ulcers. Remember to look in the interdigital spaces.
- Oedema.
- Varicose veins (ask the patient to stand up). Varicose veins are often associated with incompetent valves in the long and short saphenous veins.

Do not make the common mistake of asking the patient to stand up before having examined for varicose veins.

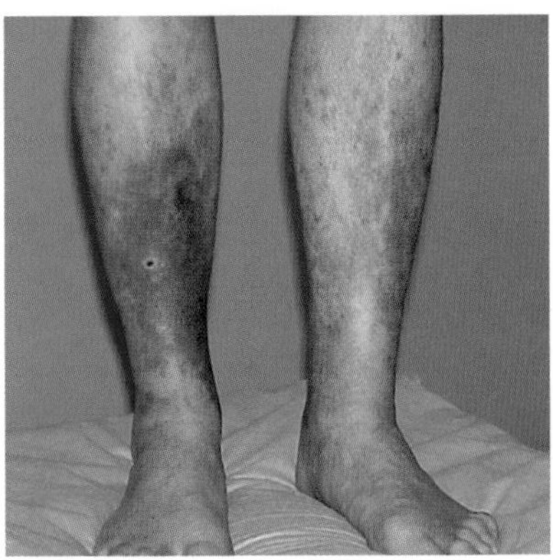

Figure 10. Lipodermatosclerosis describes areas of induration resulting from fibrosis of the subcutaneous fat, and may complicate chronic venous insufficiency.

Reproduced from www.surgicalnotes.co.uk.

Palpation and special tests

- Ask about any pain in the legs and feet.
- Assess skin temperature by running the back of your hand along the leg and the sole of the foot. Compare both legs.
- Capillary refill. Compress a nail bed for 5 seconds and let go. It should take less than 2 seconds for the nail bed to return to its normal colour.

- Peripheral pulses (compare both sides).
- Femoral pulse at the inguinal ligament.
- Popliteal pulse in the popliteal space (flex the knee).
- Posterior tibial pulse behind the medial malleolus.
- *Dorsalis pedis* pulse over the dorsum of the foot, just lateral to the extensor tendon of the great toe.

- Buerger's test:
  - lift both of the patient's legs to a 15 degree angle and note any collapse of the veins ('venous guttering'), which is indicative of arterial insufficiency
  - lift both of the patient's legs up to the point where they turn white (this is Buerger's angle); if there is no arterial insufficiency, the legs will not turn white, not even at a 90 degree angle
  - ask the patient to dangle his legs over the edge of the couch; in chronic limb ischaemia, rather than returning to its normal colour, the skin will slowly turn red like a cooked lobster (reactive hyperaemia)
- Oedema. Firm 'non-pitting' oedema is a sign of chronic venous insufficiency (compare to the 'pitting' oedema of cardiac failure).
- Varicose veins. Tenderness on palpation suggests thrombophlebitis.
- Trendelenburg's test:
  - elevate the leg to 90 degrees to drain the veins of blood
  - occlude the sapheno-femoral junction (SFJ) with two fingers
  - keep your fingers in place and ask the patient to stand up
  - remove your fingers: if the superficial veins refill, this indicates incompetence at the SFJ
- Tourniquet test:
  - elevate the leg to 90 degrees to drain the veins of blood
  - apply a tourniquet to the upper thigh
  - ask the patient to stand up: if the superficial veins below the tourniquet refill, this indicates incompetent perforators below the tourniquet
  - release the tourniquet: sudden additional filling of the veins is a sign of sapheno-femoral incompetence

[Note] The tourniquet test can be repeated further and further down the leg, until the superficial veins below the tourniquet no longer refill.

Auscultation

- Femoral arteries.
- Abdominal aorta.

After the examination

- Thank the patient.
- Ensure that he is comfortable.
- Summarise your findings and offer a differential diagnosis.
- If appropriate, indicate that you might also measure the ABPI and examine the cardiovascular system and abdomen (aortic aneurysm).

Table 5. Examination of the arterial or venous system only	
Arterial system	**Venous system**
Pallor Shininess Dystrophic nails Loss of body hair Arterial ulcers Signs of gangrene Skin temperature Capillary refill Peripheral pulses Buerger's test Auscultation of femoral arteries and aorta ABPI (if time permits, see *Station 14*)	*Atrophie blanche* Pigmentation Inflammation Eczema Lipodermatosclerosis Oedema (non-pitting) Venous ulcers Varicose veins Scars due to varicose vein surgery Trendelenburg test Perthes' test (if after the gold medal)

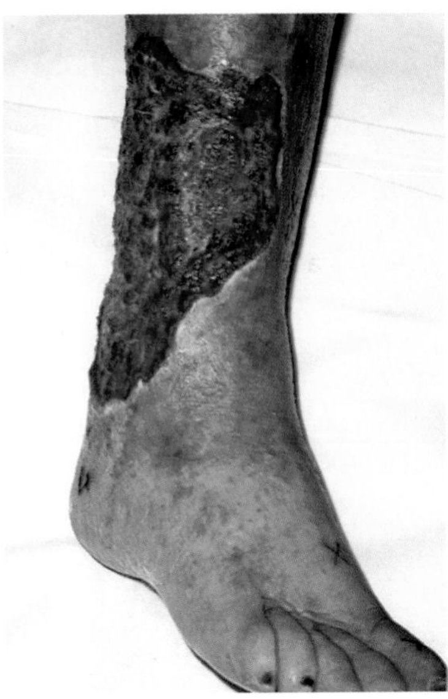

Figure 11. Large venous ulcer. Arterial and neuropathic ulcers tend to be on the sole of the foot and on pressure points, and venous ulcers on the medial and lateral aspects of the leg, above the malleoli.
Reproduced from *BMJ* (2000) **320:** 1589–91, with permission.

Ankle-brachial pressure index (ABPI)

Specifications: You are most likely to be requested to measure the ABPI for one arm and ankle only.

Calculating and interpreting ABPI

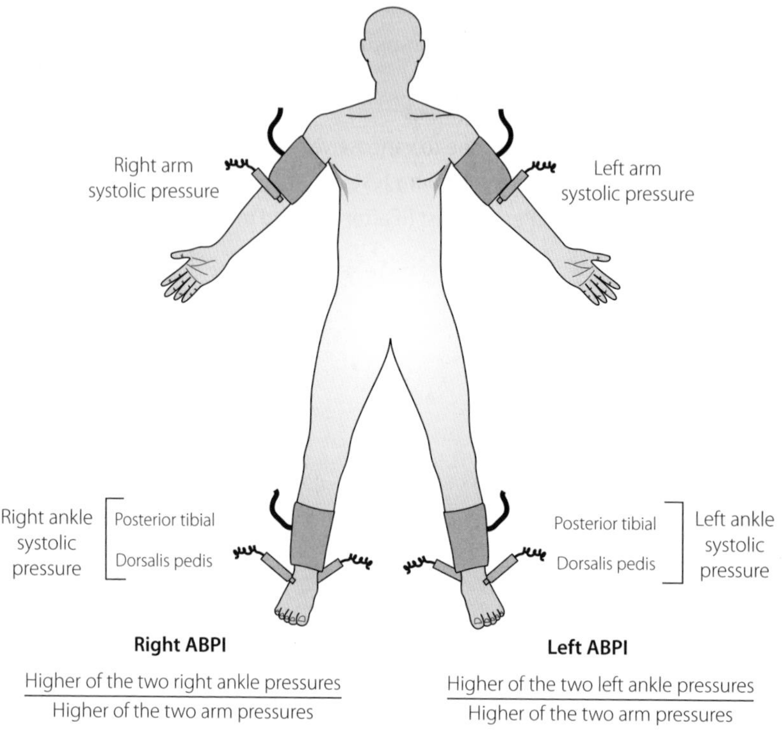

Figure 12. Calculating ABPI.

Table 6. ABPI interpretation

ABPI	Interpretation
> 0.95	Normal
0.5–0.9	Claudication pain
< 0.5	Rest pain
< 0.2	Ulceration and gangrene

Before starting

- Introduce yourself to the patient.
- Explain the procedure and ask him for consent to carry it out.
- Position him at 45° with his sleeves and trousers rolled up.
- Ensure that he is comfortable.
- State that you would allow him 5 minutes resting time before taking measurements.

The procedure

Brachial systolic pressure

- Place an appropriately sized cuff around the arm, as for any blood pressure recording.
- Locate the brachial pulse by palpation and apply contact gel at this site.
- Angle the hand-held Doppler probe at 45° to the skin and locate the best possible signal. Apply only gentle pressure, or else you risk occluding the artery.
- Inflate the cuff until the signal disappears.
- Progressively deflate the cuff and record the pressure at which the signal reappears.
- Repeat the procedure for the other arm or state that you would do so.
- Retain the higher of the two readings.

Take care not to allow the probe to slide away from the line of the artery.

Ankle systolic pressure

- Place an appropriately sized cuff around the ankle immediately above the malleoli.
- Locate the dorsalis pedis pulse by palpation or with the hand-held Doppler probe and apply contact gel at this site.
- Angle the hand-held Doppler probe at 45° to the skin and locate the best possible signal. Apply only gentle pressure, or else you risk occluding the artery.
- Inflate the cuff until the signal disappears.
- Progressively deflate the cuff, and record the pressure at which the signal reappears.
- Repeat the procedure for the posterior tibial pulse, which is posterior and inferior to the medial malleolus.
- Repeat the procedure for the dorsalis pedis and posterior tibial pulses of the other ankle or state that you would do so.
- For each ankle, retain the higher of the two readings.

After the procedure

- Clean the patient's skin of contact gel and allow him time to restore his clothing.
- Clean the hand-held Doppler probe of contact gel.
- Wash your hands.
- Calculate the ABPI and explain its significance to the patient.
- Ask the patient if he has any questions or concerns.
- Thank the patient.

Station 15 DVD

Breathlessness history

Before starting

- Introduce yourself to the patient.
- Explain that you are going to ask him some questions to uncover the nature of his breathlessness, and ask for his consent to do this.
- Ensure that he is comfortable; if not, make sure that he is.

The history

- Name, age, and occupation.

Presenting complaint

- Ask about the nature of the breathlessness. Use open questions.
- Elicit the patient's ideas and concerns.

History of presenting complaint

Ask about:

- Onset, duration, and variability of breathlessness.
- Provoking and relieving factors.
- Severity:
  - exercise tolerance: *"How far can you walk before you get breathless? How far could you walk before?"*
  - sleep disturbance: *"Do you get more breathless when you lie down? How many pillows do you use?"*
  - paroxysmal nocturnal dyspnoea: *"Do you wake up in the middle of the night feeling breathless?"*
- Associated symptoms (wheeze, cough, sputum, haemoptysis, fever, night sweats, anorexia, loss of weight, lethargy, chest pain, dizziness, pedal oedema).
- Effect on everyday life.
- Previous episodes of breathlessness.
- Smoking and alcohol.

Past medical history

- Current, past, and childhood illnesses. Ask specifically about atopy (asthma/eczema/hay fever), PE/DVT, pneumonia, bronchitis, and tuberculosis.
- Previous investigations (e.g. bronchoscopy, chest X-ray).
- Surgery.

Drug history

- Prescribed medication (especially bronchodilators, NSAIDs, β-blockers, ACE inhibitors, amiodarone, and steroids).
- Over-the-counter medication.
- Recreational drugs.
- Allergies.

Family history

- Parents, siblings, and children. Focus especially on respiratory diseases such as atopy, cystic fibrosis, tuberculosis, and emphysema (α1-antitrypsin deficiency).

Social history

- Long-haul travel.
- Exposure to tuberculosis.
- Contact with asbestos.
- Contact with work-place allergens involved in, for example, baking, soldering, spray painting.
- Contact with animals, especially cats and dogs, pigeons and budgerigars.

After taking the history

- Ask the patient if there is anything else he might add that you have forgotten to ask.
- Thank the patient.
- Summarise your findings and offer a differential diagnosis.
- State that you would like to examine the patient and carry out some investigations to confirm your diagnosis.

Common conditions most likely to come up in a breathlessness history station

Asthma:

- breathlessness, chest tightness, wheezing and coughing
- symptoms worse at night and in the early morning, and exacerbated by irritants, cold air, exercise, and emotion
- symptoms respond to bronchodilators
- there may be a history and family history of atopy

Chronic obstructive pulmonary disease:

- breathlessness, cough, wheeze
- chronic progressive disorder characterised by fixed or only partially reversible airway obstruction (cf. asthma)
- history of smoking

Pneumonia:

- breathlessness accompanied by fever, cough, and yellow sputum, and in some cases by haemoptysis and pleuritic chest pain

Tuberculosis:

- breathlessness, cough, haemoptysis, weight loss, malaise, fever, night sweats, pleural pain, symptoms of extrapulmonary disease
- more likely in certain high-risk groups such as immigrants, the homeless and the immunocompromised

Pulmonary embolism:

- breathlessness, sometimes with pleural pain and haemoptysis
- there may be predisposing factors such as recent surgery, immobility, or long-haul travel

Lung cancer:

- symptoms may include breathlessness, stridor, cough, haemoptysis, anorexia, weight loss, lethargy, pleural pain, hoarseness, Horner's syndrome, effects of distant metastases
- history of smoking in most cases

Heart failure:

- left ventricular failure leads to pulmonary oedema
- symptoms include breathlessness, orthopnoea, paroxysmal nocturnal dyspnoea, pedal oedema
- there is a cough which produces pink frothy sputum

Panic attack:

- rapid onset of severe anxiety lasting for about 20–30 minutes
- associated with chest tightness and hyperventilation

Respiratory system examination

Before starting

- Introduce yourself to the patient.
- Explain the examination and ask for his consent to carry it out.
- Position him at 45°, and ask him to remove his top(s).
- Ask him if he is in any pain or distress and ensure that he is comfortable.

The examination

General inspection

- From the end of the couch, observe the patient's general appearance (age, state of health, nutritional status, and any other obvious signs). In particular, is he visibly breathless or cyanosed? Does he have to sit up to breathe? Is his breathing audible? Are there any added sounds (cough, wheeze, stridor)?
- Note:
  - the rate, depth, and regularity of his breathing
  - any deformities of the chest (barrel chest, *pectus excavatum, pectus carinatum*) and spine
  - any asymmetry of chest expansion
  - the use of accessory muscles of respiration
  - the presence of operative scars, including in the axillae and around the back
- Next observe the surroundings. Is the patient on oxygen? If so, note the device (see *Tables 39* and *40* in *Station 107*), the concentration, and the flow rate. Look in particular for inhalers, nebulisers, peak flow meters, intravenous lines and infusions, and chest drains. If there is a sputum pot, make sure to inspect its contents.

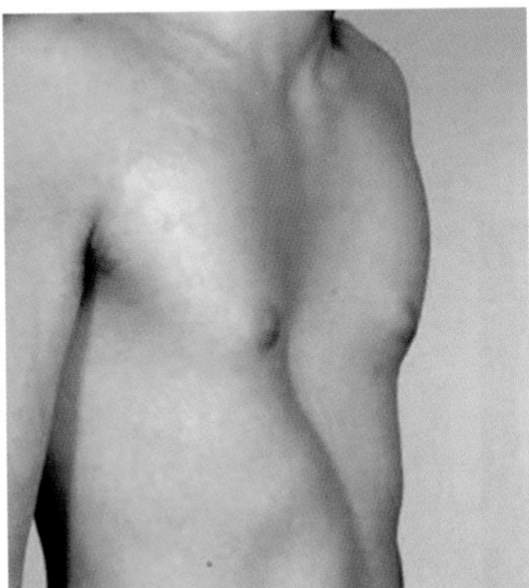

Figure 13. Respiratory system examination: *pectus excavatum.*

Inspection and examination of the hands

- Take both hands and assess them for temperature and colour. Peripheral cyanosis is indicated by a bluish discoloration of the fingertips.
- Look for tar staining and finger clubbing. When the dorsum of a finger from one hand is opposed to the dorsum of a finger from the other hand, a diamond-shaped window (Schamroth's window) is formed at the base of the nailbeds. In clubbing, this diamond shaped window is obliterated, and a distal angle is created between the fingers (see *Figure 14*). Respiratory causes of clubbing include carcinoma, fibrosing alveolitis, and chronic suppurative lung disease (see *Table 7*).
- Inspect and feel the thenar and hypothenar eminences, which can be wasted if there is an apical lung tumour that is invading or compressing the roots of the brachial plexus.
- Test for asterixis (see *Table 8*), the coarse flapping tremor of carbon dioxide retention, by asking the patient to extend both arms with the wrists in dorsiflexion and the palms facing forwards. Ideally, this position should be maintained for a full 30 seconds.
- During this time, assess the radial pulse and determine its rate, rhythm, and character. Is it the bounding pulse of carbon dioxide retention?
- Indicate that you would like to measure the blood pressure.

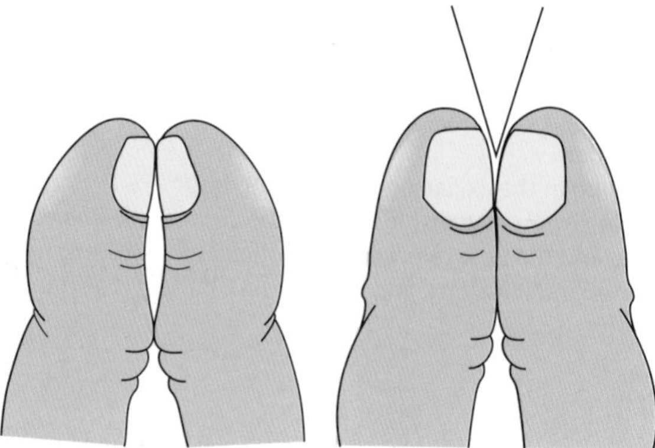

Figure 14. Clubbing. When the dorsum of a finger from one hand is opposed to the dorsum of a finger from the other hand, a diamond shaped window is formed at the base of the nailbeds. In clubbing, this diamond shaped window is obliterated, and a distal angle is created between the fingers.

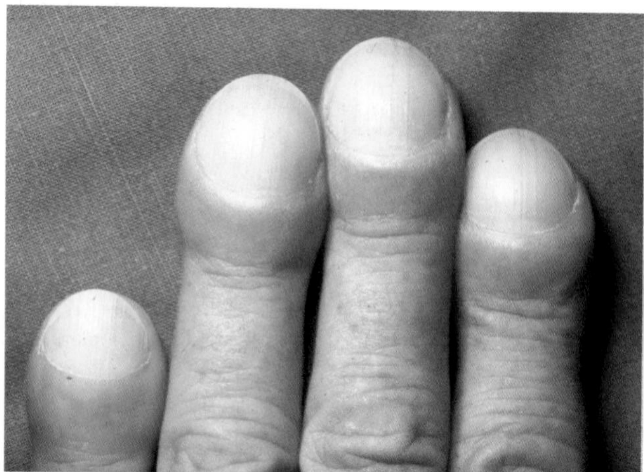

Figure 15. Finger clubbing.

Table 7. The principal causes of clubbing	
Respiratory causes	**Gastrointestinal causes**
Carcinoma	Cirrhosis
Fibrosing alveolitis	Ulcerative colitis
Chronic suppurative lung disease	Crohn's disease
Cardiac causes	Coeliac disease
Infective endocarditis	**Familial**
Cyanotic heart disease	

Table 8. The principal causes of asterixis
Hepatic failure
Renal failure
Cardiac failure
Respiratory failure
Electrolyte abnormalities (hypoglycaemia, hypokalaemia, hypomagnesaemia)
Drug intoxication, e.g. alcohol, phenytoin
CNS causes

Inspection and examination of the head and neck

- Inspect the patient's eyes. Look for a ptosis (an upper lid that encroaches upon the pupil) and for anisocoria (pupillary asymmetry). Ipsilateral ptosis, miosis, enophthalmos, and anhidrosis are strongly suggestive of Horner's syndrome, which may result from compression of the sympathetic chain by an apical lung tumour.
- Next inspect the sclera and conjunctivae for signs of anaemia.
- Ask the patient to open his mouth and inspect the underside of the tongue for the blue discoloration of central cyanosis.
- Assess the jugular venous pressure (JVP) and the jugular venous pulse form (see *Station 12*), A raised JVP is suggestive of right-sided heart failure.
- Examine the lymph nodes with the patient sitting up and from behind. Have a systematic routine for examining all of the submental, submandibular, parotid, pre- and post-auricular, occipital, anterior cervical, posterior cervical, supra- and infra-clavicular, and axillary lymph nodes (see *Station 8*).
- Palpate for tracheal deviation by placing the index and middle fingers of one hand on either side of the trachea in the suprasternal notch. Alternatively, place the index and annular fingers of one hand on either clavicular head and use your middle finger (called the *Vulgaris* in Latin) to palpate the trachea.

Palpation of the chest

 *Ask the patient if he has any chest pain.*

- Ask the patient once again if he is in any pain. Inspect the chest more carefully, looking for asymmetries, deformities, and scars.
- Inspect the precordium and palpate for the position of the cardiac apex. Difficulty palpating for the position of the cardiac apex may indicate hyperexpansion, although this is not a specific sign.

[Note] Carry out all subsequent steps on the front of the chest and, once finished, repeat them on the back of the chest. This is far more elegant than to keep asking the patient to bend forwards and backwards like a Jack-in-the-box. Pulmonary anatomy is such that examination of the back of the chest yields information about the lower lobes, whereas examination of the front of the chest yields information about the upper lobes and, on the right-side, also the middle lobe (*Figure 16*).

- Palpate for equal chest expansion, comparing one side to the other. Reduced unilateral chest expansion might be caused by pneumonia, pleural effusion, pneumothorax, and lung collapse. If there is a measuring tape, measure the chest expansion.

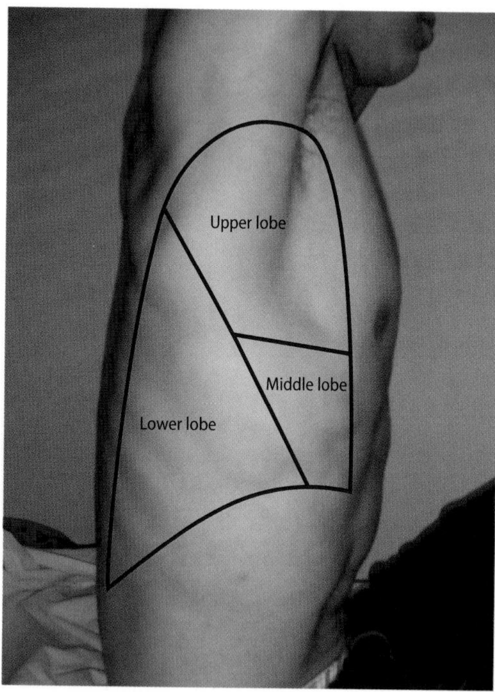

Figure 16. A right lateral view demonstrating lobar anatomy. Posterior assessment gives information about the lower lobes, whereas examination from the front looks at the upper and middle lobes (the latter only on the right).

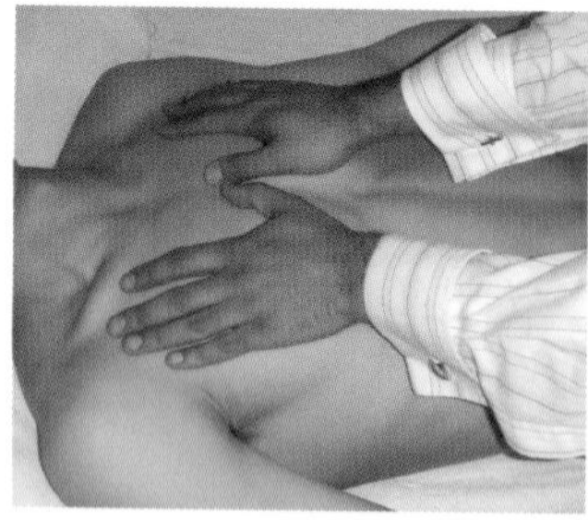
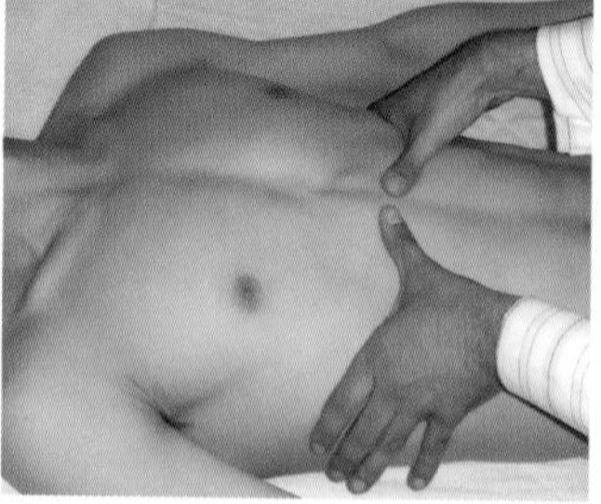
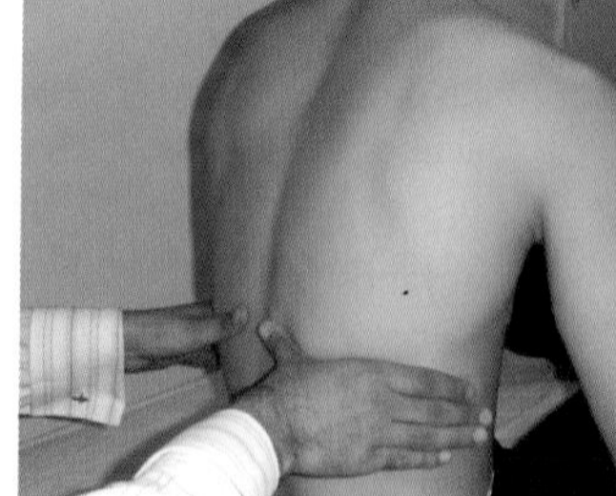

Figure 17. Palpating for equal chest expansion: upper, middle and lower lobes.

Percussion of the chest

- Percuss the chest. Start at the apex of one lung, and compare one side to the other. Do not forget to percuss over the clavicles and on the sides of the chest. For any one area, is the resonance increased or decreased? A hyper-resonant or tympanic note may indicate emphysema or pneumothorax, whereas a dull or stony dull note may indicate consolidation, fibrosis, fluid, or lung collapse. If you uncover any variation in the percussion note, be sure to map out its geographical extent.
- Test for tactile fremitus by placing the flat of the hands on the chest and asking the patient to say *"ninety nine"*.

Auscultation of the chest

- Ask the patient to take deep breaths through the mouth and, using the diaphragm of the stethoscope, auscultate the chest in the same locations as for percussion. Start at the apex of one lung, in the supraclavicular fossa, and compare one side to the other. Normal breath sounds are described as 'vesicular' and have a low pitched and rustling quality. Reduced breath sounds may indicate consolidation. Listen carefully for added sounds such as wheezes (rhonchi), crackles (crepitations), bronchial breathing, and pleural friction rubs.
- Test for vocal resonance by asking the patient to say *"ninety nine"*. Both consolidation and pleural effusions can lead to a dull percussion note, but in consolidation vocal resonance is increased whereas in pleural effusion it is decreased. Both vocal resonance and tactile fremitus (see above) provide the same sort of information.

Inspection and examination of the legs

- Inspect the legs for erythema and swelling. Palpate for tenderness and pitting oedema. A unilateral red, swollen, and tender calf suggests a DVT, whereas bilateral swelling may indicate right-sided heart failure.

After the examination

- Indicate that you would look at the observations chart, examine a sputum sample, measure the peak expiratory flow rate, and order some simple investigations such as a chest X-ray and a full blood count.
- Cover the patient up and ensure that he is comfortable.
- Thank the patient.
- Summarise your findings and offer a differential diagnosis.

Common conditions most likely to come up in a respiratory system examination station
Chronic obstructive pulmonary oedema (COPD): • signs may include breathlessness, breathing through pursed lips, cough, hyperinflated chest, cyanosis, warm hands, tar staining, asterixis, bounding pulse, rhonchi, reduced breath sounds, signs of right heart failure (*cor pulmonale*)
Cryptogenic fibrosing alveolitis: • signs may include breathlessness, dry cough, cyanosis, clubbing, reduced chest expansion, fine late inspiratory crackles, signs of right heart failure (*cor pulmonale*)
Lobectomy

Station 17

PEFR meter explanation

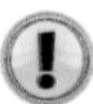 *Read in conjunction with* Station 110: Explaining skills.

Before starting

- Introduce yourself to the patient.
- Check his understanding of asthma.
- Explain the importance of using a PEFR (Peak Expiratory Flow Rate) meter and the importance of using it correctly.
- Explain that the PEFR meter is to be used first thing in the morning and at any time he has symptoms of asthma.

Explain the use of a PEFR meter

Demonstrate and ask the patient to:

- Attach a clean mouthpiece to the meter.
- Slide the marker to the bottom of the numbered scale.
- Stand or sit up straight.
- Hold the peak flow meter horizontal, keeping his fingers away from the marker.
- Take as deep a breath as possible and hold it.
- Insert the mouthpiece into his mouth, sealing his lips around the mouthpiece.
- Exhale as hard as possible into the meter.
- Read and record the meter reading.
- Repeat the procedure three to six times, recording only the highest score.
- Check this score against the peak flow chart or his previous readings.
- Check the patient's understanding by asking him to carry out the procedure.
- Ask him if he has any questions or concerns.

Interpret a PEFR reading

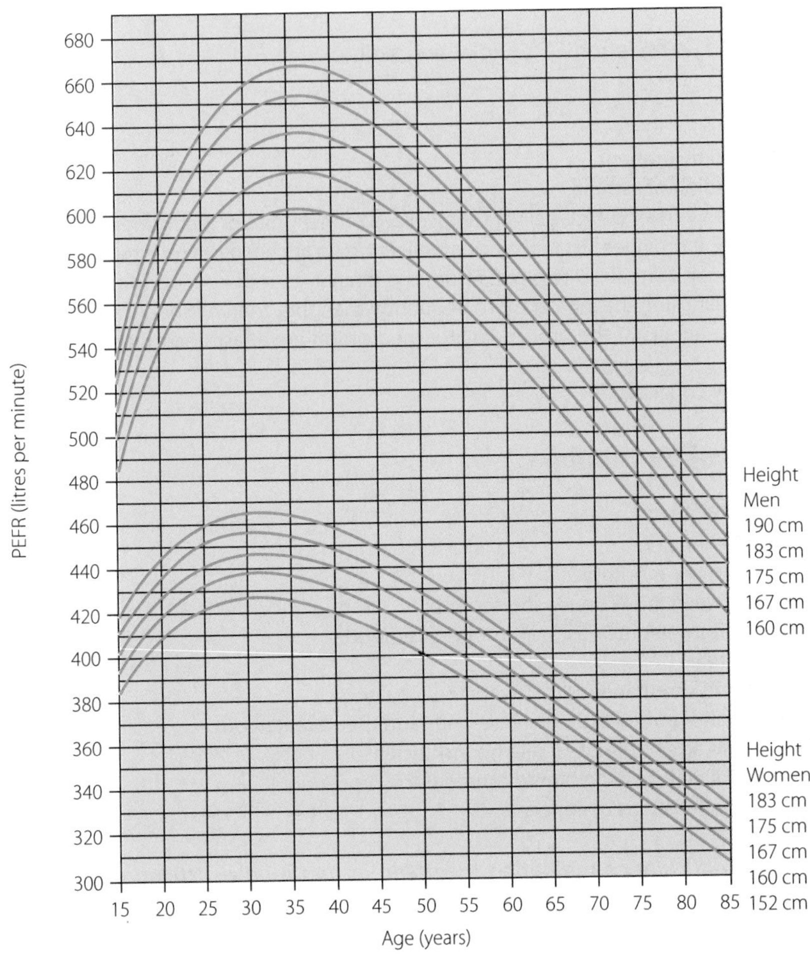

Figure 18. Expected peak flow rates in litres per minute according to age, sex, and height.

Station 18

Inhaler explanation

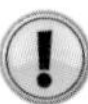 *Read in conjunction with* Station 110: Explaining skills.

Before starting

- Introduce yourself to the patient.
- Check his understanding of asthma.
- Explain to him that an inhaler device delivers aerosolised bronchodilator medication for inhalation. If used correctly, it provides fast and efficient relief from bronchospasm (or airway irritation and narrowing). He can take up to two puffs from the inhaler, as required, up to four times a day. If he finds himself using the inhaler more frequently than this, then he should speak to his doctor. Possible side-effects of the bronchodilator medication are a fast heart rate, shakiness, and headaches.
- Ask him if he has any concerns.

Instruct on the use of an inhaler

Demonstrate and ask the patient to:

- Vigorously shake the inhaler.
- Remove the cap from the mouthpiece.
- Hold the inhaler between index finger and thumb.
- Place the inhaler upright about 3–5 cm in front of his mouth.
- Breathe out completely.
- Breathe in deeply, and simultaneously activate the inhaler.
- Close his mouth and hold his breath for 10 seconds and then breathe out.
- Repeat the procedure after 1 minute if relief is insufficient.
- Check his understanding by asking him to carry out the procedure.
- Ask him if he has any questions or concerns.

 *If the patient has difficulty co-ordinating breathing in and inhaler activation, he may benefit from the added use of an aerochamber inhaler spacer.*

Drug administration via a nebuliser

A nebuliser transforms a drug solution into a fine mist for inhalation via a mouthpiece or face mask. Drugs used in nebulisers include bronchodilators, corticosteroids, and antibiotics (e.g. colistin).

Before starting

- Introduce yourself to the patient.
- Explain the need for a nebuliser and the procedure involved, and ensure consent.
- Explain the drug in the nebuliser, most likely salbutamol, and its common side-effects.
- Obtain consent.

The equipment

- An air compressor and tubing.
- A nebuliser cup.
- A mouthpiece or mask.
- A syringe.
- Drug or drug solution (e.g. salbutamol 2.5 ml) in a vial.
- Diluent (e.g. sodium chloride 0.9%) if needed.

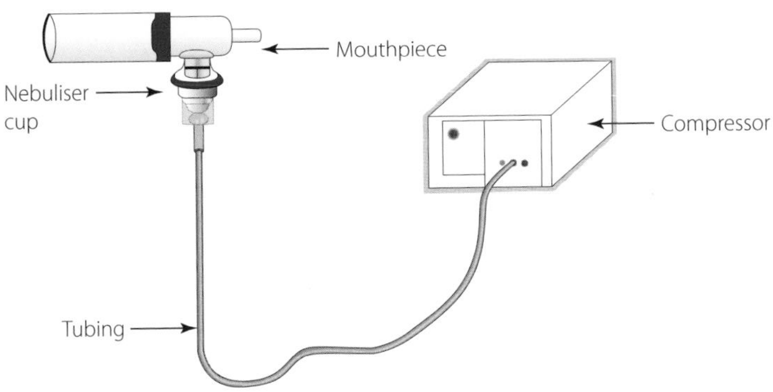

Figure 19. Nebuliser set-up.

The procedure

- Consult the prescription chart and check:
  - the identity of the patient
  - the prescription: validity, drug, dose, diluent, route of administration, date and time of starting
  - drug allergies
- Check the name, dose, and expiry date of the drug on the vial.
- Ask a colleague (registered nurse or doctor) to confirm the name, dose, and expiry date of the drug on the vial.
- Place the air compressor on a sturdy surface and plug it into the mains.

As the compressor unit delivers a set airflow rate that is most suitable for asthmatic patients, it should not be used in COPD patients. For COPD patients, connect the tubing to the oxygen outlet in the wall and set the flow rate to 8 l/min.

- Wash your hands.
- Open the vial of drug solution by twisting off the top.
- With the syringe, carefully draw up the correct amount of drug solution.
- Remove the top part of the nebuliser cup and place the drug solution into it.
- Re-attach the top part of the nebuliser cup and connect the mouthpiece or face mask to the nebuliser cup.
- Connect the tubing from the air compressor to the bottom of the nebuliser cup.
- Switch on the air compressor and ensure that a fine mist is being produced.
- Ask the patient to sit up straight.
- If using a mouthpiece, ask him to clasp it between his teeth and to seal his lips around it. If using a mask, position it comfortably and securely over his face.
- Ask him to take slow, deep breaths through the mouth and, if possible, to hold each breath for 2–3 seconds before breathing out.
- Continue until there is no drug left and the nebuliser begins to splutter (about 10 minutes).
- Turn the compressor off.
- Ask the patient to take several deep breaths and to cough up any secretions.
- Ask him to rinse his mouth with water.
- Wash your hands.
- Sign the prescription chart.

Should the patient feel dizzy, he should interrupt the treatment and rest for about 5 minutes. After resuming the treatment, he should be instructed to breathe more slowly through the mouthpiece.

After the procedure

- Tell the examiner that you would clean and disinfect the equipment.
- Sign the drug chart and record the diluent used, and the date, time, and dose of the drug in the medical records.
- Indicate that you would have your checking colleague countersign it.
- Ask the patient if he has any questions or concerns.
- Ensure that he is comfortable.

Abdominal pain history

Before starting

- Introduce yourself to the patient.
- Explain that you are going to ask him some questions to uncover the cause of his abdominal pain, and ask for his consent to do this.
- Ensure that he is comfortable.

Ensure that the patient is nil by mouth. Acute abdomen is a surgical complaint and the patient must therefore be kept nil by mouth until the need for surgery has been excluded.

The history

- Name, age, and occupation.

Presenting complaint and history of presenting complaint

- For any pain, try to determine:
  - site
  - radiation
  - character, for example, sharp, dull, aching, or burning
  - severity
  - onset and progression
  - timing and duration
  - aggravating and alleviating factors
  - associated symptoms and signs
- Ensure that you ask about:
  - fever
  - loss of weight or anorexia
  - dysphagia
  - indigestion
  - nausea, vomiting, and haematemesis
  - diarrhoea or constipation
  - melaena or rectal bleeding
  - steatorrhoea
  - jaundice
  - genitourinary symptoms: frequency, dysuria, haematuria
  - menses (menarche, menopause, length of menstrual periods, amount of bleeding, pain, intermenstrual bleeding, last menstrual period)
  - effect on everyday life

Past medical history

- Previous episodes of abdominal pain.
- Current, past, and childhood illnesses.
- Surgery.

Drug history

- Prescribed medications. Ask specifically about corticosteroids, NSAIDs, antibiotics, and the contraceptive pill.
- Over-the-counter medication.
- Recreational drugs.
- Allergies.

Family history

- Parents, siblings, and children. Ask specifically about colon cancer, irritable bowel syndrome, inflammatory bowel disease, jaundice, peptic ulcer, and polyps.

Social history

- Alcohol consumption.
- Smoking.
- Recent travel.
- Employment, past and present.
- Housing.
- Contact with jaundiced patients.

After taking the history

- Ask the patient if there is anything that he might add that you have forgotten to ask.
- Ask the patient if he has any questions or concerns.
- Thank the patient.
- State that you would carry out a full abdominal examination and order some key investigations such as urinalysis, serum analysis, and an abdominal X-ray, as appropriate.
- Summarise your findings and offer a differential diagnosis.

Conditions most likely to come up in an abdominal pain history station

Appendicitis:

- more common in younger age groups
- diffuse central pain that then shifts into the right iliac fossa
- aggravated by movement, touch, coughing
- associated with nausea and vomiting, fever, anorexia

Gastro-oesophageal reflux disease:

- retrosternal burning
- clear relationship with food and alcohol, but no relationship with effort
- aggravated by lying down and alleviated by sitting up and by antacids such as Gaviscon or milk
- may be associated with odynophagia and nocturnal asthma

Peptic ulceration:

- severe epigastric pain, during meals in the case of gastric ulcers, and between meals and at night in the case of duodenal ulcers
- aggravated by spicy food, alcohol, stress
- associated with bloating, heartburn, nausea and vomiting, anorexia, haematemesis, melaena
- predisposed to by NSAIDs, alcohol, and smoking

Biliary colic:

- constant but episodic epigastric or right upper quadrant pain that may radiate to the back and shoulders
- can be provoked by eating a large, fatty meal
- associated with nausea and vomiting and diarrhoea
- presence of fever may indicate biliary tract infection (cholecystitis)
- risk factors for gall stones are fat, forty, female, and pregnant or fertile ('the 4 Fs'), the contraceptive pill, and HRT

Acute pancreatitis:

- acute, severe epigastric pain radiating to the back
- may be alleviated by sitting forward ('pancreatic position') or by remaining still
- associated with nausea and vomiting, diarrhoea, anorexia, fever

Ureteric colic:

- severe pain in the loin that radiates to the groin
- often colicky but may be constant
- associated with nausea and vomiting
- predisposed to by dehydration

Diverticulitis:

- left iliac fossa pain and tenderness
- aggravated by movement
- associated with fever, nausea, anorexia, constipation, diarrhoea
- more common in the elderly

Colorectal cancer:

- signs and symptoms may include change in bowel habit, tenesmus, change in stool shape, rectal bleeding, melaena, bowel obstruction leading to constipation, abdominal pain, abdominal distension, and vomiting, fatigue, anorexia, weight loss

Irritable bowel syndrome:

- chronic abdominal pain or discomfort
- associated with frequent diarrhoea or constipation, bloating, urgency for bowel movements, tenesmus

Remember that basal pneumonia, diabetic ketoacidosis, and an inferior myocardial infarct can also present as abdominal pain.

Abdominal examination

Before starting

- Introduce yourself to the patient.
- Ask the patient for permission to examine his abdomen.
- Say to the examiner that you would normally expose the patient from nipples to knees, but that in this case you are going to limit yourself to exposing the patient to the groins.
- Position the patient so that he is lying flat on the couch, with his arms at his side and his head supported by a pillow.
- Ensure that the patient is comfortable.

The examination

General inspection

- From the end of the couch, observe the patient's general appearance (age, state of health, nutritional status, and any other obvious signs).
- Next observe the surroundings, looking in particular for the presence of a nasogastric tube, intravenous infusion, urinary catheter, drain, or stoma bag.
- Inspect the abdomen for its contours and any obvious distension, localised masses, scars, and skin changes. Ask the patient to lift his head up and to cough. This makes hernias more visible and, if the patient has difficulty complying with your instructions, suggests peritonism.

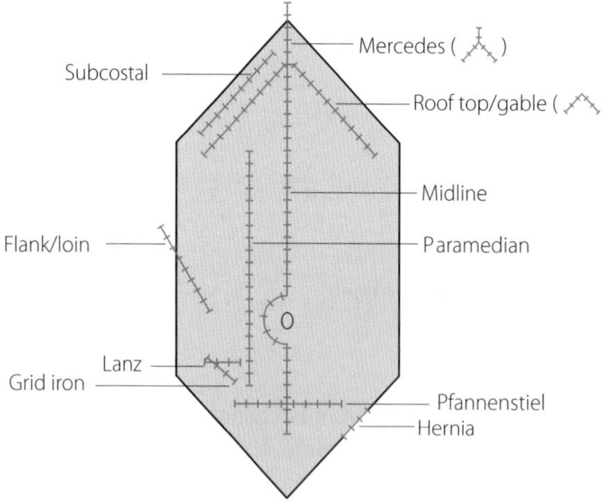

Figure 20. Abdominal scars.

Inspection and examination of the hands

- Take both hands, noting their temperature and looking for:
  - clubbing
  - palmar erythema (liver disease)
  - nail signs: leukonychia (hypoalbuminaemia; see *Figure 21*) and koilonychia (iron deficiency; see *Figure 22*)
  - Dupuytren's contracture (cirrhosis; see *Figure 23*)
- Test for asterixis or 'liver flap' (hepatic failure) by showing the patient how to extend both arms with the wrists dorsiflexed and the palms facing forwards. Ask him to hold this posture for at least 10 and ideally 30 seconds.

- Next, feel the pulse for at least 15 seconds and measure the respiratory rate.
- Moving up, inspect the arms for bruising, scratch marks, injection track marks, and tattoos.

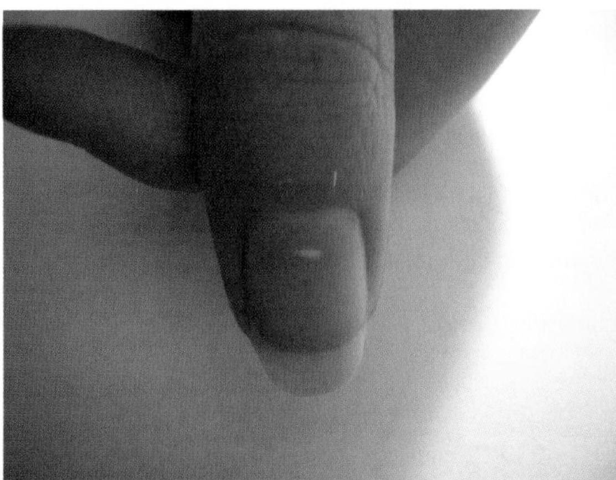

Figure 21. Leukonychia.

Reproduced from http://commons.wikimedia.org with permission.

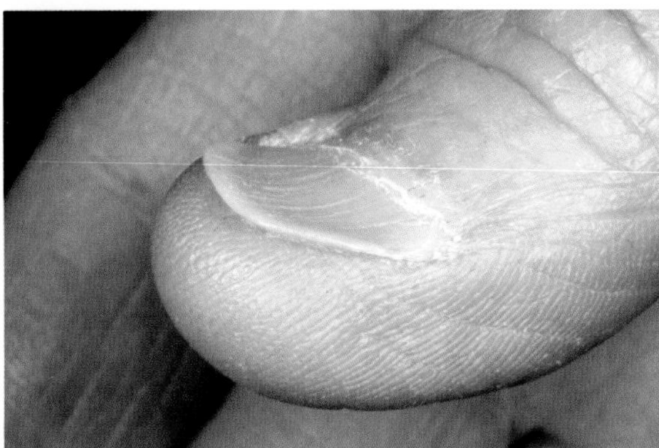

Figure 22. Koilonychia.

Reproduced from www.dermnet.com with permission.

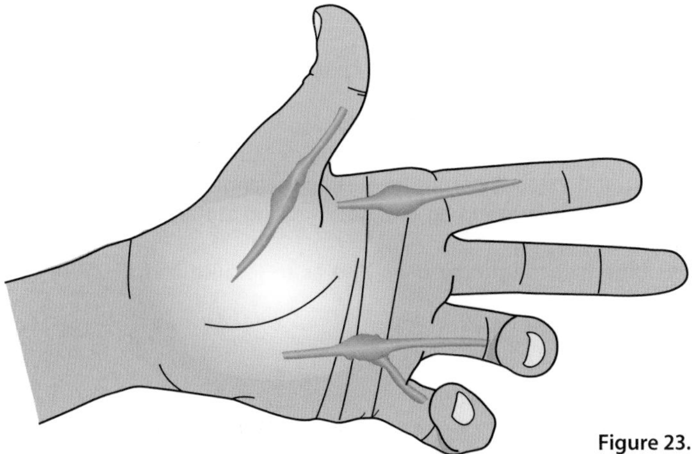

Figure 23. Dupuytren's contracture.

Inspection and examination of the head, neck, and upper body

- Ask the patient to look up and then inspect the sclera for jaundice.
- Gently retract the eyelid and inspect the conjunctiva for anaemia.
- Ask the patient to open his mouth, and note any odour on the breath (alcohol, *foetor hepaticus*, ketones). Inspect the mouth, looking for signs of dehydration, furring of the tongue (loss of appetite), angular stomatitis (nutritional deficiency), atrophic glossitis (iron deficiency, vitamin B12 deficiency, folate deficiency; see *Figure 24*), ulcers (Crohn's disease), and the state of the dentition.
- If you suspect alcoholism or an eating disorder, feel for enlargement of the parotid glands.
- Assess the jugular venous pressure (JVP).
- Palpate the neck for lymphadenopathy, making sure to take in the left supraclavicular fossa (Virchow's node, gastric carcinoma).
- Examine the upper body for gynaecomastia (cirrhosis), caput medusae, and spider naevi (chronic liver disease).

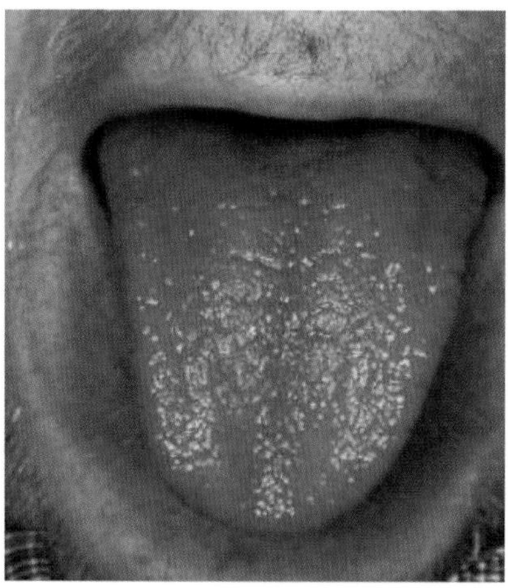

Figure 24. Atrophic glossitis. Note the loss of filliform papillae.
Reproduced from www.joplink.net – photograph by Dr Echenique-Eligondo.

Palpation of the abdomen

Before you begin, ask the patient to identify any area of pain or tenderness.

- Sit or kneel beside the patient and use the palmar surface of your fingers to lightly palpate in all nine regions of the abdomen (*Figure 25*), beginning with the region furthest away from any pain or tenderness. By flexing and extending your metacarpophalangeal joints, palpate for tenderness, rebound tenderness, guarding, and rigidity. Keep looking at the patient's face for any signs of discomfort.
- Repeat the procedure, this time palpating more deeply so as to localise and describe any masses.

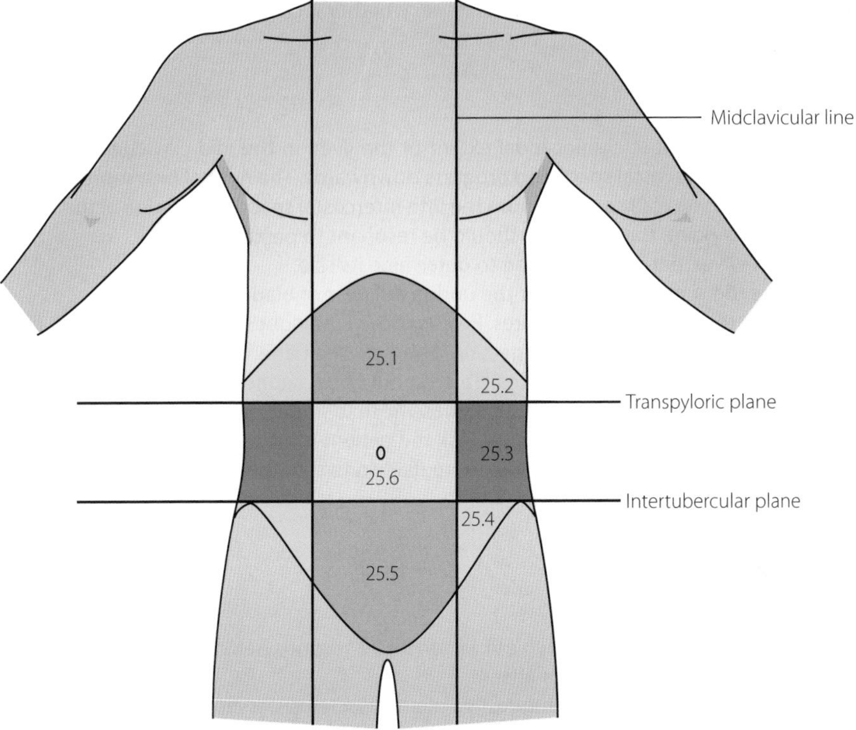

Figure 25. Regions of the abdomen.
25.1 Epigastric
25.2 Left hypochondriac
25.3 Left lumbar
25.4 Left iliac fossa
25.5 Suprapubic/hypogastric
25.6 Umbilical

Palpation of the organs

- *Liver* – Ask the patient to breathe in and out and, starting in the right iliac fossa, feel for the inferior liver edge using the radial aspect of your index finger. Each time the patient inspires, move your hand closer to the costal margin and press your fingers firmly into the abdominal wall. The inferior liver edge may be felt as the liver descends upon inspiration, and can be described in terms of regularity, nodularity, and tenderness.
- *Gallbladder* – Palpate for tenderness over the tip of the right ninth rib.
- *Spleen* – Palpate for the spleen as for the liver, once again starting in the right iliac fossa. Press the tips of your fingers firmly against the abdominal wall so that your hand is pointing up and leftwards. If the spleen is enlarged, the splenic notch may be 'caught' as the spleen descends upon inspiration.
- *Kidneys* – Position the patient close to the edge of the bed and ballot each kidney using the technique of deep bimanual palpation. Place one hand flat over the anterior aspect of the flank (right hand for left kidney, left hand for right kidney), and press down whilst using the other hand to push the kidney up from below.
- *Aorta* – Palpate the descending aorta with the tips of your fingers on either side of the midline, just above the umbilicus. Pressing your fingers firmly into the abdominal wall, assess whether

the aorta is pulsatile and whether it is expansile, i.e. whether it causes the fingers of your right and left hands to move apart.

Percussion

- *Liver* – Percuss out the entire craniocaudal extent of the liver. In the mid-clavicular line, start above the right fifth intercostal space and progress downwards. The normal liver represents an area of dullness which typically extends from the fifth intercostal space to the edge of the costal margin. Beyond this point, the abdomen should be resonant to percussion.
- *Spleen* – As for the liver, percuss the spleen to determine its size.
- *Bladder* – Percuss the suprapubic area for the undue dullness of bladder distension.
- *'Shifting dullness'* – this sign indicates ascites. Percuss down the right side of the abdomen. If an area of dullness is detected, keep two fingers on it and ask the patient to roll over onto his left. After about 30 seconds, re-percuss the area which should now sound resonant. The change in the percussion note reflects the redistribution of ascitic fluid under the effect of gravity.
- *'Fluid thrill'* – this sign indicates severe ascites. Ask the patient to place his hand along the mid-line of his abdomen. Then place one hand on one flank, and flick the opposite flank with your other hand in an attempt to elicit a thrill.

Auscultation

Auscultate over:

- The mid-abdomen for bowel sounds (*Table 9*). Listen for 30 seconds before concluding that they are normal, hyperactive, hypoactive, or absent.
- The abdominal aorta for aortic bruits suggestive of arteriosclerosis or an aneurysm.
- 2.5 cm above and lateral to the umbilicus for renal artery bruits suggestive of renal artery stenosis.

Table 9. Principal causes of altered bowel sounds

Hypoactive	• Constipation • Drugs such as anticholinergics and opiates • General anaesthesia • Abdominal surgery • Paralytic ileus (absent bowel sounds)
Hyperactive	• Diarrhoea of any cause • Inflammatory bowel disease • GI bleeding • Mechanical bowel obstruction (high pitched bowel sounds)

After the examination

- Cover up the patient and thank him. Enquire about and address any concerns that he may have.
- Indicate to the examiner that you would normally test for pedal oedema, examine the hernia orifices and the external genitalia, and carry out a digital rectal examination. You would also look at the observations chart, dipstick the urine, and consider investigations such as ultrasound scan, FBC, LFTs, U&Es, clotting screen, pregnancy test, and urine drug screen.
- Summarise your findings and offer a differential diagnosis.

Conditions most likely to come up in an abdominal examination station
Chronic liver disease: • may result from alcoholic liver disease, viral hepatitis, right heart failure, haemochromatosis, Wilson's disease, amongst others • signs may include clubbing, palmar erythema, leukonychia, metabolic flap, hyperventilation, bruising, jaundice, gynaecomastia, spider naevi, caput medusae, scratch marks, hepatomegaly, ascites, pedal oedema, Dupuytren's contracture (alcohol), tattoos (hepatitis C), signs of right heart failure such as raised JVP and pedal oedema, bronzing of the skin (haemochromatosis), Kayser–Fleischer rings (Wilson's disease)
Splenomegaly: • causes include portal hypertension (usually complicating liver cirrhosis), lymphoproliferative and myeloproliferative diseases, haemolytic anaemias, and infections such as infectious mononucleosis and malaria
Polycystic kidney
Renal transplant
Scars
Hernias (see *Station 23*)

Rectal examination

Rectal examination is commonly indicated in cases of rectal or GI bleeding (suspected or actual), severe constipation, faecal or urinary incontinence, anal or rectal pain, suspected enlargement of the prostate gland, and urethral discharge or bleeding. It can also be used to screen for cancers of the rectum, colon, and prostate.

Specifications: A plastic model in lieu of a patient.

Before starting

- Introduce yourself to the patient.
- Explain the procedure to him, emphasising that it might be uncomfortable but that it should not be painful, and ask for his consent to carry it out.
- Ask for a chaperone.
- Ensure privacy.
- Ask the patient to lower his trousers and underpants.
- Ask him to lie on his left side, to bring his buttocks to the side of the couch, and to bring his knees up to his chest.

The examination

- Put on a pair of gloves.
- Gently separate the buttocks and inspect the anus and surrounding skin. In particular, look out for skin tags, excoriations, ulcers, fissures, external haemorrhoids, prolapsed haemorrhoids, and mucosal prolapse.
- Lubricate the index finger of your right hand.
- Position the finger over the anus, as if pointing to the genitalia.
- Ask the patient to bear down so as to relax the anal sphincter.
- Gently insert the finger into the anus, through the anal canal, and into the rectum (*Figure 26*). Note any pain upon insertion.

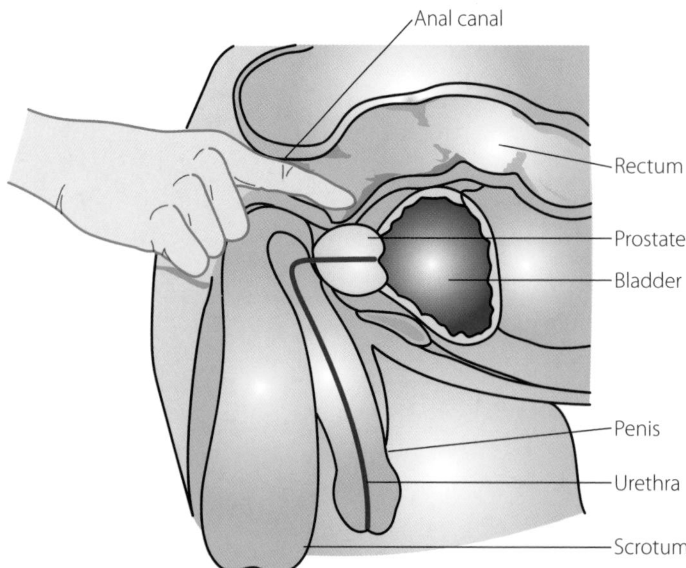

Figure 26. Digital rectal examination.

- Test anal tone by asking the patient to squeeze your finger.
- Rotate the finger so as to palpate the entire circumference of the anal canal and rectum. Feel for any masses, ulcers, or induration and for faeces in the rectum. If there are any faeces in the rectum, assess their consistency.
  - In males pay specific attention to the size, shape, surface, and consistency of the prostate gland. Assess whether the midline groove is palpable.
  - In females, the cervix and uterus may be palpable.
- Remove the finger and examine the glove. In particular look at the colour of any stool, and for the presence of any mucous or blood.
- Remove and dispose of the gloves.

After the examination

- Clean off any lubricant or faeces on the anus or anal margin.
- Give the patient time to put his clothes back on.
- Ensure that he is comfortable.
- Address any questions or concerns that he may have.
- Present your findings to the examiner, and offer a differential diagnosis.

Conditions most likely to come up in a rectal examination station
Benign prostatic hypertrophy (BPH): • in BPH the prostate is enlarged in size (>3.5 cm) and slightly distorted in shape, but it is still rubbery and firm, with a smooth surface and a palpable midline groove
Prostate carcinoma • in prostate carcinoma, the prostate is also enlarged and asymmetrical, but this time it is hard and irregular/nodular and the midline groove may no longer be palpable

Hernia examination

Inguinal anatomy

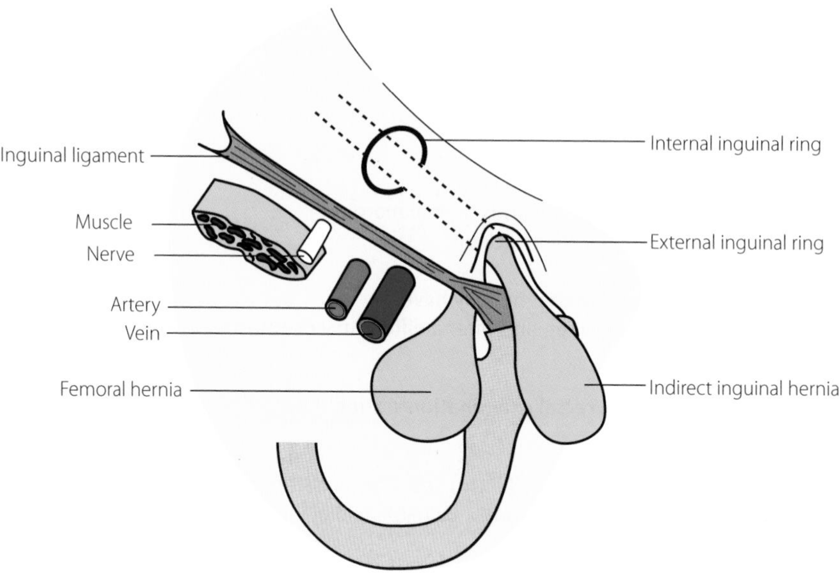

Figure 27. The inguinal canal runs along the inguinal ligament, from the internal (deep) ring to the external (superficial) ring. The inguinal ligament stretches from the anterior superior iliac spine to the pubic tubercle. The internal ring lies approximately 1.5 cm superior to the femoral pulse, itself in the midline of the inguinal ligament. The external ring lies immediately superior and medial to the pubic tubercle.

Definition of a hernia

A hernia is defined as the protrusion of an organ or part thereof through a deficiency in the wall of the cavity in which it is contained. There are many different types of hernia but the ones that are most likely to be examined and discussed in an OSCE are indirect and direct inguinal hernias and femoral hernias. Their principal differentiating features are summarised in *Table 10*. The differential diagnosis of a lump in the groin is listed in *Table 11*.

Table 10. Principal differentiating features of indirect and direct inguinal and femoral hernias

Indirect hernia	Direct hernia	Femoral hernia
• Neck of hernia is superior to the inguinal ligament/pubic tubercle and lateral to the inferior epigastric vessels • Accounts for 80% of inguinal hernias • Irreducible • Can strangulate	• Neck of hernia is superior to the inguinal ligament/ pubic tubercle and medial to the inferior epigastric vessels • Accounts for 20% of inguinal hernias • Easily reducible • Rarely strangulates	• Neck of hernia is inferior and lateral to the inguinal ligament pubic tubercle • Is more common in females • Often irreducible • Frequently strangulates

Table 11. Differential diagnosis of a lump in the groin

Superior to the inguinal ligament	Inferior to the inguinal ligament
• Indirect or direct inguinal hernia • Incisional hernia • Sebaceous cyst • Lipoma • Undescended testis	• Femoral hernia • Lymph node • Sebaceous cyst • Lipoma • Saphena varix • Femoral artery aneurysm • Psoas abscess (rare) • Undescended testis • Scrotal mass (see *Station 26*)

Before starting

- Introduce yourself to the patient.
- Explain the examination and ask for his consent to carry it out.
- Ask for a chaperone.
- Ask the patient to lie on the couch and to expose his abdomen from the umbilicus to the knees.
- Ensure that he is comfortable.
- Warm up your hands.

Ensure the patient's dignity at all times.

The examination

Inspection and palpation

- Inspect the groins (both sides!) for an obvious lump. If a lump is visible, determine its location in relation to its surrounding anatomical landmarks. Also determine its size, shape, colour, consistency, and mobility. Is it tender to touch? Can it be transilluminated? (See *Station 8: Examination of a superficial mass*.)
- Look for old surgical scars (incisional hernia).
- Ask the patient to stand up and look again.

Cough impulse and cough tests

(The patient is still standing.)

- Ask the patient to cough and look again.
- Test the lump for a cough impulse. Place two fingers over the lump and ask the patient to cough once more.
- If you are satisfied that the lump is an inguinal hernia, ask the patient to reduce the lump. Once the lump is fully reduced, place two fingers over the internal ring and ask the patient to cough.
  - If the lump does not reappear it is an indirect inguinal hernia. Release your fingers and ask the patient to cough again.
  - If the lump reappears medially it is a direct inguinal hernia.
- Once again ask the patient to reduce the lump. This time place two fingers over the *external* ring and ask the patient to cough.

  - If the lump does not reappear it is a direct inguinal hernia. Release your fingers and ask the patient to cough again.
  - If the lump reappears laterally it is an indirect inguinal hernia.
- Percuss the lump for resonance (bowel involvement).
- Auscultate the lump for bowel sounds (bowel involvement).

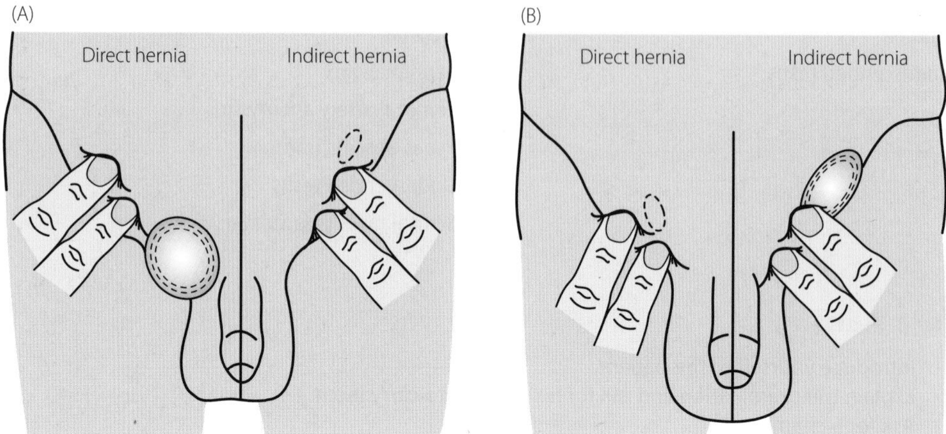

Figure 28. The cough test with two fingers over the internal ring (A) and then over the external ring (B).

After the examination

- Indicate that you would also examine the femoral pulses, inguinal lymph nodes, and scrotum.
- Cover up the patient.
- Ensure that he is comfortable.
- Thank him.
- Summarise your findings and offer a differential diagnosis. Don't fret over your diagnosis as even experienced surgeons are notoriously poor at differentiating between indirect and direct inguinal hernias. Apart from inguinal and femoral hernias, other (more rare) types of hernia are epigastric hernias that occur in the epigastric area in the midline, spigellian or semilunar hernias that occur on the outer border of the rectus muscles, umbilical and paraumbilical hernias that occur at or around the navel, and incisional hernias that occur at the site of an old surgical incision.
- Wash your hands.

Nasogastric intubation

Specifications: A mannequin in lieu of a patient.

Choice of NG tube

Nasogastric (NG or Ryle's) tubes can be used for feeding or drug administration, to decompress the stomach, to obtain a sample of gastric fluid, or to drain the stomach's contents (e.g. after an overdose or if emergency surgery is required). If the tube is being used for aspiration or drainage, a gauge of 10 or greater is required. If not, a fine bore tube should be preferred.

The equipment

- A pair of non-sterile gloves.
- An NG tube of appropriate size.
- K-Y jelly.
- Xylocaine spray.
- A glass of water with a straw.
- Tape.
- Stethoscope.
- A 20 ml syringe and some pH paper.
- A spigot or catheter bag.
- A vomit bowl.

Before starting

- Introduce yourself to the patient.
- Explain the need for an NG tube and the procedure for inserting it, and ensure consent.
- Position the patient upright and ask about nostril preference/examine the nostrils.
- Ensure that the patient is comfortable.

The procedure

- Gather the equipment.
- Wash your hands and don the gloves.
- Measure the length of NG tube to be inserted by placing the tip of the tube at the nostril and extending the tube behind the ear and then to two fingerbreadths above the umbilicus.
- Lubricate the tip of the NG tube with K-Y jelly.
- Spray the back of the throat with xylocaine or state that you would do so.
- Insert the NG tube into the preferred nostril and slide it along the floor of the nose into the nasopharynx.
- Ask the patient to tilt his head forward and to swallow some water through a straw as you continue to advance the tube through the pharynx and oesophagus and into the stomach. Each time the patient swallows, advance the tube a little bit further.
- If the patient coughs or gags, slightly withdraw the tube and leave him some time to recover.
- Insert the tube to the required length.
- Ensure that the tip of the tube is in the stomach.
  - Inject 20 ml of air into the tube and listen over the epigastrium with your stethoscope.
  - Pull back on the plunger to aspirate stomach contents. Test the aspirate with pH paper to confirm its acidity (pH < 6). If a fine-bore tube has been inserted, it may not be possible to aspirate stomach contents.
  - Request a chest X-ray or indicate that you would do so.
- Tape the tube to the nose and to the side of the face.
- Attach a spigot or catheter bag to the NG tube.

After the procedure

- Ask the patient if he has any questions or concerns.
- Ensure that he is comfortable.
- Thank him.
- Make an entry in the patient's notes.

[Note] The principal complications of NG tube insertion are aspiration and tissue trauma.

Urological history

Before starting

- Introduce yourself to the patient.
- Explain that you are going to ask him some questions to uncover the nature of his urological complaint, and ask for consent to do this.
- Ensure that he is comfortable.

The history

- Name, age, and occupation.

Presenting complaint and history of presenting complaint

- Ask about the main presenting complaint. Ask open questions.
- Elicit the patient's ideas, concerns, and expectations.
- Determine the time course of events and the severity of the problem.
- Ask specifically about:
  - pain: for any pain, ask about site, radiation, intensity, character, onset, duration, relieving and aggravating factors, and associated factors
  - fever
  - frequency: *"Are you passing water more often than usual?"*
  - nocturia: *"Do you find yourself waking up in the middle of the night to pass water?"*
  - urgency: *"When you need to pass water, how long can you wait?"*
  - incontinence: *"Are there times when it can no longer wait and you end up going there and then?"*
  - dysuria: *"When you pass water, is there any pain or burning?"*
  - haematuria: *"When you pass water, is there any blood in your urine? Does it colour all of your urine or only some of it?"*
  - hesitancy, poor stream and terminal dribbling (if male): *"When you are standing at the toilet do you have to wait before you are able to pass water? Is the jet as strong as it ever was? What about after, does urine continue to trickle out?"*
  - back pain, leg weakness, weight loss, nausea, anorexia
  - vaginal/urethral discharge, genital sores
  - testicular masses, testicular pain
  - sexual dysfunction
  - sexual contacts

Past medical history

- Past urological problems.
- Ask specifically about UTI, renal colic, diabetes mellitus, hypertension, and gout.
- Current, past, and childhood illnesses.
- Surgery.

Drug history

- Prescribed medication including anticholinergics and anticoagulants.
- Over-the-counter medication.
- Recreational drugs.
- Allergies.

Family history

- Parents, siblings, and children. In particular, has anyone in the family had a similar problem?
- Ask specifically about polycystic kidney disease and bladder cancer.

Social history

- Employment. Has the patient ever worked with chemicals or dyes?
- Housing.
- Travel.
- Alcohol consumption.
- Smoking.

After taking the history

- Ask the patient if there is anything he might add that you have forgotten to ask about.
- Thank the patient.
- State that you would carry out abdominal and genital examinations and order some key investigations, e.g. urine dipstick, urine microscopy and culture, U&Es, PSA levels, transrectal ultrasound, cystoscopy, KUB X-ray.
- Summarise your findings and offer a differential diagnosis.

Conditions most likely to come up in a urological history station

Urinary tract infection:

- most common in young females
- common symptoms are frequency, urgency, dysuria, haematuria, and a pressure above the pubic bone
- if the infection is above the bladder, there may be fever, nausea, and back pain
- there may be history of recent sexual intercourse

Benign prostatic hypertrophy:

- most common in elderly males
- common symptoms are frequency, nocturia, urgency, incontinence, hesitancy, poor stream and intermittency, and terminal dribbling

Prostate carcinoma:

- most common in elderly males
- symptoms, when present, are similar to those seen in benign prostatic hypertrophy with the possible addition of dysuria, haematuria, sexual dysfunction, weight loss, and bone pain
- there may be a family history

Bladder carcinoma:

- three to four times more common in males than in females
- more common in the elderly
- painless haematuria is characteristic, but there may also be dysuria and/or frequency
- associated with smoking and occupational exposure to chemicals and dyes

Renal calculus:

- more common in males than in females
- severe pain in the loin that radiates to the groin
- the pain is often colicky but it may be constant
- the pain may be associated with nausea and vomiting
- haematuria is a common finding
- dehydration is a common predisposing factor

Male genitalia examination

Specifications: You may be asked to examine the male genitalia on a real patient or, more likely, on a pelvic mannequin.

Before starting

- Introduce yourself to the patient.
- Explain the examination and ask for his consent to carry it out.
- Ask for a chaperone.
- Ask him to lie on the couch and expose his groin area.
- Ensure that he is comfortable.

Ensure the patient's comfort and dignity at all times.

The examination

General inspection

- From the end of the couch observe the patient's general appearance. The patient's age can give you an indication of the most likely pathology.
- In particular, note the distribution of facial, axillary, and pubic hair.
- Look for gynaecomastia.

Inspection and examination of the male genitalia

- Warm your hands.
- Ensure that the patient is not in pain.

Penis

- Inspect the penis for lesions and ulcers.
- Retract the foreskin and examine the *glans penis* and the external urethral meatus. Is there a discharge? Can a discharge be expressed?
  - If there is a discharge, indicate that you would swab it for microscopy and culture.

Scrotum

- Inspect the scrotum. Are the testicles present? Is their lie normal? If a testicle is absent, is it retracted or undescended? If you find a scar, the absent testicle may have been surgically removed.
- Fix upon the patient's face and palpate:
  - the testis
  - the epididymis
  - the spermatic cord
- If you locate a mass, try to get above it. If you cannot, it is likely to be a hernia so test for a cough impulse (see *Station 23*). Determine the size, shape and consistency of the mass.
- Next, transilluminate the mass using a pen torch. Is it a cyst or a solid mass? If it is a cyst, is it a hydrocoele or an epididymal cyst? If it is a solid mass, is it tender? Is it testicular or epididymal?
- If you suspect a varicocoele, a collection of varicosities in the pampiniform venous plexus, examine the patient in the standing position and test for a cough impulse. **Note that varicocoeles are almost invariably left-sided.**

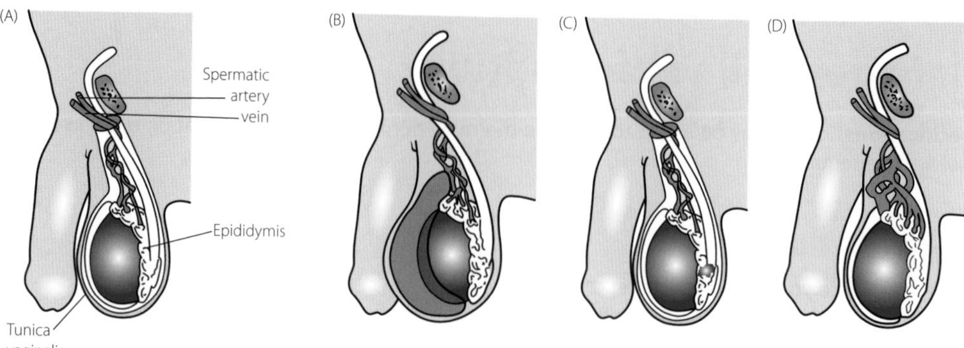

Figure 29. Normal testis and appendages (A), hydrocoele (B), epididymal cyst (C), and varicocoele (D).

Examination of the lymphatics

- Palpate the inguinal nodes in the inguinal crease. Remember that only the penis and scrotum drain to the inguinal nodes, as the testicles drain to the para-aortic lymph nodes.

After the examination

- Cover up the patient.
- Thank the patient.
- Ensure that he is comfortable.
- Summarise your findings and offer a differential diagnosis.

Conditions most likely to come up in a male genitalia examination	
Hydrocoele: • collection of fluid in the tunica vaginalis surrounding the testis • presents as unilateral (or less commonly bilateral) scrotal swelling • not tender • fluctuant • transilluminant	**Varicocoele:** • dilated veins along the spermatic cord • almost invariably left-sided • 'bag of worms' upon palpation • there may be a cough impulse • likely to disappear upon lying down
Epididymal cyst: • arises in the epididymis • epididymal cysts may be multiple and bilateral • unlike in a hydrocoele, the testis is palpable quite separately from the cyst • smooth and fluctuant • transilluminant	**Direct inguinal hernia** (see *Station 23*)

Male catheterisation

Specifications: A male anatomical model in lieu of a patient.

Before starting

- Introduce yourself to the patient.
- Explain the procedure and ask for his consent to carry it out.
- Position him flat on the couch with legs apart and groin exposed.

The equipment

On a clean trolley, gather:

- A catheterisation pack.
- Saline solution.
- Sterile gloves.
- A 10 ml pre-filled syringe containing 2% lignocaine gel.
- A 12–16 french Foley catheter.
- A catheter bag.
- A 10 ml syringe containing sterile water.
- Adhesive tape.

The procedure

- Gather the equipment.
- Check the expiry date of the catheter.
- Open the catheter pack aseptically onto a trolley, attach the yellow bag to the side of the trolley, and pour saline solution into the receiver.
- If pre-filled syringes are not provided with the pack, draw up 10 ml sterile water and 10 ml lignocaine gel into separate syringes.
- Wash and dry your hands.
- Put on sterile gloves.
- Drape the patient.
- Place a collecting vessel in the patient's *entre-jambes*.
- With your non-dominant hand, hold the penis with a sterile swab.
- With your dominant hand, retract the foreskin and clean the area around the urethral meatus with saline-soaked swabs. So as not to break sterility, hold the swabs with plastic prongs, and use one set of prongs per swab.
- Coat the end of the catheter with lignocaine gel and instil 10 ml of lignocaine gel into the urethra. Hold the urethral meatus closed.
- Indicate that the anaesthetic needs about 5 minutes to work.
- Hold the penis so that it is vertical.
- Holding the catheter by its sleeve, gently and progressively insert it into the urethra. Upon feeling resistance from the prostate, hold the penis horizontally so as to facilitate insertion.
- Once a stream of urine is obtained, inject 10 ml of sterile water to inflate the catheter's balloon, continually ensuring that this does not cause the patient any pain.
- Gently retract the catheter until a resistance is felt.
- Attach the catheter bag.
- Reposition the foreskin.
- Tape the catheter to the thigh.

After the procedure

- Ensure that the patient is comfortable.
- Thank the patient.
- Discard any rubbish.
- Record the date and time of catheterisation, type and size of catheter used, volume of water used to inflate the balloon, and volume of urine in the catheter bag.

Examiner's questions

Indications for catheterisation:

- hygienic care of bedridden patients
- monitoring of urine output
- acute urinary retention
- chronic obstruction
- collection of a specimen of uncontaminated urine
- irrigation of the bladder
- imaging of the urinary tract

Contraindications:

- pelvic trauma
- previous stricture
- previous failure to catheterise
- severe phimosis

Complications:

- paraphimosis (from failure to reposition the foreskin)
- urethral perforation and creation of false passages
- bleeding
- infection
- urethral strictures

Female catheterisation

Specifications: A female anatomical model in lieu of a patient.

Before starting

- Introduce yourself to the patient.
- Explain the procedure and ask for her consent to carry it out.
- Ask her to undress from the waist down and place a sheet over her.

The equipment

On a clean trolley, gather:

- Two pairs of sterile gloves.
- A catheterisation pack.
- Saline solution.
- A 12–16 french Foley catheter.
- A 10 ml pre-filled syringe containing 2% lignocaine gel.
- A 10 ml syringe containing sterile water.
- A catheter bag.
- Adhesive tape.

The procedure

- Gather the equipment.
- Open the catheter pack aseptically onto a trolley, attach the yellow bag to the side of the trolley, and pour antiseptic solution into the receiver.
- If pre-filled syringes are not provided with the pack, draw up 10 ml sterile water and 10 ml lignocaine into separate syringes.
- Wash and dry your hands.
- Put on both pairs of gloves (practise this – it's not easy).
- Ask the patient to remove her sheet and lie flat on the couch, bringing her heels to her buttocks and then letting her knees flop out.
- Drape the patient.
- Place a collecting vessel in the patient's *entre-jambes*.
- Use your non-dominant hand to separate the labia minora.
- Clean the area around the urethral meatus with saline-soaked swabs.
- Coat the end of the catheter with lignocaine gel and instil 5 ml of lignocaine into the urethra.
- Indicate that the anaesthetic needs about 5 minutes to work.
- Discard the outer pair of gloves.
- Holding the catheter by its sleeve, gently and progressively insert it into the urethra.
- Once a stream of urine is obtained, inject 10 ml of sterile water to inflate the catheter's balloon, continually ensuring that this does not cause the patient any pain.
- Gently retract the catheter until a resistance is felt.
- Attach the catheter bag.
- Tape the catheter to the thigh.

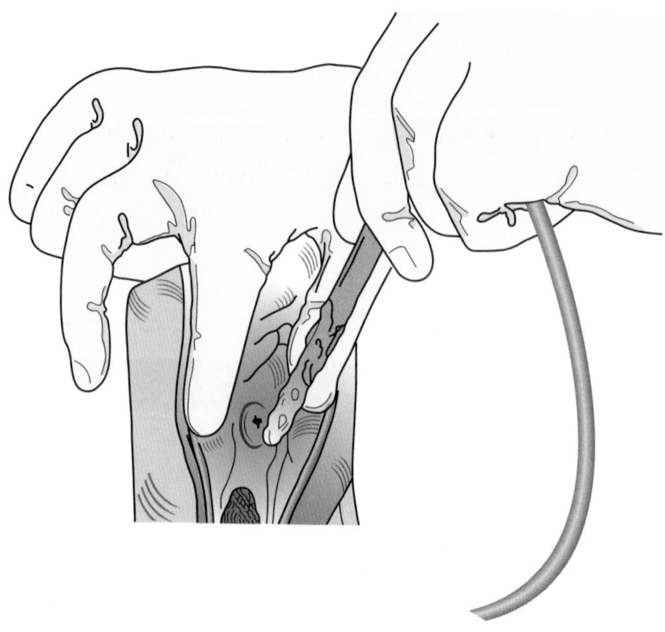

Figure 30. Preparing to insert the catheter.

After the procedure

- Ensure that the patient is comfortable.
- Thank the patient.
- Discard any rubbish.
- Record the date and time of catheterisation, type and size of catheter used, volume of water used to inflate the balloon, and volume of urine in the catheter bag.

History of headaches

'I'm very brave generally', he went on in a low voice: 'only today I happen to have a headache'.

Lewis Carroll, *Through the Looking Glass*

Before starting

- Introduce yourself to the patient.
- Explain that you are going to ask him some questions to uncover the nature of his headaches, and ask for his consent to do this.
- Ensure that he is comfortable.

The history

- Name, age, and occupation.

Presenting complaint and history and presenting complaint

First use open questions to get the patient's history, and elicit his ideas, concerns, and expectations.

Then ask specifically about:

- **S**ite. Ask the patient to point at the site of the pain.
- **O**nset.
- **C**haracter, for example, sharp, dull, throbbing, band-like constriction.
- **R**adiation.
- **A**ssociated factors.
  - Nausea and vomiting.
  - Visual disturbances such as double vision and fortification spectra.
  - Photophobia.
  - Fever, chills.
  - Weight loss.
  - Rash.
  - Scalp tenderness.
  - Neck pain, stiffness.
  - Myalgia.
  - Rhinorrhoea, lacrimation.
  - Altered mental status.
  - Neurological deficit (weakness, numbness, 'pins and needles').
- **T**iming and duration.
- **E**xacerbating and relieving factors, for example, activity, stress, eye strain, caffeine, alcohol, dehydration, hunger, certain foods, coughing/sneezing).
- **S**everity. Ask the patient to rate the pain on a scale of 1 to 10, and to determine the effect that it is having on his life.

Socrates (470–399 BC)

Whither haste ye, O men? Yea, verily ye know not that ye are doing none of the things ye ought …

Past medical history

- Current, past, and childhood illnesses.
- Ask specifically about headache, migraine, hypertension, cardiovascular disease, and travel sickness as a child.
- Surgery.

Drug history

- Prescribed medication. Ask specifically about withdrawal from NSAIDs, opioids, glyceryl trinitrate, and calcium channel blockers.
- Over-the-counter medication.
- Recreational drugs.
- Allergies.

Family history

- Parents, siblings, and children.
- Ask about migraine and travel sickness.

Social history

- Employment, past and present.
- Housing.
- Mood. Depression is a common cause of headaches.
- Smoking.
- Alcohol use. Alcohol is a common cause of headaches.
- Diet: tea and coffee, cheese and yoghurt, chocolate.

After taking the history

- Ask the patient if there is anything he might like to add that you have forgotten to ask about.
- Ask him if he has any questions or concerns.
- Thank him.
- Summarise your findings and offer a differential diagnosis.
- State that you would like to carry out a physical examination and some investigations to confirm your diagnosis and exclude life-threatening causes of headaches (see box below).

Conditions most likely to come up in a history of headaches station

Tension headaches:

- constant pressure, 'as if the head were being squeezed in a vice'
- pain typically last 4–6 hours but this is highly variable
- may be precipitated by stress, eye strain, sleep deprivation, bad posture, irregular meal times

Cluster headaches ('suicide headaches'):

- excruciating unilateral headache that is of rapid onset
- located in the periorbital or temple area, may radiate to the neck or shoulder
- associated with autonomic symptoms such as ptosis, conjunctival injection, lacrimation
- each headache lasts from 15 minutes to 3 hours
- headaches most often occur in 'clusters': once or more every day, often at the same time of day, for a period of several weeks

Migraines:

- unilateral, dull, throbbing headache lasting from 4 to 72 hours
- may be aggravated by activity
- associated with nausea, vomiting, photophobia, phonophobia
- about half experience prodromal symptoms such as altered mood, irritability, or fatigue several hours or days before the headache
- about one-third experience an aura, commonly consisting of visual disturbances or neurological symptoms, before or along with the headache
- frequency of headaches varies considerably, but average is about 1–3 a month

Cranial arteritis:

- unilateral pain in the temporal region
- associated with scalp tenderness, jaw claudication, blurred vision, and tinnitus
- three times more common in females
- mean age of onset is 70 years
- urgent treatment is required to prevent sudden loss of vision

Cervical spondylosis:

- occipital headaches associated with cervical pain
- cervical pain may radiate to the base of the skull, shoulder, or hand and fingers
- may be associated with weakness, numbness, or pins and needles in the arms and hands

Meningitis:

- severe and bilateral headache
- may be associated with high fever, neck stiffness, photophobia, phonophobia, altered mental status

Subarachnoid haemorrhage:

- thunderclap headache ('like being kicked in the head') that is of very rapid onset
- may be associated with vomiting, altered mental status, neck stiffness, photophobia, visual disturbances, seizures

Raised intracranial pressure

- dull, throbbing headache associated with vomiting, ocular palsies, visual disturbances, altered mental status
- may be worse in the morning and may wake the patient up from sleep
- aggravated by coughing and head movement
- alleviated by standing

Sinusitis:

- dull and constant headache or facial pain over the sinuses
- may be associated with flu-like symptoms and facial tenderness
- may be aggravated by bending over or lying down

Trigeminal neuralgia:

- intense unilateral facial pain ('like stabbing electric shocks') lasting from seconds to minutes
- may occur several times a day
- triggered by common activities such as eating, talking, shaving, and tooth-brushing
- may be associated with a trigger area on the face

History of 'funny turns'

Before starting

- Introduce yourself to the patient.
- Explain that you are going to ask him some questions to uncover the cause of his collapse, and ask for his consent to do this.
- Ensure that he is comfortable.

The history

- Name, age, and occupation.

Presenting complaint and history of presenting complaint

First use open questions to get the patient's story, and elicit their ideas, concerns and expectations.

Think about the common causes of a funny turn, as these should inform your line of questioning.

Ask about:

- If the patient remembers falling.
- The circumstances of the fall:
  - had the patient just arisen from bed? (postural hypotension)
  - did the patient suffer an intense emotion? (vasovagal syncope)
  - had the patient been coughing or straining? (situational syncope)
  - had the patient been turning or extending his neck? (carotid sinus syncope)
  - had the patient been exercising? (arrhythmia)
  - did the patient have any palpitations, chest pain, or shortness of breath? (arrhythmia)
- Any loss of consciousness and its duration.
- Prodromal symptoms such as aura, change in mood, strange feeling in the gut, sensation of *déjà vu*.
- Fitting, frothing at the mouth, tongue biting, incontinence.
- Headache or confusion, or amnesia upon recovery.
- Injuries sustained.
- Previous episodes.

Past medical history

- Current, past, and childhood illnesses. Ask specifically about epilepsy, hypertension, heart problems, stroke, diabetes (autonomic neuropathy), cervical spondylosis, and arthritis.
- Surgery.

Drug history

- Prescribed medication. Drugs such as antipsychotics, tricyclic antidepressants, and antihypertensives can cause postural hypotension. Insulin can cause hypoglycaemia.
- Over-the-counter medication.
- Recreational drugs.
- Recent changes in medication.

Family history

- Parents, siblings, and children.
- Ask specifically about epilepsy and heart problems.

Social history

- Smoking.
- Alcohol use.
- Employment, past and present.
- Housing.
- Effect of falls on patient's life.

After taking the history

- Ask the patient if there is anything he might add that you have forgotten to ask about.
- Ask him if he has any questions or concerns.
- Thank him.
- Summarise your findings and offer a differential diagnosis.
- State that you would like to carry out a physical examination and some investigations to confirm your diagnosis.

Conditions most likely to appear in a history of 'funny turns' station	
Simple faint: • loss of consciousness lasting from a few seconds to a few minutes is preceded by nausea, sweatiness, dizziness or tightness in the throat • provoked by stressful, anxiety-provoking, or painful situations (vasovagal syncope), by coughing or straining (situational syncope), or by applying pressure upon the carotid sinus, for example, by wearing a tight collar, turning the head, or shaving (carotid sinus syncope)	**Postural hypotension:** • loss of consciousness preceded by dizziness, light-headedness, confusion, or blurry vision • provoked by postural change • causes include hypovolaemia (e.g. dehydration, bleeding, diuretics, vasodilators), drugs (e.g. tricyclic antidepressants, antipsychotics, alpha blockers), and certain medical conditions (e.g. diabetes, Addison's disease)

Arrhythmia (cardiac syncope):	**Generalised tonic-clonic seizure:**
• may be either a bradycardia or tachycardia • may be provoked by exertion • may be associated with palpitations, chest pain, shortness of breath, fatigue • history of heart disease/risk factors for heart disease are very likely • patient should be hospitalised and placed on a cardiac monitor to rule out ventricular tachycardia, which can result in sudden death • less commonly, cardiac syncope can be caused by an obstructive cardiac lesion such as aortic or mitral stenosis	• sudden loss of consciousness accompanied by fitting, frothing at the mouth, tongue biting, incontinence • seizure lasts for about 2 minutes • seizure is followed by confusion and amnesia • seizure may be preceded by an aura which may involve déjà vu, dizziness, unusual emotions, altered sense perceptions, or other symptoms **Transient ischaemic attack:** • most frequent symptoms include loss of vision, aphasia, unilateral hemiparesis, and unilateral paraesthesia • symptoms last for a few seconds to a few minutes and never for more than 24 hours (by definition) • loss of consciousness can occur, although it is very uncommon

Cranial nerve examination

Specifications: You may be asked to limit your examination to certain cranial nerves only, e.g. I–VI, VII–XII.

Before starting

- Introduce yourself to the patient.
- Explain the examination and ask for his consent to carry it out.
- Ensure that he is comfortable.

The examination

The olfactory nerve (CN I)

- Ask the patient if he has noticed a change in his sense of smell or taste. If he has, indicate that you would perform an olfactory examination by asking the patient to smell different scents, such as mint or coffee.

The optic nerve (CN II)

(See *Station 47: Vision and the eye examination* for more details.)

- Ask the patient whether he wears glasses. If he does, ask him to put them on.
- Test visual acuity on a Snellen chart either from a distance of 6 or 3 metres.
- Test near vision by asking the patient to read test types (or a page in a book).
- Indicate that you could use Ishihara plates to test colour vision specifically.
- Test the visual fields by confrontation. Sit directly opposite the patient, at the same level as him. Ask him to look straight at you and to cover his right eye with his right hand. Cover your left eye with your left hand, and test the visual field of his left eye with your right hand. Bring a wiggly finger into the upper left quadrant, asking the patient to say when he sees the finger. Repeat for the lower left quadrant. Then swap hands and test the upper and lower right quadrants. Now ask the patient to cover his left eye with his left hand. Cover your right eye with your right hand and test the visual field of his right eye with your left hand. Bring a wiggly finger into the upper right quadrant, asking the patient to say when he sees the finger. Repeat for the lower right quadrant. Then swap hands and test the upper and lower left quadrants.
- Indicate that you could use a red hat pin to uncover the blind spot and the presence of a central scotoma.
- Indicate that you could examine the eyes by direct fundoscopy.

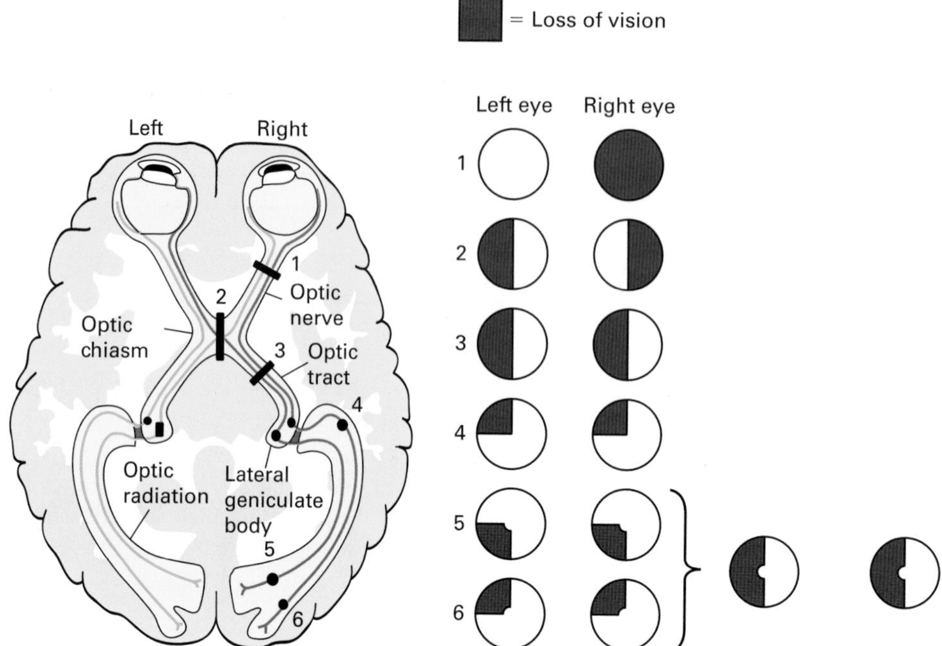

Figure 31. Visual field defects and their origins.

The oculomotor, trochlear, and abducens nerves (CN III, IV, and VI)

(See *Station 47: Vision and the eye examination* for more details.)

- Inspect the eyes, paying particular attention to the size and symmetry of the pupils, and excluding a visible ptosis (Horner's syndrome; see *Figure 32*) or squint.
- Test the direct and consensual pupillary light reflexes. Explain that you are going to shine a bright light into the patient's eye and that this may feel uncomfortable. Bring the light in onto his left eye and look for pupil constriction. Bring the light in onto his left eye once again, but this time look for pupil constriction in his *right eye* (consensual reflex). Repeat for the right eye.
- Perform the swinging flashlight test. Swing the light from one eye to another and look for sustained pupil constriction in both eyes. Intermittent pupil constriction in one eye (Marcus Gunn pupil) suggests a lesion of the optic nerve anterior to the optic chiasm.
- Perform the cover test. Ask the patient to fixate on a point and cover one eye. Observe the movement of the uncovered eye. Repeat the test for the other eye.
- Examine eye movements. Ask the patient to keep his head still and to follow your finger with his eyes. Ask him to report any pain or double vision at any point. Draw an 'H' shape with your finger. Observe for nystagmus at the extremes of gaze.
- Test the accommodation reflex. Ask the patient to follow your finger in to his nose. As the eyes converge, the pupils should constrict.

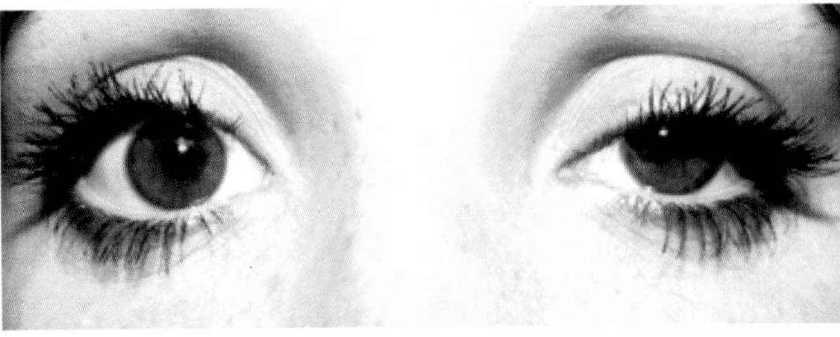

Figure 32. Horner's syndrome. Characteristic features are ipsilateral ptosis, miosis, apparent enophthalmos, and anhydrosis and vasodilatation on the same side of the face.

Reproduced from Otolaryngology – Houston at www.ghorayeb.com with permission.

The trigeminal nerve (CN V)

Sensory part

- Using cotton wool, test light touch in the three branches of the trigeminal nerve. Compare both sides.
- Indicate that you could test the corneal reflex, but that this is likely to cause the patient some discomfort.

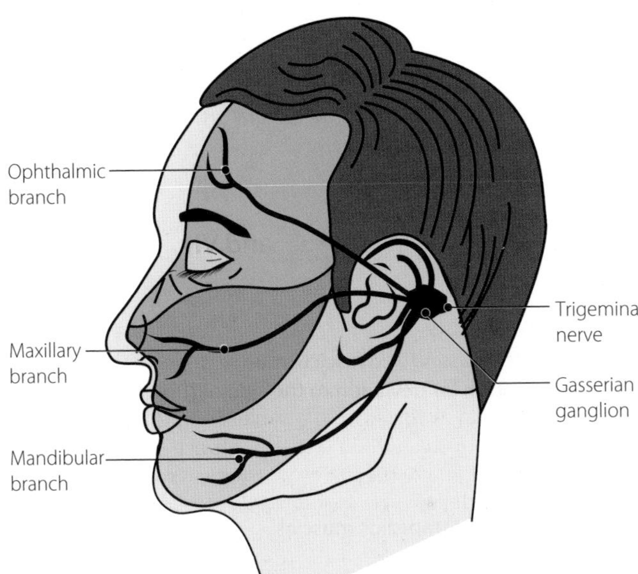

Figure 33. The three branches of the trigeminal nerve. 'Trigeminal' means 'three twins'.

Motor part

- Test the muscles of mastication (the temporalis, masseter, and pterygoid muscles) by asking the patient to:
  - clench his teeth (palpate his temporalis and masseter muscles bilaterally)
  - open and close his mouth against resistance (place your fist under his chin)
- Indicate that you could test the jaw jerk. Ask the patient to let his mouth fall open slightly. Place your fingers on the top of his mandible and tap them lightly with a tendon hammer.

The facial nerve (CN VII)

- Look for facial asymmetry. Note that the nasolabial folds and the angle of the mouth are especially indicative of facial asymmetry.

Sensory part

- Indicate that you could test the anterior two-thirds of the tongue for taste.

Motor part

- Test the muscles of facial expression by asking the patient to:
  - lift his eyebrows as far as they will go
  - close his eyes as tightly as possible (try to open them)
  - blow out his cheeks
  - purse his lips or whistle
  - show his teeth

The acoustic nerve (CN VIII)

(See *Station 46: Hearing and the ear examination* for more details.)

- Test hearing sensitivity in each ear by occluding one ear and rubbing your thumb and fingers together in front of the other.
- Indicate that you could carry out the Rinne and Weber tests and examine the ears by auroscopy (see *Station 46*).

The glossopharyngeal nerve (CN IX)

- Indicate that you could test the gag reflex by touching the tonsillar fossae on both sides with an orange stick, but that this is likely to cause the patient some discomfort.

The vagus nerve (CN X)

- Ask the patient to phonate (say 'aah') and, aided by a pen torch, look for deviation of the uvula to the opposite side of the lesion. Use a tongue depressor if necessary.

The hypoglossal nerve (CN XII)

- Aided by a pen torch, inspect the tongue for wasting and fasciculation.
- Ask the patient to stick out his tongue and look for deviation to the side of the lesion. Now ask him to wiggle it from side to side.

The accessory nerve (CN XI)

- Look for wasting of the sternocleidomastoid and trapezius muscles.
- Ask the patient to:
  - shrug his shoulders against resistance
  - turn his head to either side against resistance

After the examination

- Thank the patient.
- Ensure that he is comfortable.
- If appropriate, state that you would order some key investigations, e.g. a CT or MRI.
- Summarise your findings and offer a differential diagnosis.

Conditions most likely to appear in a cranial nerve examination station

Third nerve palsy:

- the eye is depressed and abducted (down and out)
- elevation, adduction, and depression are limited, but abduction and intortion are normal
- there is a ptosis (drooping of the upper eyelid)
- the pupil may be dilated and unreactive to light or accommodation

Bell's (facial nerve) palsy:

- facial drooping and paralysis on the affected half
- if the forehead muscles are spared, it is a central rather than a peripheral palsy

Horner's syndrome:

- signs of Horner's syndrome are ptosis, miosis, enophthalmos, and facial anhydrosis

Cavernous sinus syndrome:

- the cavernous sinus contains the carotid artery and its sympathetic plexus, CN III, IV, and VI and the ophthalmic and maxillary branches of CN V
- signs of a cavernous sinus lesion may include (generally unilateral) proptosis, chemosis, ophthalmoplegia, and loss of sensation in the first and second divisions of the trigeminal nerve

Cerebellopontine angle syndrome:

- lesions in the area of the cerebellopontine angle can cause compression of CN V, VII, and VIII
- signs may include palsies of CN V and VII, nystagmus, ipsilateral deafness, and ipsilateral cerebellar signs

Bulbar palsy:

- lower motor neurone lesion in the medulla oblongata leads to bilateral impairment of function of CN IX–XII
- signs include speech difficulties, dysphagia, wasting and fasciculation of the tongue, absent palatal movements, absent gag reflex

Pseudo-bulbar palsy:

- upper motor neurone lesion in the corticobulbar pathways in the pyramidal tract leads to impairment of function of CN IX–XII and also CN V and VII
- signs include speech difficulties, dysphagia, conical and spastic tongue, brisk jaw jerk, emotional lability

Station 32

Motor system of the upper limbs examination

Before starting

- Introduce yourself to the patient.
- Explain the examination and ask for his permission to carry it out.
- Position him and ask him to expose his arms.
- Ask if he is currently experiencing any pain.

The examination

Inspection

- Look for abnormal posturing.
- Look for abnormal movements such as tremor, fasciculation, dystonia, athetosis.
- Assess the muscles of the hands, arms, and shoulder girdle for size, shape, and symmetry. You can also measure the circumference of the arms.

Tone

- Ensure that the patient is not in any pain.
- Ask the patient to relax the muscles in his arms.
- Test the tone in the upper limbs by holding the patient's hand and simultaneously pronating and supinating and flexing and extending the forearm. If you suspect increased tone, ask the patient to clench his teeth and re-test. Is the increased tone best described as spasticity (clasp-knife) or as rigidity (lead pipe)? Spasticity suggests a pyramidal lesion, rigidity suggests an extra-pyramidal lesion.

Power

- Test muscle strength for shoulder abduction, elbow flexion and extension, wrist flexion and extension, finger flexion, extension, abduction and adduction, and thumb abduction and opposition. Compare muscle strength on both sides, and grade it on the MRC muscle strength scale:
  0 No movement.
  1 Feeble contractions.
  2 Movement, but not against gravity.
  3 Movement against gravity, but not against resistance.
  4 Movement against resistance, but not to full strength.
  5 Full strength.

Table 12. Important root values in the upper limb – muscle strength

Movement	Root value
• Shoulder abduction	C5
• Elbow flexion	C6
• Elbow extension	C7
• Wrist extension	C6, C7
• Wrist flexion	C7, C8
• Finger extension	C7 (radial nerve)
• Finger flexion	C8
• Finger abduction/adduction	T1 (ulnar nerve)
• Thumb abduction/opposition	T1 (median nerve)

Reflexes

- Test biceps, supinator, and triceps reflexes with a tendon hammer (see *Figure 34*). Compare both sides. If a reflex cannot be elicited, ask the patient to clench his teeth and re-test.

Table 13. Important root values in the upper limb – reflexes	
• Biceps	C5, C6
• Supinator	C6
• Triceps	C7

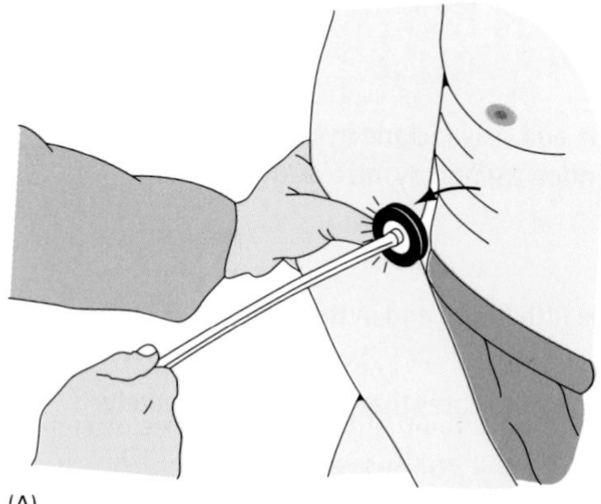
(A)

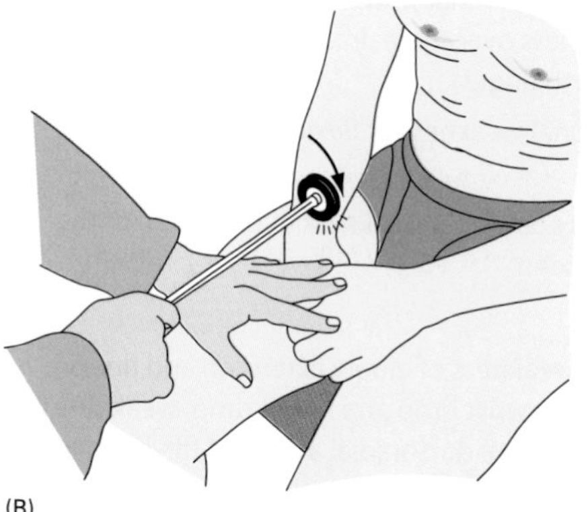
(B)

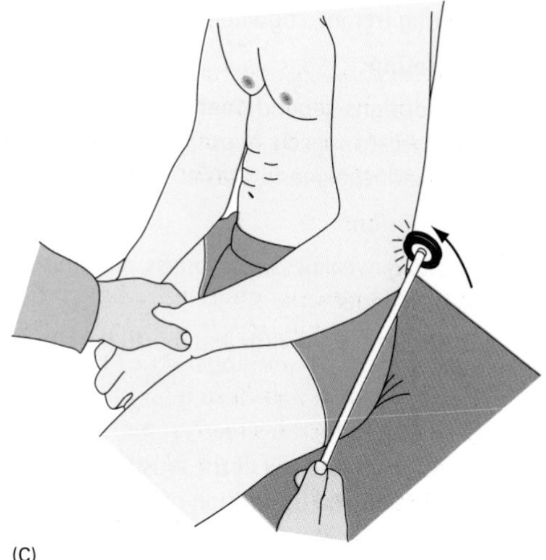
(C)

Figure 34. Testing (A) biceps, (B) suppinator, and (C) triceps reflexes.

Cerebellar signs

- Test for intention tremor, dysynergia, and dysmetria (past-pointing) by asking the patient to carry out the finger-to-nose test.
  - Place your index finger at about 2 feet from the patient's face. Ask him to touch the tip of his nose and then the tip of your finger with the tip of his index finger. Once he is able to do this, ask him to do it as fast as he can. And remember that he has two hands!
- Then test for dysdiadochokinesis.
  - Ask the patient to clap and then show him how to clap by alternating the palmar and dorsal surfaces of one hand. Once he is able to do this, ask him to do it as fast as he can. Ask him to repeat the test with his other hand.

After the examination

- Thank the patient.
- Ensure that he is comfortable.
- Ask to carry out a full neurological examination.
- If appropriate, indicate that you would order some key investigations, e.g. CT, MRI, nerve conduction studies, electromyography, etc.
- Summarise your findings and offer a differential diagnosis.

Conditions most likely to come up in a motor system of the upper limbs examination
Parkinson's disease: • motor signs include forward-flexed posture, mask-like facial expression, speech difficulties, resting tremor, cogwheel rigidity, bradykinesia
Cerebellar lesion: • motor signs depend on the anatomy of the lesion, and may include nystagmus, slurred or staccato speech, hypotonia, hyporeflexia, intention tremor, dysmetria, dysynergia, dysdiadochokinesis, ataxia
Ulnar nerve lesion: • wasting, weakness, numbness, and tingling in the fifth finger and in the medial half of the fourth finger • curling up of the fifth and fourth fingers ('ulnar claw') indicates that the nerve is severely affected
Median nerve lesion: • a lesion at the level of the wrist produces wasting of the thenar muscles, weakness of abduction and opposition of the thumb, and numbness over the palmar aspect of the thumb, index finger, third finger, and lateral half of the fourth finger • a lesion at the level of the forearm produces additional weakness of flexion of the distal and middle phalanges • a lesion at the level of the elbow or above produces additional weakness of pronation of the forearm and ulnar deviation of the wrist on wrist flexion
Radial nerve lesion: • a lesion at the level of the axilla or above produces weakness of elbow extension and flexion, weakness of wrist and finger extension with attending wrist drop and finger drop, weakness of thumb abduction and extension, and sensory loss over the dorsoradial aspect of the hand and the dorsal aspect of the radial 3½ fingers (usually circumscribed to a small, triangular area over the first dorsal web space) • inferior lesions are likely to spare triceps (elbow extension), brachioradialis (elbow flexion), and extensor carpi radialis longus (wrist extension and radial abduction, but only one of five wrist extensors)
Radiculopathy, affecting a single root nerve (see *Table 13*)
Hemiplegia/hemiparesis: • paralysis or weakness on one side of the body accompanied by decreased movement control, spasticity, and hyper-reflexia (upper motor neurone syndrome)
Myopathy: • symmetrical weakness predominantly affecting proximal muscle groups • in contrast to neuropathy, in myopathy muscle atrophy and hyporeflexia occur very late

Sensory system of the upper limbs examination

Before starting

- Introduce yourself to the patient.
- Explain the examination and ask for his permission to carry it out.
- Position him so that he is comfortably seated and ask him to expose his arms and to position them so that the palms are facing towards you.
- Ask if he is currently experiencing any pain.

The examination

To examine the sensory system, test light touch, pain, vibration sense, and proprioception.

Do not forget to inspect the arms before you start. In particular, look for muscle wasting, fasciculation, scars and other obvious signs.

- Light touch (not light rub). Ask the patient to close his eyes and to say 'yes' each time he is touched with a wisp of cotton wool. Apply the cotton wool to his sternum as a test. Then apply it to each of the dermatomes of the arm, moving from the hand and up along the arm. Remember to compare both sides as you go along.
- Pain. Ask the patient to close his eyes and apply a sharp object – ideally a neurological pin – to the sternum and then to each of the dermatomes of the arm, as above. Compare both sides as you go along. If there is any loss of or difference in sensation, map out the area affected.

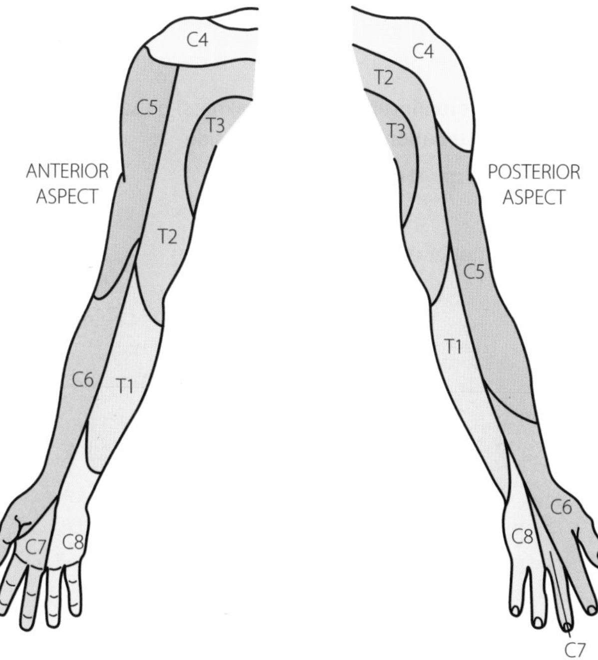

Figure 35. Dermatomes of the arm.

- Vibration. Ask the patient to close his eyes and apply a vibrating 128 Hz or 256 Hz tuning fork (not the smaller 512 Hz tuning fork used in hearing tests) to the sternum and then over the bony prominences of the arm, starting with the interphalangeal joint of the thumb and moving up to the wrist and then the elbow. Compare both sides as you go along.
- Proprioception. Ensure that the patient does not suffer from arthritis or from some other painful condition of the hand. Ask him to close his eyes. Hold the distal interphalangeal joint of his index finger between the thumb and index finger of one hand. With the other hand, move the distal phalanx up and down at the joint, asking him to identify the direction of each movement, e.g. *"I'm going to move your finger up and down. Is this up or down?" "What about this? And that?"* Compare both sides.

After the examination

- Thank the patient.
- Ensure that he is comfortable.
- Ask to carry out a full neurological examination.
- Summarise your findings and offer a differential diagnosis.

Conditions most likely to come up in a sensory examination of the upper limbs station
Mononeuropathy: • lesion affecting a single nerve, e.g. ulnar, median, or radial nerve (see *Station 32*)
Polyneuropathy: • lesion affecting multiple nerves in a glove and stocking distribution, such as in diabetic neuropathy
Radiculopathy: • lesion affecting a single root nerve, e.g. C6
Brown–Séquard syndrome: • numbness to touch and vibration and loss of proprioception (and weakness) on same side of the lesion, and loss of pain and temperature sensation on the opposite side • caused by lateral hemisection or injury of the spinal cord
Syringomyelia: • loss of pain and temperature sensation but not of other sensory modalities

Motor system of the lower limbs examination

Before starting

- Introduce yourself to the patient.
- Explain the examination and ask for his permission to carry it out.
- Position him and ask him to expose his legs.
- Ask if he is currently experiencing any pain.

The examination

Inspection

- Look for deformities of the foot.
- Look for abnormal posturing.
- Look for fasciculation.
- Assess the muscles of the legs for size, shape, and symmetry. You can also measure the circumference of the quadriceps or calves.

Tone

- Ensure that the patient is not in any pain.
- Ask the patient to relax the muscles in his legs.
- Test the tone in the legs by rolling the leg on the bed, by flexing and extending the knee, and/or by abruptly lifting the leg at the knee.

Power

- Test muscle strength for hip flexion, extension, abduction and adduction, knee flexion and extension, plantar flexion and dorsiflexion of the foot and big toe, and inversion and eversion of the forefoot. Compare muscle strength on both sides, and grade it on the MRC scale for muscle strength:
  0 No movement.
  1 Feeble contractions.
  2 Movement, but not against gravity.
  3 Movement against gravity, but not against resistance.
  4 Movement against resistance, but not to full strength.
  5 Full strength.

Table 14. Important root values in the lower limb – muscle strength	
• Hip flexion	L1, L2
• Hip extension	S1
• Hip adduction	L2
• Knee flexion	L5, S1
• Knee extension	L3, L4
• Foot dorsiflexion	L4, L5
• Foot plantar flexion	S1
• Big toe dorsiflexion	L5

Reflexes

- Test the knee jerk and ankle jerk with a tendon hammer (see *Figure 36*). Test the knee jerk by raising and supporting the knee with one arm and striking the patellar tendon with the other. To test the ankle jerk, abduct and externally rotate the hip and flex the knee and ankle. Then strike at the Achilles' tendon. Compare both sides. If a reflex cannot be elicited, ask the patient to clench his teeth and re-test.

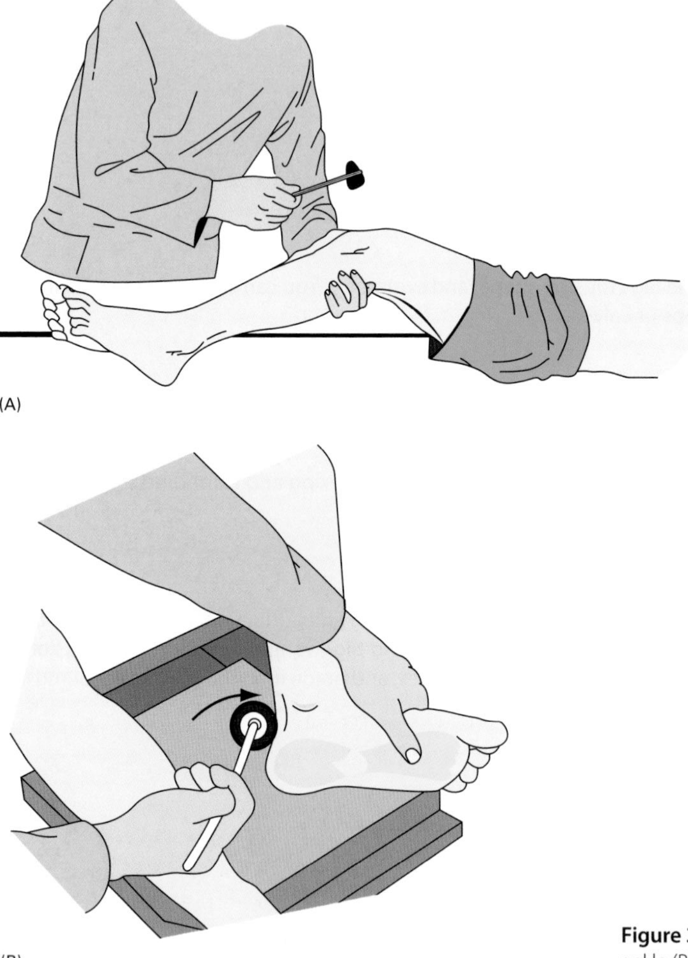

Figure 36. Testing the knee (A) and ankle (B) reflexes.

- Test for clonus by holding up the ankle and rapidly dorsiflexing the foot.
- Test for the Babinsky sign (extensor plantar reflex) by scraping the side of the foot with the sharp end of a tendon hammer or with an orange stick. The sign is positive if there is extension of the big toe at the MTP joint, so-called 'upgoing plantars'.

Table 15. Important root values in the lower limb – reflexes	
Knee jerk	L3, L4
Ankle jerk	S1

Cerebellar signs

- Carry out the heel-to-shin test.
  - Lie the patient on a couch. Ask him to run the heel of one leg down the shin of the other, and then to bring the heel back up to the knee and to start again. Ask him to repeat the test with his other leg.

Gait

- If he can, ask the patient to walk to the end of the room and to turn around and walk back. (See *Station 36: Gait, co-ordination, and cerebellar function examination*.)

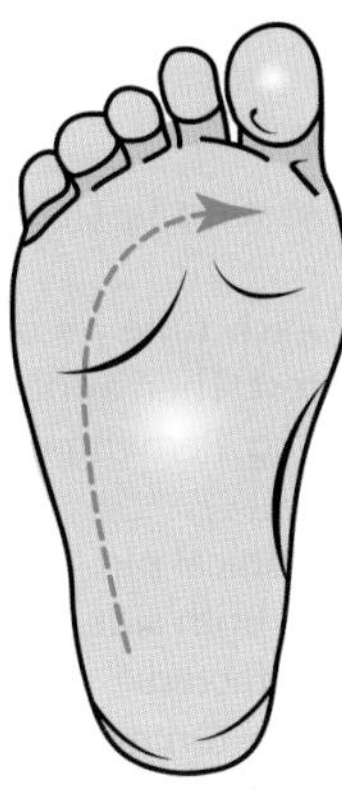

Figure 37. Testing for the Babinsky or extensor plantar sign.

After the examination

- Thank the patient.
- Ensure that he is comfortable.
- Ask to carry out a full neurological examination.
- If appropriate, indicate that you would order some key investigations, e.g. CT, MRI, nerve conduction studies, electromyography, etc.
- Summarise your findings and offer a differential diagnosis.

Conditions most likely to come up in a motor system of the lower limbs examination station	
Mononeuropathy: • lesion affecting a single nerve, most commonly the common peroneal nerve (resulting in foot drop) **Polyneuropathy:** • lesion affecting multiple nerves in a glove and stocking distribution as in diabetic neuropathy **Radiculopathy:** • lesion affecting a single root nerve (see *Table 15*) **Hemiplegia/hemiparesis:** • paralysis or weakness on one side of the body accompanied by decreased movement control, spasticity, and hyperreflexia (upper motor neurone sydrome)	**Cauda equina lesion:** • signs include unilateral or bilateral lower limb motor and/or sensory deficits • the ankle jerks are usually absent on both sides • upper motor neurone signs such as Babinsky sign and clonus are absent **Myopathy:** • symmetrical weakness predominantly affecting proximal muscle groups • in contrast to neuropathy, in myopathy muscle atrophy and hyporeflexia occur very late

Sensory system of the lower limbs examination

Before starting

- Introduce yourself to the patient.
- Explain the examination and ask for his permission to carry it out.
- Position him on a couch and ask him to expose his legs.
- Ask if he is currently experiencing any pain.

The examination

To examine the sensory system, test light touch, pain, vibration sense, and proprioception.

- Do not forget to inspect the legs before you start. In particular, look for muscle wasting, fasciculation, scars, and any other obvious signs.
- Light touch (not light rub). Ask the patient to close his eyes and to say 'yes' each time he is touched with a wisp of cotton wool. Apply the cotton wool to his sternum as a test. Then apply it to each of the dermatomes of the leg, moving from the foot and up along the leg. Remember to compare both sides as you go along.
- Pain. Ask the patient to close his eyes and apply a sharp object – ideally a neurological pin – to the sternum and then to each of the dermatomes of the leg, as above. Compare both sides as you go along. If there is any loss of or difference in sensation, map out the area affected.
- Vibration. Ask the patient to close his eyes and apply a vibrating 128 Hz or 256 Hz tuning fork (not the smaller 512 Hz tuning fork used in hearing tests) to the sternum and then over the bony prominences of the leg, starting with the interphalangeal joint of the big toe. Compare both sides as you go along.

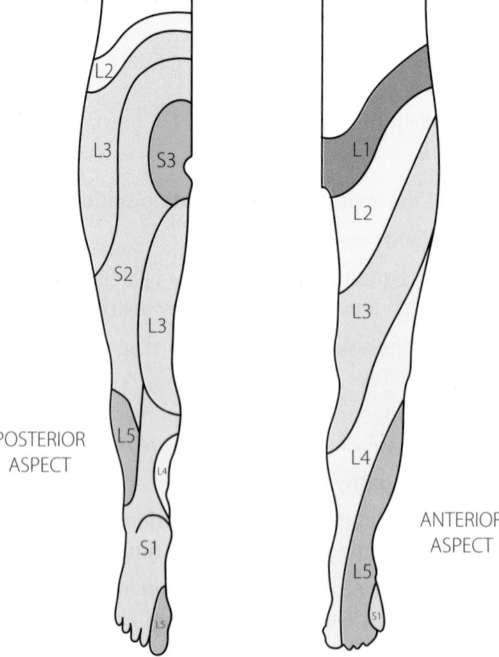

Figure 38. Dermatomes of the leg.

- Proprioception. Ensure that the patient does not suffer from arthritis, gout, or some other painful condition of the foot. Ask him to close his eyes. Hold the interphalangeal joint of his big toe between the thumb and index finger of one hand. With the other hand, move the distal phalanx up and down at the joint, asking him to identify the direction of each movement, e.g. *"I'm going to move your toe up and down. Is this up or down?" "What about this? And that?"* Compare both sides. If the patient is able to stand, you can also perform Romberg's test (see *Station 36: Gait, co-ordination, and cerebellar function examination*).

After the examination

- Thank the patient.
- Ensure that he is comfortable.
- Ask to carry out a full neurological examination.
- If appropriate, indicate that you would order some key investigations, e.g. CT, MRI, nerve conduction studies, electromyography, etc.
- Summarise your findings and offer a differential diagnosis.

Conditions most likely to come up in a sensory system of the lower limbs examination station
Mononeuropathy: • lesion affecting a single nerve
Polyneuropathy: • lesion affecting multiple nerves as in alcoholic or diabetic neuropathy
Radiculopathy: • lesion affecting a single root nerve (see *Figure 38*)
Cauda equina lesion: • signs include unilateral or bilateral lower limb motor and/or sensory deficits, including 'saddle anaesthesia' (loss of sensation in the area of the buttocks and perineum)
Hemisensory loss: • loss of sensation including light, pain, temperature, vibration, and proprioception on one side of the body • normally accompanied by hemiplegia/hemiparesis with attendant spasticity and hyperreflexia (upper motor neurone syndrome)
Brown–Séquard syndrome: • numbness to touch and vibration and loss of proprioception (and weakness) on same side of the lesion, and loss of pain and temperature sensation on the opposite side • caused by lateral hemisection or injury of the spinal cord
Posterior column disease: • loss of proprioception and vibration but not of other sensory modalities

Station 36

Gait, co-ordination, and cerebellar function examination

Before starting

- Introduce yourself to the patient.
- Explain the examination and ask for his consent to carry it out.
- Ask if he is currently experiencing any pain.

Examination of gait

- Inspection. Inspect the patient in the sitting position, noting any abnormalities of posture. Ask him to stand up and ensure that he is steady on his feet. Truncal ataxis suggests a midline cerebellar lesion. Inspect posture from both front and side.
- Gait and arm swing. Ask him to walk to the end of the room and to turn around and walk back. If he normally uses a stick or frame, he should not be prevented from doing so. Note the gait and also the arm swing and any difficulty in standing or turning.
- Heel-to-toe test. Ask him to walk heel-to-toe, 'as if on a tightrope'. Ataxia on a narrow-based gait suggests a cerebellar or vestibular lesion.
- Romberg's test. Ask him to stand unaided with his feet together, his arms by his sides and his eyes closed. If he sways and threatens to lose his balance, the test is said to be positive, indicating posterior column disease.

You must be in a position to steady the patient should he threaten to fall.

Examination of co-ordination

- Resting tremor. Ask the patient to sit down, to rest his hands in his lap, and to close his eyes. Resting tremor is a sign of Parkinson's disease.
- Intention tremor. Ask the patient to do something, e.g. remove his watch or write a sentence.
- Muscle tone in the arms. Examine muscle tone in the elbow (flexion and extension) and wrist (flexion and extension, abduction and adduction) joints. Compare both sides.
- Dysdiadochokinesis. Ask the patient to clap and then show him how to clap by alternating the palmar and dorsal surfaces of one hand. Once he is able to do this, ask him to do it as fast as he can. Ask him to repeat the test with his other hand.
- Finger-to-nose test. Place your index finger at about 2 feet from the patient's face. Ask him to touch the tip of his nose and then the tip of your finger with the tip of his index finger. Once he is able to do this, ask him to do it as fast as he can. And remember that he has two hands! Look for intention tremor and dysmetria (past-pointing), both signs of cerebellar disease.
- Fine finger movements. Ask the patient to oppose his thumb with each of his other fingers in turn. Once he is able to do this, ask him to do it as fast as he can. Again, remember that he has two hands.
- Muscle tone in the legs. Ask the patient to lie down on a couch and, if possible, to relax the muscles in his legs. Test the tone in his legs by rolling the leg on the bed, by flexing and extending the knee, and/or by abruptly lifting the leg at the knee.
- Heel-to-shin test. Ask the patient to run the heel of one leg down the shin of the other, and then to bring the heel back up to the knee and to start again. Ask him to repeat the test with his other leg.

Assessment of cerebellar function

- If you are specifically asked to assess cerebellar function, carry out the above plus test eye movements (nystagmus) and ask the patient to say 'baby hippopotamus' (slurred/staccato speech). If you are then asked to list cerebellar signs, simply remember the acronym DANISH:
  - **D**ysdiadochokinesis and dysmetria (finger overshoot)
  - **A**taxia
  - **N**ystagmus – test eye movements
  - **I**ntention tremor
  - **S**lurred/staccato speech – ask the patient to say 'baby hippopotamus' or 'British constitution'
  - **H**ypotonia/hyporeflexia

After the examination

- Ask the patient if he has any questions or concerns.
- Thank the patient.
- Ensure that he is comfortable.
- Ask to carry out a full neurological examination.
- Summarise your findings and offer a differential diagnosis.

Conditions most likely to come up in a gait and co-ordination examination
Hemiplegic gait: • the pelvis tilts upwards, the hip is abducted, and the leg is swung forwards in a semi-circular movement • the leg is stiff and extended but the arm may be held in flexion and adduction with minimal swing
Scissor gait: • a spastic gait seen in cerebral palsy and resulting from muscle contractures • the hips, knees, and ankles are flexed, producing a crouching and tiptoeing appearance • in addition, the hips are adducted and internally rotated, such that the knees cross or hit each other in a scissor-like movement
Festinating gait: • seen in Parkinson's disease • short shuffling steps with stiff arms and legs and stooped posture; difficulty starting and turning
Ataxic gait: • seen in spinal and cerebellar lesions and in alcohol intoxication • unsteady, broad-based gait with a lurching quality
Neuropathic gait: • seen in peripheral neuropathies • weak foot dorsiflexors result in a high-stepping gait with foot-slapping; the high-stepping is an attempt to prevent the foot from dragging and being injured; also called 'high-stepping gait' or 'foot-slapping gait'

Trendelenburg gait: • seen in weakness of the hip abductors or in an inability or reluctance to abduct the hip, e.g. due to a fractured neck of femur or to arthritic pain • the pelvis tilts to the unaffected side in the stance phase; as a result, the trunk lurches to the affected side in an attempt to maintain a level pelvis • bilateral Trendelenburg results in a typical waddling gait
Antalgic gait: • seen in arthritis and trauma • avoidance of motions that trigger pain • often quick, short, and light footsteps • not to be confused with a Trendelenburg gait
Myopathic gait: • in muscular diseases the proximal pelvic girdle muscles are most affected, such that the patient is unable to stabilise the pelvis in the stance phase • the pelvis drops to the side of the leg being raised, and this results in a broad-based, waddling gait

Speech assessment

The patient is likely to find the assessment difficult and distressing, so remember to be especially empathetic. In particular, do not rush the examination or keep on interrupting the patient, but move at a pace that feels comfortable for him.

Table 16. Definitions

Dysphonia	Impairment of ability to vocalise speech.
Dysarthria	Impairment of ability to articulate speech.
Dysphasia	Impairment of ability to comprehend or express language.
Expressive dysphasia (Broca's area, in the inferolateral dominant frontal lobe) and receptive dysphasia (Wernicke's area, in the posterior superior dominant temporal lobe) often co-exist.	

Before starting

- Introduce yourself to the patient.
- Explain the assessment and obtain his consent to carry it out.
- Ask him to try to describe his current problems.

The assessment

Orientation in time and place

Time

Name: (year) (season) (month) (date) (day)

Place

Name: (country) (county/region) (town) (hospital) (floor)

Dysphasia

Expressive

Assess whether the patient has difficulty in finding the right words whilst in conversation with you.

Nominal

Ask the patient to name some common objects such as a watch, pen, or penny coin; then to name the components of some of these objects, e.g. hour hand, winder, strap. Note that nominal dysphasia is a common form of expressive dysphasia.

Receptive

Assess whether the patient has difficulty understanding you by asking him to carry out some simple instructions such as 'shut your eyes', 'touch your nose', and 'point to the door'.

Dysarthria

Ask the patient to repeat some of the following: 'British constitution', 'West Register Street', 'Baby hippopotamus', 'Biblical criticism', and 'Artillery'.

Assess the structures involved in phonation and articulation by asking the patient to repeat:

- 'Me, me, me' Lips
- 'La, la, la' Tongue
- 'Khu, gut' Palate
- 'Ah' Palate, larynx, and expiratory muscles

Dysphonia

- Make a note of the patient's volume of speech, which may be low if there is weakness of the vocal cords or respiratory muscles. Ask the patient to cough, and look out for 'bovine' cough.

Dyslexia

- Correct the patient's vision and ask him to read a short paragraph from a newspaper or magazine, and bear in mind that not all people who can't read are dyslexic!

Dyscalculia

- Ask the patient to carry out simple sums and subtractions.

Dysgraphia

- Ask the patient to write a sentence.

After the assessment

- Ask the patient if he has any questions or concerns.
- Thank the patient.
- Summarise your findings, offer a differential diagnosis, and state the probable area of the lesion.

Conditions most likely to come up in a speech assessment station
Dsyphasia: • expressive dysphasia results from damage to Broca's area in the left inferior frontal region • there is 'telegraphic speech' characterised by reduction in word range and non-fluent speech with errors of grammar and syntax • receptive dysphasia results from damage to Wernicke's area in the left superior posterior temporal lobe • comprehension is poor and speech, although fluent, may be meaningless • global dysphasia results from damage to both Broca's area and Wernicke's area • there is both poor comprehension and lack of fluency
Dysarthria (slurred speech): • can result from lesions of the tongue, lips, or mouth; bilateral upper motor neurone lesions of the corticobulbar tract (pseudobulbar or spastic dysarthria, 'hot potato speech'); bulbar palsy (nasal speech with slurring of labial and lingual consonants); cerebellar lesions (scanning or staccato speech); Parkinson's disease (monotonous speech with a soft voice); or myasthenia gravis (nasal speech with hoarseness and vocal fatigue), amongst others
Dysphonia: • results from vocal cord pathology, as in laryngitis, or from damage to the vagal nerve supply to the vocal cords • bovine cough results from inability to abduct vocal cords
Dyslexia, dyscalculia, dysgraphia: • result from lesions of the dominant parietal lobe

General psychiatric history

Specifications: The instructions for this station are likely to ask you to focus on one part of the history, e.g. presenting complaint and history of presenting complaint, social history, personal history.

In taking a psychiatric history, it is especially important to put the patient at ease and to be seen to be sensitive, tactful, and empathetic.

Before starting

- Introduce yourself to the patient.
- Ensure that he is comfortable. Make some general comments to put him at ease and build a rapport.

The history

- Name, age, and mode of referral (if not already provided).

Presenting complaint and history of presenting complaint

- Ask mainly open questions, e.g. *Can you tell me why you've come to the hospital today?* Try to form a diagnostic hypothesis and to validate or falsify it by asking further questions (logico-deductive approach).
- Ask about:
  - the onset and duration of symptoms
  - the effect the symptoms are having on the patient's everyday life
  - any treatments so far
- If you have not done so already, ask screening questions about mood, anxiety, obsessions, abnormal beliefs, and abnormal perceptions (see *Station 39: Mental state examination*).

Past psychiatric history

- Previous episodes of illness.
- Previous treatments and their outcomes.
- Previous admissions, formal and informal.
- History of neglect or self-harm.
- History of violence.

Past medical history

- Current illness:
  - acute illness
  - chronic illness
  - vascular risk factors
- Past and childhood illnesses, including head injury.
- Surgery.

Drug history/current treatments

- Psychological treatments.
- Prescribed medication.

- Recent changes in prescribed medication.
- Over-the-counter drugs.
- Allergies.

Substance use

- Alcohol.
- Tobacco.
- Illicit drugs.

[Note] Further questioning to establish dependence may be required if alcohol use and/or illicit drug use is high (see *Station 42: Alcohol history*).

Family history

- Determine if anyone in the family has suffered from psychiatric illness or attempted suicide, e.g. *"Has anyone in the family ever had a nervous breakdown?"*
- Partner: age or age at death, occupation, health.
- Children: age or age at death, occupation, health.
- Quality of relationships and atmosphere in the home.
- Recent events in the family.

Social history

- Self-care.
- Social support.
- Housing.
- Finances.
- Typical day.
- Interests and hobbies.
- Predominant mood and premorbid personality.

Personal history

- Birth.
- Developmental milestones.
- Childhood: emotional problems, serious illnesses, prolonged separation from parents.
- Educational achievement.
- Occupational history.
- Forensic history.
- Psychosexual history: past and present partners (including same sex partners), quality of relationships, frequency of sexual intercourse, sexual problems, physical or sexual abuse.
- Forensic history, e.g. *"Have you ever had problems with the police or with the law?"*
- Religious or spiritual orientation, e.g. *"Do you believe there is something beyond us, like God?"*

After taking the history

- Ask the patient if there is anything he might add that you have forgotten to ask about.
- Indicate that you could check the patient's psychiatric records (if any) and take an informant history, for example, from a relative, friend, carer, police officer, GP, or other healthcare professional.
- Summarise your findings and offer a differential diagnosis.
- Thank the patient.

Common conditions most likely to appear in a psychiatric history station

- Depressive disorder
- Anxiety disorder, e.g. agoraphobia, social phobia, panic disorder, generalised anxiety disorder
- Mixed depression–anxiety
- Obsessive–compulsive disorder
- Eating disorder
- Mania and bipolar affective disorder
- Schizophrenia and other delusional disorders

NB. For descriptions of these conditions, see *Table 17* at the end of *Station 39*.

Mental state examination

Specifications: The instructions for this station are likely to ask you to focus on one part of the mental state examination only, or to omit cognitive assessment. In some places, the patient–actor might by replaced by a real patient on a video recording.

Before starting

- Introduce yourself to the patient.
- Explain that you would like to explore his thoughts and feelings, and ask him if this is OK.
- Take out a pen and pad.

Assessing the mental state

The mental state can be assessed under 7 main headings:
1. Appearance and behaviour.
2. Speech.
3. Mood.
4. Abnormal thoughts.
5. Abnormal experiences.
6. Cognition.
7. Insight.

Appearance and behaviour

Begin by asking the patient some open questions, and focusing your attention on his *appearance and behaviour*.

- Level of consciousness.
- Appearance: body build, posture, general physical condition, grooming and hygiene, dress, physical stigmata such as scars, piercings, and tattoos.
- Inappropriate behaviour and attitude to the examiner. In particular note: facial expression, degree of eye contact, and quality of rapport.
- Motor activity/disorders of movement, e.g. agitation, retardation, tremor, dystonias, mannerisms.

Speech

Note:

- Amount, rate, volume, and tone of speech, e.g. logorrhoea (large amount of speech), pressure of speech (increased rate of speech), poverty of speech (small amount of speech), speech retardation (decreased rate of speech), mutism (no speech).
- Form of speech, e.g. circumstantiality, tangentiality, clang associations, puns, rhymes, neologisms, perseverations. In circumstantiality, speech is organised and goal-oriented but cramped by excessive or irrelevant detail and parenthetical remarks. In tangentiality, speech is organised but not goal-oriented in that it is only very indirectly related to the questions being asked.

Mood

Note or ask about:

- Current mood state and severity. If there is the suggestion of depression, ask the patient to rate his mood on a scale of 1 to 10, with 1 being the worst that he has ever felt and 10 being normal.
- Biological symptoms: sleep, appetite, libido, energy.
- Ideas of harm to self, e.g. *"People with problems similar to those that you have been describing often feel that life is no longer worth living. Have you felt that life is no longer worth living?"* If yes, then this should be explored further: *"Have you ever thought of killing yourself?" "Have you made any plans?" "Would you carry out those plans?" "What stops/would stop you?"*.
- Ideas of harm to others.
- Anxiety and anxiety symptoms, e.g. butterflies, giddiness, clamminess, palpitations, difficulty catching breath. If there is the suggestion of an anxiety disorder, this should be explored further.

You are likely to fail this station if you do not ask about ideas of harm in an at-risk patient.

Abnormal thoughts

Note or ask about:

- Stream of thought, e.g. pressure of thought, poverty of thought, thought blocking.
- Form of thought, e.g. flight of ideas, loosening of associations, over-inclusive thinking.
- Content of thought.
  - Preoccupations, ruminations, obsessions, and compulsive acts, e.g. for obsessions, *"Do certain things keep coming into your mind even though you try hard to keep them out?"* And for compulsive acts, *"Do you ever find yourself spending a lot of time doing the same thing over and over again even though you've already done it well enough?"*
  - Phobias, e.g. *"Do you have any special fears, like some people are afraid of spiders or snakes?"*
  - Delusions and overvalued ideas. For obvious reasons, you cannot easily ask directly about delusions. Begin by an introductory statement and general questions, such as *"I would like to ask you some questions that might seem a little bit strange. These are questions that we ask to everyone who comes to see us. Is that all right with you? Do you have any ideas that your friends and family do not share?"* Explore any delusions and in particular ask about their onset, their effect on the patient's life, and the patient's explanation for them (degree of insight). If necessary, ask specifically about common delusional themes, e.g. delusions of persecution, reference, control, guilt, grandeur.

Abnormal experiences

Ask about:

- Illusions and hallucinations. Again begin by an introductory statement and general questions, such as *"I gather that you have been under quite some pressure recently. When people are under pressure they sometimes find that their imagination plays tricks on them. Have you had any such experiences? Have you seen things which other people cannot see? Have you heard things which other people cannot hear?"* Ask about all five modalities and explore any positive findings for content, onset, frequency, duration, and effect on the patient's life. Exclude pseudohallucinations and hypnogogic and hypnopompic hallucinations. For auditory hallucinations of voices, determine if there is more than one voice, and if the voices talk to the patient (second person) or about him (third person). If the voices talk to him, do they command him to do dangerous things and, importantly, is he likely to act on these commands? If the voices talk about him, do they comment on his every thought and action (running commentary)? Other forms of auditory hallucinations are *écho de la pensée* and *gedankenlautwerden*, both first rank symptoms of schizophrenia.

Differentiating between true hallucinations and pseudo-hallucinations

A pseudo-hallucination may differ from a true hallucination in that:

- it is perceived to arise from the mind (inner space) rather than the sense organs (outer space)
- it is less vivid
- it is less distressing
- the patient may have some degree of control over it

True hallucinations tend to be a feature of functional disorders, whereas pseudo-hallucinations tend to be a feature of personality disorder. This is, however, not a hard and fast rule.

- Depersonalisation and derealisation, e.g. for depersonalisation *'Have you ever felt unreal?'* And for derealisation, *'Have you ever felt that things around you are unreal?'*

Cognition

Generally speaking, a quick and informal cognitive assessment can be carried out by recording the following:

- Orientation in time, place, and person
- Attention and concentration, e.g. serial sevens test, spelling 'world' backwards. Record the time taken and the number of errors
- Memory:
  - short-term memory: ask the patient to name and remember three objects, then carry out the serial sevens test, then ask him to recall the three objects
  - recent memory: ask him how he came to the clinic this morning/afternoon
  - remote memory: ask him where he was born, where he grew up, etc.
- Grasp: ask the patient to name the prime minister and reigning monarch.

If cognitive impairment is suspected, you can carry out the Folstein Mini-Mental State Examination (MMSE). The MMSE is scored out of 30. Scores of less than 22 are indicative of significant cognitive impairment, while scores of 22 to 25 are indicative of moderate cognitive impairment. The result is invalid if the patient is delirious or has an affective disorder.

Insight

To determine degree of insight, ask the patient:

- *"Do you think there is anything wrong with you?"*

If no,

- *"Why did you come to hospital?"*

If yes,

- *"What do you think is wrong with you?"*
- *"What do you think the cause of it is?"*
- *"Do you think you need treatment?"*
- *"What are you hoping treatment will do for you?"*

After the mental state examination

- Thank the patient.
- Ensure that he is comfortable.
- Summarise your findings. Note that mood should be reported as subjective mood and objective mood. Do not omit to comment upon risk.
- Offer a differential diagnosis.

Table 17. Principal features of key psychiatric disorders
See ICD-10 or DSM-IV for detailed diagnostic criteria.

Depressive disorder	See *Station 40*
Mania	• Garish clothing, accessories, and makeup • Hyperactive, flirtatious, hypervigilant, assertive, and/or aggressive behaviour • Pressured speech; abnormalities of the form of speech • Euphoric or irritable or labile mood • Grandiose thoughts with flight of ideas and loosening of associations; mood congruent delusions • Hallucinations • Poor concentration • Poor insight
Schizophrenia	• Delusions • Hallucinations • Disorganised speech • Disorganised or catatonic behaviour • Negative symptoms
Agoraphobia	Persistent irrational fear of places difficult or embarrassing to escape from, such as places that are confined, crowded, or far from home. Increased reliance on trusted companions for accompaniment or, in severe cases, restriction to the home.
Social phobia	Persistent irrational fear of being scrutinised by others and of being embarrassed or humiliated, either in most social situations or in specific social situations such as public speaking.
Specific phobia	Persistent irrational fear of one or more objects or situations. Common specific phobias include heights, darkness, enclosed spaces, storms, animals, flying, driving, blood, injections, and dental and medical procedures.
Panic disorder	Panic attacks are characterised by rapid onset of severe anxiety lasting for about 20–30 minutes. They may occur in the phobic anxiety disorder listed above or in other disorders such as OCD, PTSD, and organic disorders. In panic disorder, panic attacks occur recurrently and unexpectedly. There is fear of the implications and consequences of an attack, e.g. having a heart attack, losing control, 'going crazy'. Anticipatory fear of panic attacks develops and may itself lead to further panic attacks and to significant behavioural changes such as the development of agoraphobia.

continued

Table 17. Principal features of key psychiatric disorders – *continued*

Generalised anxiety disorder	Long-standing free-floating anxiety that may fluctuate but that is neither situational (phobic anxiety disorders) nor episodic (panic disorder). There is apprehension about a number of events far out of proportion to the actual likelihood or impact of the feared events. Other common symptoms include symptoms of autonomic arousal, irritability, poor concentration, muscle tension, tiredness, and sleep disturbances.
Obsessive compulsive disorder (OCD)	An obsessional thought is a recurrent idea, image, or impulse that is perceived as being senseless, that is unsuccessfully resisted, and that results in marked anxiety and distress. A compulsive act is a recurrent stereotyped behaviour that is not useful or enjoyable but that reduces anxiety and distress. It is usually perceived as being senseless and is unsuccessfully resisted. A compulsive act may be a response to an obsessive thought or according to rules that must be applied rigidly.
Post-traumatic stress disorder (PTSD)	A protracted and sometimes delayed response to a highly threatening or catastrophic experience characterised by numbing, detachment, flashbacks, nightmares, partial or complete amnesia for the event, avoidance of (and distress at) reminders of the event, and prominent anxiety symptoms. Associated psychiatric disorders are very common, especially depressive disorders, anxiety disorders, and alcohol and substance misuse.
Adjustment disorder	A protracted response to a significant life change or life event characterised by depressive symptoms and/or anxiety symptoms that are not severe enough to meet a diagnosis of depressive disorder or anxiety disorder, but that nevertheless lead to an impairment of social functioning.
Somatisation disorder (Briquet's syndrome)	A long history of multiple and severe physical symptoms that cannot be accounted for by a physical disorder or other psychiatric disorder. Compare to factitious disorders such as Münchausen syndrome and to malingering.
Hypochondriacal disorder (hypochondriasis)	A fear or belief of having a serious physical disorder despite medical reassurance to the contrary.
Eating disorders	See *Station 43*.
Alcohol dependence	See *Station 42*.

Depression history

For this station, it is especially important to put the patient at ease and to be sensitive, tactful, and empathetic.

Before starting

- Introduce yourself to the patient.
- Explain that you are going to ask him some questions about his feelings, and ask for his consent to do this.
- Ensure that he is comfortable.
- Unless this information has been provided, ask for his name, age, and occupation.

The interview

- First ask open questions about the patient's current mood, listening attentively and gently encouraging him to open up.
- Ask about the onset of illness, and about its triggers and causes.

Ensure that you ask about:

- The core features of depression:
  - depressed mood
  - loss of interest
  - fatiguability
- Other common features of depression:
  - poor concentration
  - poor self-esteem and self-confidence
  - guilt
  - pessimism/hopelessness
- The somatic features of depression:
  - sleep disturbance
  - early morning waking
  - morning depression
  - loss of appetite and/or weight loss
  - loss of libido
  - anhedonia
  - agitation and/or retardation
- Screen for possible anxiety, hallucinations, delusions, and mania, so as to exclude other possible psychiatric diagnoses.
- Take brief past medical, drug, family, and social history. Remember that drugs and alcohol are a common cause of depression.
- Assess the severity of the illness and its effect on the patient's life.

Ask about suicidal ideation (also see Station 41: Suicide risk assessment*). You may fail this station if you don't!*

Asking about suicidal ideation

Asking about suicide can feel uncomfortable for some. Use a formulation such as, *"People with problems similar to those that you have been describing often feel that life is no longer worth living. Have you felt that life is no longer worth living?"* If yes, then this should be explored further: *"Have you ever thought of killing yourself?" "Have you made any plans?" "Would you carry out those plans?" "What stops/would stop you?"*

After finishing

- Ask the patient if there is anything he might add that you have forgotten to ask about.
- Thank him.
- Summarise your findings and suggest a further course of action, for example, further assessment of suicidal risk (see *Station 41*), follow-up by the Community Mental Health Team, intensive support from the Crisis Team, admission to a psychiatric unit.

Station 41 DVD

Suicide risk assessment

And so it was I entered the broken world
To trace the visionary company of love, its voice
An instant in the wind (I know not whither hurled)
But not for long to hold each desperate choice.

From *Broken Tower*, by Hart Crane (b. 1899; d. 1932, by suicide)

Before starting

- Introduce yourself to the patient.
- Establish rapport.

The assessment

Ask about:

- The history of the current episode of self-harm (if any) to determine degree of suicidal intent (higher intent/lower intent – guidelines only):
  - what was the precipitant for the attempt? (serious precipitant/trivial precipitant)
  - was it planned? (planned/unplanned)
  - what was the method of self-harm, and did he expect this to be lethal? (violent method/non-violent method)
  - did he make a will or leave a suicide note? (suicide note/no suicide note)
  - was he alone? (alone/not alone)
  - did he take any precautions against discovery? (precautions/no precautions)
  - was he intoxicated?
  - did he seek help after the attempt? (sought help/did not seek help)
  - how did he feel when help arrived? (angry or disappointed/relieved)
- Assess risk factors for suicide:
  - previous suicide attempt(s)
  - recent life crisis
  - male sex, especially if between the ages of 25–44
  - divorced, widowed, or single
  - unemployed or in certain occupations, e.g. medicine, farming
  - poor level of social support
  - physical illness
  - psychiatric illness
  - substance misuse
  - family history of depression, substance misuse, or suicide
- Mental state: assess current mood and exclude psychosis.
- Will he be returning to the same situation? What has changed? Are there any important protective factors?
- Ask about current suicidal ideation. Has he made any plans?

After the assessment

- Thank the patient.
- Summarise your findings, state the patient's suicide risk, and suggest a plan of action (e.g. further investigations, psychiatric assessment, crisis team, hospitalisation …).
- Indicate that you would discuss this plan of action with a senior or specialist colleague.

Alcohol history

Before starting

- Introduce yourself to the patient.
- Establish rapport.
- Explain to the patient that you would like to ask him some questions to evaluate his drinking habits, and ask for his consent to this. As he may be reluctant to give his consent, it is important that you be particularly gentle and tactful.

The alcohol history

Ask about:

- Alcohol intake:
  - amount
  - type
  - place
  - timing
  - onset and duration
- Features of alcohol dependence:
  1. compulsion to drink/craving
  2. primacy of drinking over other activities
  3. stereotyped pattern of drinking, e.g. narrowing of drinking repertoire
  4. increased tolerance to alcohol, i.e. needing more and more to produce same effect
  5. withdrawal symptoms, e.g. anxiety, sweating, tremor ('the shakes'), nausea, fits, *delirium tremens*
  6. relief drinking to avoid withdrawal symptoms, e.g. 'eye opener' first thing in the morning
  7. reinstatement after abstinence

NB. For a diagnosis of alcohol dependence to be made, DSM-IV requires at least three from a similar list of seven features occuring at any time during a 12-month period.

Medical history

Ask about depression and the common medical complications of alcohol abuse, e.g. peptic ulceration, pancreatitis, ischaemic heart disease, liver disease, peripheral neuropathy.

Drug history

Note that:

- Illicit drug use is common in alcoholics.
- Alcohol potentiates the effects of certain drugs such as phenytoin.

Family history

Social history

Cover employment, housing, marital problems, financial problems, and legal (forensic) problems.

After finishing

- Give the patient feedback on his drinking habits (e.g. number of units drunk versus recommended number of units) and, if appropriate, suggest ways for him to cut down his alcohol use.
- Ask him if he has any questions or concerns.
- Thank him for his cooperation.

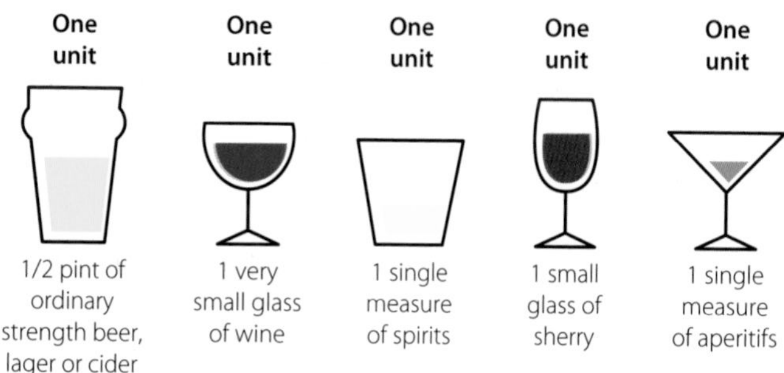

Figure 39. Equivalences for one unit of alcohol. Note that one bottle of wine is equivalent to approximately 10 units, and one bottle of spirits to approximately 30 units.

Motivational interviewing

Scenario A

Doctor: According to your blood tests, you appear to be drinking rather too much alcohol.

Patient: I suppose I do enjoy the odd drink.

Doctor: Are you sure it is just the odd drink? Alcohol is very bad for you and I think that if you are drinking too much then you really need to stop.

Patient: You sound like my wife.

Doctor: Well, she's right you know. Alcohol can cause liver and heart problems and many other things besides. So you really need to stop drinking, OK?

Patient: Yes, doctor, thank you. (Patient never returns.)

Scenario B (using motivational interviewing)

Doctor: We all enjoy a drink now and then, but sometimes alcohol can do us a lot of harm. What do you know about the harmful effects of alcohol?

Patient: Quite a bit, I'm afraid. My best friend, well he used to drink a lot. Last year he spent three months in hospital. I visited him often, but most of the time he wasn't with it. Then he died from internal bleeding.

Doctor: I'm sorry to hear that, alcohol can really do us a lot of damage.

Patient: It does a lot of damage to the liver, doesn't it?

Doctor: That's right, but it doesn't just do harm to our body, it also does harm to our lives: our work, our finances, our relationships.

Patient: Funny you should say that. My wife's been at my neck…

(…)

Doctor: So, you've told me that you're currently drinking about 16 units of alcohol a day. This has placed severe strain on your marriage and on your relationship with your daughter Emma, not to mention that you haven't been to work since last Tuesday and have started to fear for your job. But what you fear most is ending up lying on a hospital bed like your friend Tom. Is that a fair summary of things as they stand?

Patient: Things are completely out of hand, aren't they? If I don't stop drinking now, I might lose everything I've built over the past 20 years: my job, my marriage, even my daughter.

Doctor: I'm afraid you might be right.

Patient: I really need to quit drinking.

Doctor: You sound very motivated to stop drinking. Why don't we make another appointment to talk about the ways in which we might support you? (…)

Excerpted from *Psychiatry* 2e, by Neel Burton (Wiley-Blackwell, 2010)

Eating disorders history

Before starting

- Introduce yourself to the patient.
- Explain that you are going to ask some questions about her eating habits, and ask for her consent to do this.
- Ensure that she is comfortable.
- If this information is not provided, ask for her name, age, and occupation.

The history

Weight and perception of weight

Determine:

- Her current weight and height.
- The amount of weight that she has lost, and over what period.
- Whether the weight loss has been intentional.
- Whether she still considers that she is overweight.
- How often she weighs herself/looks at herself in the mirror.

Diet and compensatory behaviours

Ask about:

- Amount and type of food eaten in an average day.
- Binge eating.
- Vomiting.
- The use of laxatives, purgatives, diuretics, appetite suppressants, and stimulants.
- Physical exercise.

Other

Ask about:

- Menstrual periods.
- Effect on patient's life:
  - relationships
  - medical complications, e.g. anaemia, peptic ulceration, constipation
  - psychiatric complications, especially substance misuse, depression, and self harm
- Past medical, drug, and family history (briefly and only if you have time left).

After finishing

- Ask the patient if there is anything she might add that you have forgotten to ask about.
- Determine the patient's level of insight into her problem.
- Thank the patient, offer feedback, and suggest a further course of action, e.g. informant history from the mother, physical examination, investigations, dietary advice, psychotherapy, antidepressants, hospitalisation.

Table 18. Anorexia nervosa vs. bulimia nervosa
DSM-IV diagnostic criteria
Anorexia A. Refusal to maintain normal body weight at more than 85% of expected body weight. B. Intense fear of gaining weight or becoming fat. C. Disturbed perception of body weight or shape. D. In postmenarchal females, amenorrhoea for at least three consecutive cycles (if not on the oral contraceptive pill).
Bulimia A. Recurrent episodes of binge eating. B. Recurrent inappropriate compensatory behaviour to prevent weight gain. C. Episodes of binge eating and compensatory behaviour occur at least twice a week for a period of 3 months. D. Self-evaluation is unduly influenced by body shape and weight. E. Disturbance does not occur exclusively during periods of anorexia nervosa.

Capacity and its assessment

In this station, you may be asked to carry out a formalised assessment of competence to decide on the ability of a patient to give informed consent (see *Station 111*). Alternatively, you may simply be asked to discuss the subject.

The first thing to note is that the terms capacity and competence are often used interchangeably but, strictly speaking, capacity is the legal presumption that adult persons have the ability to make decisions, whereas competence is a clinical determination of a patient's ability to make decisions about his treatment.

Issues about capacity frequently arise in three groups of patients: children and adolescents, patients with learning difficulties, and patients with mental illness. A person has capacity so long as he has the ability to understand and retain relevant information for long enough to reach a *reasoned* decision, **regardless of the actual decision reached**. An adult person should be presumed to have the competence to make a particular decision until a judgement about capacity can be made. This judgement can only be made about present capacity, not about past or future capacity, and it should only be made for a specific decision, as different decisions require different levels of capacity, as established by the case of Re. C (1994). If capacity is lacking or cannot be established (e.g. in an emergency situation), treatment can be justified under the common law *Principle of Necessity*, as established by the case of Re. F (1990). The doctor in charge has the responsibility to act in the best interests of the patient, and in accordance with a responsible and competent body of opinion, as established by the case of *Bolam v. Friern Hospital Management Committee* (1957) (the 'Bolam test'). Nevertheless, it is good practice for him to involve colleagues, carers, and relatives in the decision-making. In difficult situations, or if there are differences of opinion about the patient's best interests, the doctor should consult a senior colleague or seek legal advice. In England and Wales, the Mental Capacity Act 2005 provides for a Court of Protection to help with difficult decisions. Note that, in some cases, a child (a person under the age of 16) can be competent to consent to treatment if he or she fully understands the treatment proposed, as established by the case of *Gillick v. West Norfolk and Wisbech Area Health Authority* (1985) ('Gillick competency').

Assessing capacity

1. Ensure that the patient understands:
    - what the intervention is
    - why the intervention is being proposed
    - the alternatives to the intervention, including no intervention
    - the principal benefits and risks of the intervention and of its alternatives
    - the consequences of the intervention and of its alternatives
2. Ensure that the patient retains the information for long enough to weigh it in the balance and reach a reasoned decision, whatever that decision might be. In some cases, the patient may not have the cognitive ability or emotional maturity to reach a reasoned decision, or may be unduly affected by mental illness.
3. Ensure that the patient is not subject to coercion or threat.

It is important to bear in mind that a patient's capacity can be enhanced by, for example:

- making your explanations easier to understand, e.g. using diagrams
- seeing the patient at his best time of day
- seeing the patient with a friend or relative
- improving the patient's environment, e.g. finding a quiet side-room
- adjusting the patient's medication, e.g. decreasing the dose of sedative drugs

Common law and the Mental Health Act

Treatment under common law

Common law is the law that is based on previous court rulings (case law, such as Re. C), in contradistinction to the law that is enacted by parliament (statute law, such as the Mental Health Act). Under common law, adults have a right to refuse treatment, even when doing so may result in permanent physical injury or death. If a competent adult refuses consent or lacks the capacity to provide consent, no one can provide consent on his behalf, not even his next of kin. That having been said, treatment without consent can be given under common law.

- If serious harm or death is likely to occur and there is doubt about the patient's capacity at the time and no advance directive (or 'living will') has been made; and the clinician is able to justify that he or she is acting in the patient's best interests and in accordance with established medical practice ('Bolam's test').
- In an emergency to prevent serious harm to the patient or to others or to prevent a crime.

The Mental Health Act

In England and Wales, the Mental Health Act 1983 (amended in 2007) is the principal Act governing not only the compulsory admission and detention of people to a psychiatric hospital, but also their treatment, discharge from hospital, and aftercare. People with a mental disorder as defined by the Act can be detained under the Act in the interests of their health or safety or in the interests of the safety of others. To minimize the potential for abuse, the Act specifically excludes as mental disorder dependence on alcohol or drugs. Note that Scotland is governed by the Mental Health (Care and Treatment) (Scotland) Act 2003 and Northern Ireland by the Mental Health (Northern Ireland) Order 1986.

Two of the most common 'Sections' of the Mental Health Act used to admit people with a mental disorder to a psychiatric hospital are the so-called Sections 2 and 3.

Section 2

Section 2 allows for an admission for assessment and treatment that can last for up to 28 days. An application for a Section 2 is usually made by an Approved Mental Health Professional (AMHP) with special training in mental health, and recommended by two doctors, one of whom must have special experience in the diagnosis and treatment of mental disorders. Under a Section 2, treatment can be given, but only if this treatment is aimed at treating the mental disorder or conditions directly resulting from the mental disorder (so, for example, treatment for an inflamed appendix cannot be given under the Act, although treatment for deliberate self-harm probably can be). A Section 2 can be 'discharged' or revoked at any time by the Responsible Clinician (usually the consultant psychiatrist in charge), by the hospital managers, or by the nearest relative. Furthermore, a patient under a Section 2 can appeal against the Section, in which case his or her appeal is heard by a specially constituted tribunal. The claimant is represented by a solicitor who helps him or her to make a case in favour of discharge to the tribunal. The tribunal is by nature adversarial, and it falls upon members of the detained patient's care team to argue the case for continued detention. This can be quite trying for both the claimant and his or her care team, and it can at times undermine the claimant's trust in his or her care team. Section 2 is broadly equivalent to Section 26 of the Mental Health (Care and Treatment) (Scotland) Act 2003, except that Section 26 cannot be used to admit a patient to hospital. Instead, Section 26 tags onto Section 24 (Emergency admission to hospital) or Section 25 (Detention of patients already in Hospital).

Section 3

A patient can be detained under a Section 3 after a conclusive period of assessment under a Section 2. Alternatively, he or she can be detained directly under a Section 3 if his or her diagnosis has already been established by the care team and is not in reasonable doubt. Section 3 corresponds to an admission for treatment and lasts for up to 6 months. As for a Section 2, it is usually applied for by an AMHP with special training in mental health and approved by two doctors, one of whom must have special experience in the diagnosis and treatment of mental disorders. Treatment can only be given under a Section 3 if it is aimed at treating the mental disorder or conditions directly resulting from the mental disorder. After the first 3 months, any treatment requires either the consent of the patient being treated or the recommendation of a second doctor. A Section 3 can be discharged at any time by the Responsible Clinician (usually the consultant psychiatrist in charge), by the hospital managers, or by the nearest relative. Furthermore, the patient under a Section 3 can appeal against the Section, in which case his or her appeal is heard by a specially constituted tribunal, as explained above. If the patient still needs to be detained after six months, the Section 3 can be renewed for further periods. Section 3 is broadly similar to Section 18 of the Health (Care and Treatment) (Scotland) Act 2003.

Aftercare

If a patient has been detained under Section 3 of the Mental Health Act, he or she is automatically placed under a 'Section 117' at the time of his or her discharge from the Section 3. Section 117 corresponds to 'aftercare' and places a duty on the local health authority and local social services authority to provide the patient with a care package aimed at rehabilitation and relapse prevention. Although the patient is under no obligation to accept aftercare, in some cases he or she may also be placed under a 'Supervised Community Treatment' or 'Guardianship' to ensure that he or she receives aftercare. Under Supervised Community Treatment, the patient is made subject to certain conditions and if these conditions are not met, he or she can be recalled into hospital.

Other civil Sections

Commonly used civil Sections of the Mental Health Act are summarised in *Table 19*.

Police Sections

Section 135 enables the removal of a person from his premises to a place of safety, and is valid for 72 hours. Section 136 enables the removal of a person from a public place to a place of safety by a police officer, and is also valid for 72 hours. The person must appear to the police officer to have a mental disorder.

Criminal Sections

The principal criminal Sections are Sections 35 and 36, and Sections 37 and 41.

Sections 35 and 36 mirror Sections 2 and 3 (above), but are used for persons suffering from a mental disorder and awaiting trial for a serious offence. Section 35 can be enacted by a Crown Court or Magistrates' Court on the evidence of a Section 12 approved doctor. Section 36 can only be enacted by a Crown Court on the evidence of two doctors, one of whom must be Section 12 approved. In contrast to Section 36, Section 35 does not enable treatment, and is used solely for the purpose of remanding a person to hospital for a report on his or her mental state. Both Sections 35 and 36 have an initial duration of 28 days, but can be extended for up to 28 days at a time for up to 12 weeks.

Table 19. Commonly used Sections of the Mental Health Act

Section	Description	Duration	Treatment	Application/ recommendation	Discharge/ renewal
2	Admission for assessment	28 days	Can be given, but note that the MHA only authorizes treatment of the mental disorder itself or conditions directly resulting from the mental disorder	Application by AMHP or nearest relative. Recommendation by two doctors (at least one must be Section 12 approved)	Patient may appeal to tribunal. Can be discharged by RC, hospital managers, or nearest relative. Usually converted to Section 3 if longer period of detention is required
3	Admission for treatment	6 months	Can be given for first 3 months, then consent or second opinion is needed	Application by AMHP or nearest relative. Recommendation by two doctors (at least one must be Section 12 approved)	Patient may appeal to tribunal. Can be discharged by RC, hospital managers, or nearest relative. Can be renewed if needed
4	Emergency admission for assessment (usually used in lieu of a Section 2)	72 hours	Consent needed unless treatment is being given under common law	Application by AMHP or nearest relative. Recommendation by any doctor	Patient cannot appeal. Can be discharged by RC only
5(2)	Emergency holding order (patient already admitted to hospital on an informal basis)	72 hours	Consent needed unless treatment is being given under common law	Recommendation from the doctor or AC in charge of the patient's care or their nominated deputy	Patient cannot appeal. Can be discharged by RC only
5(4)	Emergency holding order (patient already admitted to hospital on an informal basis)	6 hours	Consent needed unless treatment is being given under common law	Recommendation from a registered mental nurse	Patient cannot appeal
117	Automatically applies if a patient has been detained under Section 3. Under Section 117 it is the duty of the local health authority and the local social services authority to provide aftercare. Unlike under Supervised Community Treatment, there is no obligation for the patient to accept it.				

AC, Approved Clinician; AMHP, Approved Mental Health Professional; RC, Responsible Clinician, usually the consultant in charge. Section 12 approval is usually granted to psychiatrists having obtained Membership of the Royal College of Psychiatrists (MRCPsych) or having more than 3 years of relevant experience.

Section 37 is used for the detention and treatment of persons suffering from a mental disorder and convicted of a serious offence which is punishable by imprisonment. It is enacted by a Crown Court or Magistrates' Court on the evidence of two Section 12 approved doctors. Section 37 has an initial duration of 6 months, and can be either discharged or extended. Sometimes a Section 41 or 'restriction order' is added onto a Section 37, such that leave and discharge can only be granted with the approval of the Ministry of Justice.

Consent to treatment

Patients on a long-term treatment order can be treated with standard psychiatric drugs with or without consent for up to 3 months, after which an additional order is required for their continued treatment. This additional order is a Section 58, which requires either the patient's consent or a second opinion.

Mental disorders and driving

The following advice applies to mania, schizophrenia and other schizophrenia-like psychotic disorders, and more severe forms of anxiety and depression.

Patients should stop driving during a first episode or relapse of their illness, because driving while ill can seriously endanger lives. In the UK, the patient must notify the Driver and Vehicle Licensing Authority (DVLA). Failure to do so makes it illegal for them to drive and invalidates their insurance. The DVLA then sends the patient a medical questionnaire to fill in, and a form asking for permission to contact their psychiatrist. The patient's driving licence can generally be reinstated if the psychiatrist can confirm that:

- their illness has been successfully treated with medication for a certain amount of time, typically at least 3 months
- the patient is conscientious about taking his medication
- the side-effects of the medication are not likely to impair the patient's driving
- the patient is not misusing drugs

People who suffer from substance misuse or dependence should also stop driving, as should some people who suffer from other mental disorders such as dementia, learning disability, or personality disorder.

Further information can be obtained from the DVLA website at www.dvla.gov.uk. Note that the rules for professional driving are different from and more strict than those described above.

Hearing and the ear examination

Before starting

- Introduce yourself to the patient.
- Explain the examination and ask for his consent to carry it out.
- Sit him so that he is facing you and ensure that he is comfortable.

The history

- Name, age, and occupation, if this information has not already been provided.
- Ask the patient if there has been any loss of hearing.

If there has been loss of hearing, assess its:

- Characteristics (bilaterality, onset, duration, severity, impact on the patient's life).
- Associated features (tinnitus, vertigo, pain, discharge, weight loss).
- Possible causes (noise exposure, trauma, infection, antibiotics, family history).
- Impact on the patient's life.
- Previous ear problems.

The examination

Hearing

Test hearing by whispering into the ear at various distances, whilst distracting or occluding the other ear. As whispering into people's ears may no longer be considered politically correct, you may prefer rubbing your fingers together instead.

Tuning fork tests

Use a 512 Hz tuning fork, and not the larger 128 Hz or 256 Hz tuning forks used for neurological examinations.

- The Rinne test. Place the base of the vibrating tuning fork on the mastoid process of each ear. Once the patient can no longer 'hear' the vibration, move the tuning fork in front of the ear. If the tuning fork can be heard, air conduction is better than bone conduction, and there is therefore no conductive hearing loss. The test is said to be *positive*. If the tuning fork cannot be heard, there is a conductive hearing loss, and the test is said to be *negative*.

The false negative Rinne test: if the Rinne test is performed on a deaf ear, it may appear negative because the vibration is transmitted to the opposite ear.

- The Weber test. Place the vibrating tuning fork in the midline of the skull. If hearing is normal, or if hearing loss is symmetrical, the vibration should be heard equally in both ears.

Note:

- If there is conductive deafness in one ear, the vibration is best heard *in that same ear* (since there is no background interference).
- If there is sensorineural deafness in one ear, the vibration is best heard in the other ear.

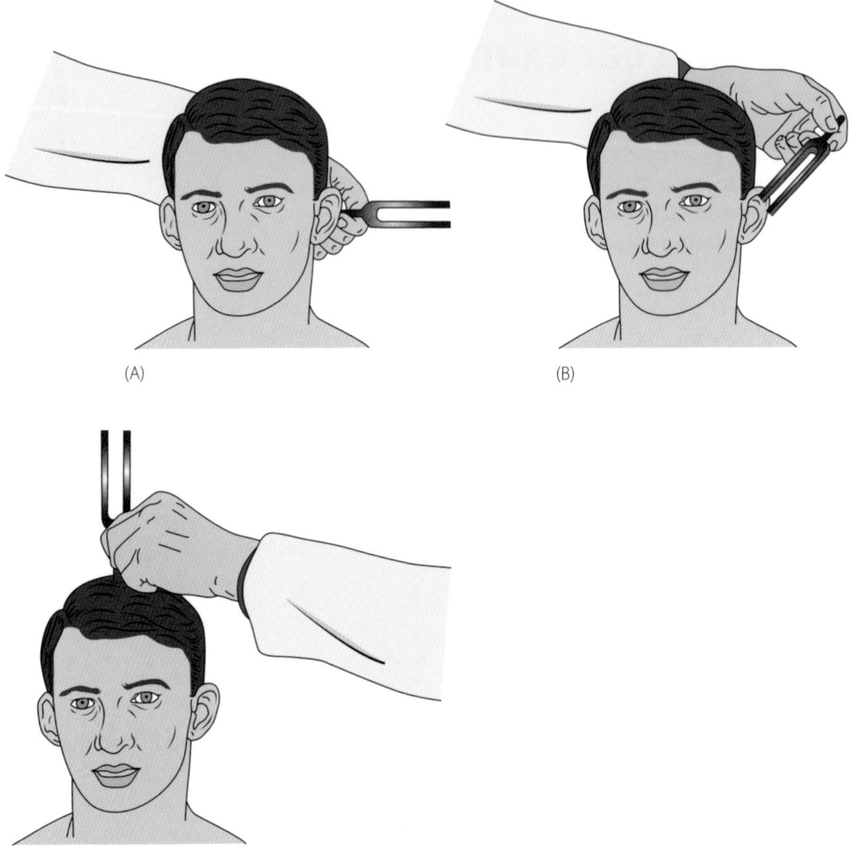

Figure 40. The Rinne (A, B) and Weber (C) tests.

Auroscopy

- Examine the pinnae for size, shape, deformities, pre-auricular sinuses.
- Look behind the ears for any scars.
- Palpate the pre-auricular, post-auricular, and infra-auricular lymph nodes.
- Affix a speculum of appropriate size onto the auroscope.
- Gently pull the pinna upwards and backwards so as to straighten the ear canal and, holding the auroscope like a pen (see *Figure 41*), introduce it into the external auditory meatus.

 *If examining the right ear, use your right hand to hold the auroscope. If examining the left ear, use your left hand.*

- Through the auroscope, inspect the ear canal (discharge, foreign body, wax, exotosis, otitis externa) and the tympanic membrane (normal anatomy, colour (normally pearly grey), shape (normally concave), light relex (normally present), effusions, cholesteatomata, perforations, grommets).

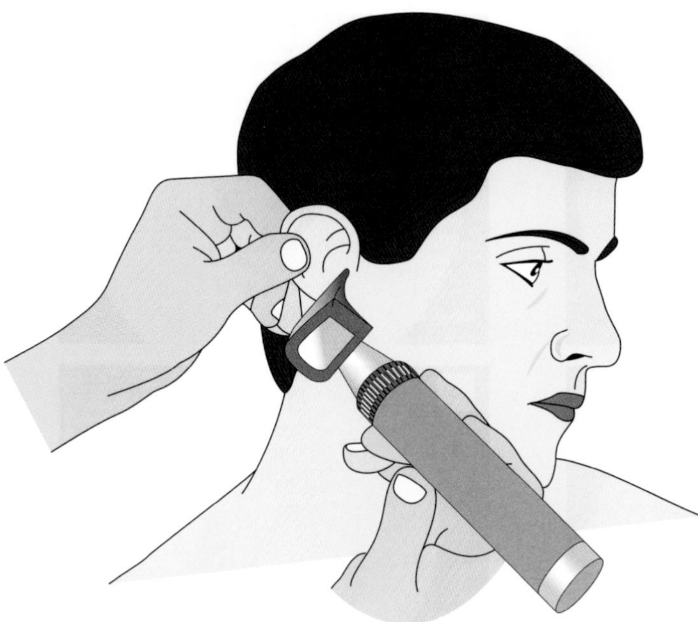

Figure 41. Holding the auroscope.

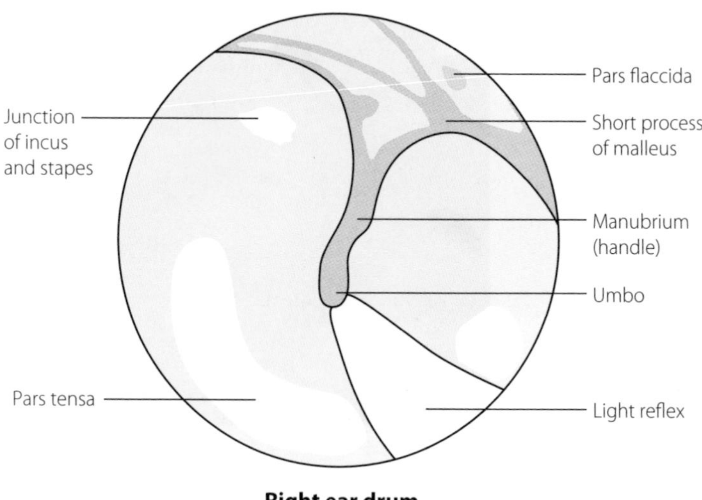

Figure 42. The normal right ear drum.

After examining the ear

- Ask the patient if he has any questions or concerns.
- Thank the patient.
- Summarise your findings and offer a differential diagnosis, e.g. ear wax, otitis media, perforated ear drum.

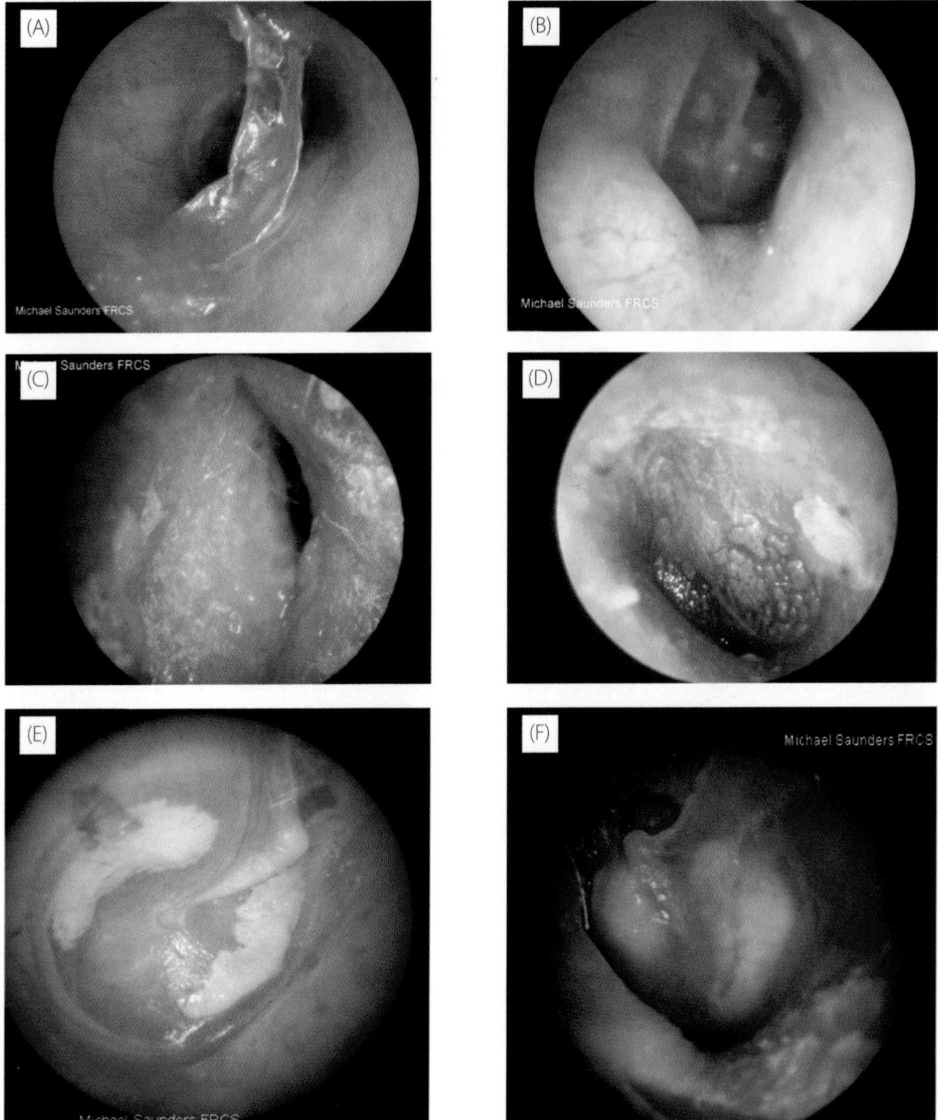

Figure 43. Common ear problems.

(A) Wax: excess or impacted wax, can occlude the ear canal.
(B) Exostoses: bony swellings in the ear canal due to chronic cold water exposure, can cause pain and predispose to infection or occlusion of the ear canal.
(C) Otitis externa: inflammation of the outer ear and ear canal, associated with pain, can cause swelling and discharge and occlusion of the ear canal – pain is typically exacerbated by pulling on the pinna or pushing on the tragus.
(D) Acute otitis media: inflammation of the middle ear due to infection, associated with pain, redness and bulging of the tympanic membrane, disintegration of the light reflex, effusions, perforation.
(E) Tympanosclerosis: calcium deposits in the ear drum due to trauma or infection, can lead to impairment of hearing.
(F) Cholesteatoma: destructive growth of keratinising squamous epithelium in the middle ear, often due to a tear or retraction of the ear drum, can lead to impairment of hearing.

Reproduced with permission from Michael Saunders, Bristol Royal Infirmary.

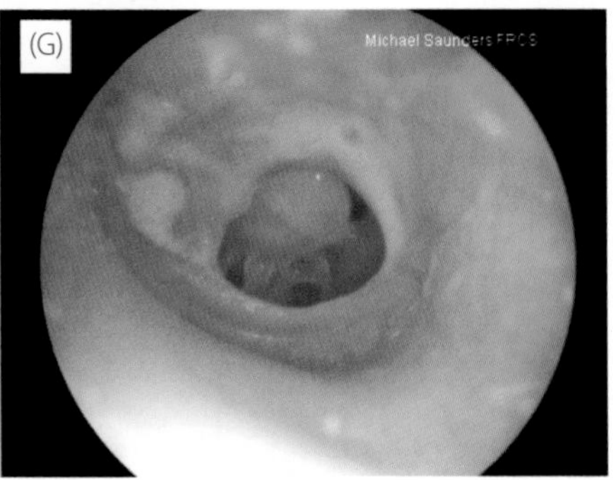

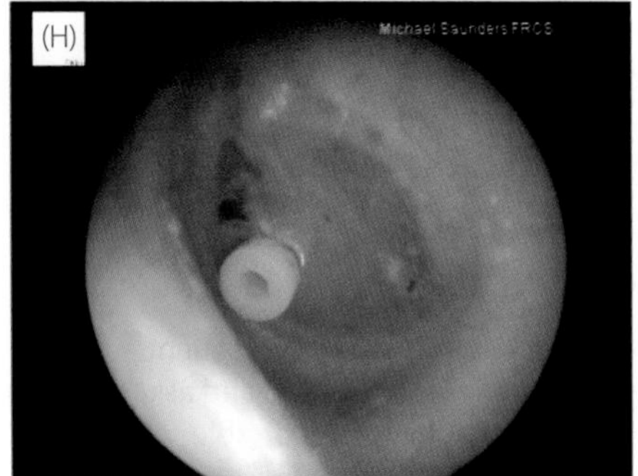

Figure 43. Common ear problems – *continued.*

(G) Perforation.
(H) Grommet: small tube inserted in chronic otitis media to drain and ventilate the middle ear.

Reproduced with permission from Michael Saunders, Bristol Royal Infirmary.

Conditions most likely to come up in a hearing and the ear examination
Conductive hearing loss: • commonly caused by wax, foreign bodies, exostoses, otitis externa, otitis media, trauma or damage to the ear drum or ossicles
Sensorineural hearing loss: • may be caused by noise exposure, degenerative changes (presbyacusis), trauma, infection, aminoglycoside drugs such as gentamicin, Ménière's disease, acoustic neuroma

Vision and the eye examination (including fundoscopy)

Before starting

- Introduce yourself to the patient.
- Explain the examination and ask for his consent to carry it out.
- Ensure that he is comfortable.

The examination

1. Visual acuity

- *Snellen chart.* Assess each eye individually, either from a distance of 6 m or 3 m, correcting for any refractive errors (glasses, pinhole). If the patient cannot read the Snellen chart, either move him closer or ask him to count fingers. If he fails to count fingers, test whether he can see hand movements and, if he cannot, test whether he can see light.
- *Test types* (or fine print). Assess each eye individually, correcting for any refractive errors.
- *Ishihara plates.* Indicate that you could use Ishihara plates to test colour vision specifically.

2. Visual fields

- *Confrontation test.* Test the visual fields by confrontation. Sit directly opposite the patient, at the same level as him. Ask him to look straight at you and to cover his right eye with his right hand. Cover your left eye with your left hand, and test the visual field of his left eye with your right hand. Bring a wiggly finger into the upper left quadrant, asking the patient to say when he sees the finger. Repeat for the lower left quadrant. Then swap hands and test the upper and lower right quadrants. Now ask the patient to cover his left eye with his left hand. Cover your right eye with your right hand and test the visual field of his right eye with your left hand. Bring a wiggly finger into the upper right quadrant, asking the patient to say when he sees the finger. Repeat for the lower right quadrant. Then swap hands and test the upper and lower left quadrants.
- *Mapping of central visual field defects.* Indicate that you could use a red pin to delineate the patient's blind spot and any central visual field defects.
- *Visual inattention test.* Ask the patient to fix his gaze upon you and simultaneously bring a moving finger into each of the patient's right and left visual fields. In some parietal lobe lesions, only the ipsilateral finger is perceived by the patient.

3. Pupillary reflexes

- *Inspection.* Inspect the eyes, paying particular attention to the size and symmetry of the pupils, and excluding a visible ptosis or squint.
- Test the direct and consensual pupillary light reflexes. Explain that you are going to shine a bright light into the patient's eye and that this may feel uncomfortable. Bring the light in onto his left eye and look for pupil constriction. Bring the light in onto his left eye once again, but this time look for pupil constriction in his *right eye* (consensual reflex). Repeat for the right eye.
- Perform the swinging flashlight test. Swing the light from one eye to another and look for sustained pupil constriction in both eyes. Intermittent pupil constriction in one eye (Marcus Gunn pupil) suggests a lesion of the optic nerve anterior to the optic chiasm.
- Test the accommodation reflex. Ask the patient to follow your finger in to his nose. As the eyes converge, the pupils should constrict.

4. Eye movements

- Perform the cover test. Ask the patient to fixate on a point and cover one eye. Observe the movement of the uncovered eye. Repeat the test for the other eye.
- Examine eye movements. Ask the patient to keep his head still and to follow your finger with his eyes. Ask him to report any pain or double vision at any point. Draw an 'H' shape with your finger.
- *Nystagmus*. Look out for nystagmus at the extremes of gaze. You can do this as part of eye movements or separately by fixing the patient's head and asking him to track your finger through a cross pattern.

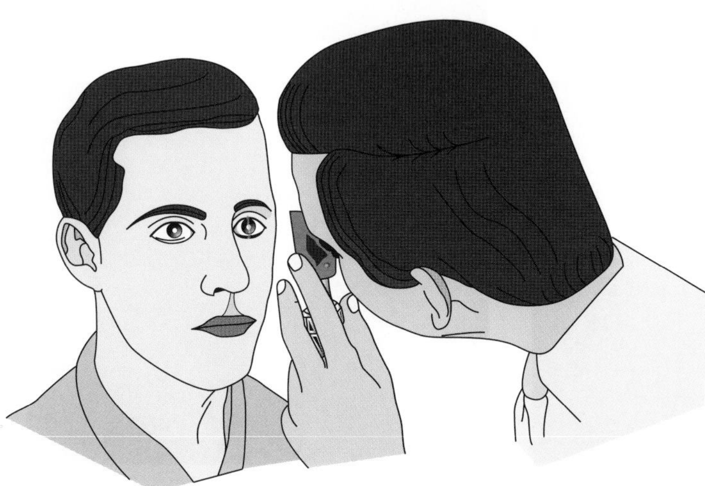

Figure 44. Holding the ophthalmoscope.

5. Fundoscopy

Explain the procedure, mentioning that it may be uncomfortable. Darken the room and ask the patient to fixate on a distant object (or to 'look over my shoulder'). State to the examiner that, ideally, the pupils should have been dilated using a solution of 1% cyclopentolate.

- *Red reflex*. Test the red reflex in each eye from a distance of about 10 cm. An absent red reflex is usually caused by a cataract.
- *Fundoscopy*. Use your right eye to examine the patient's right eye, and your left eye to examine the patient's left eye. If you use your left eye to examine the patient's right eye, you may appear more caring than the examiner might like to see. Look at the optic disc, the blood vessels, and the macula. To find the macula, ask the patient to look directly into the light. Describe any features according to protocol, e.g. *"There are soft exudates at 3 o'clock, two disc diameters away from the disc"*.

If the station is examining fundoscopy alone, the patient is likely to be replaced by a model in which the retinas are very easy to visualise. Before the exam, it is a good idea to look at as many retinas as you can, both in patients and in textbooks/on the internet.

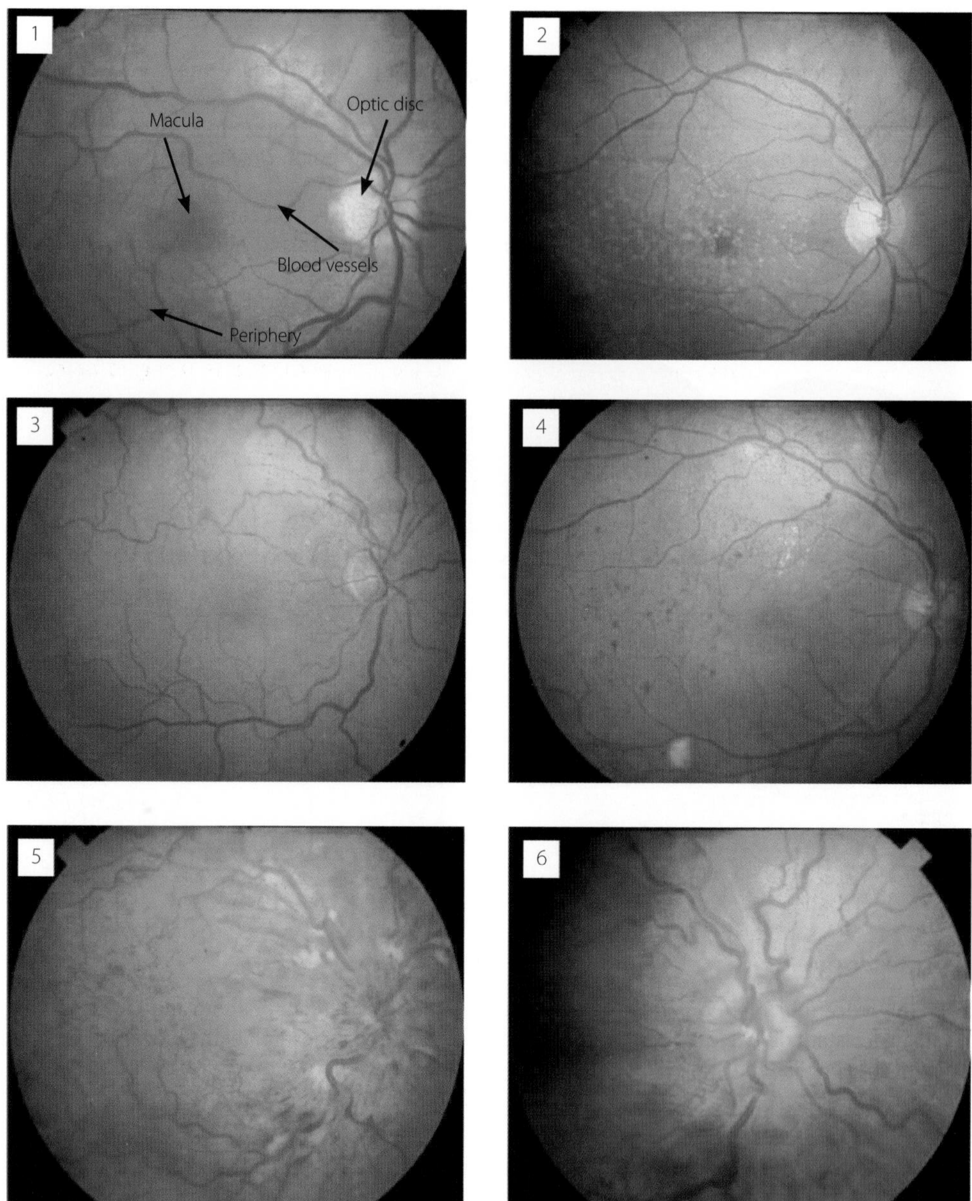

Figure 45. Findings on fundoscopy of the right eye.

1. Normal.
2. Senile macular degeneration.
3. Hypertensive retinopathy.
4. Pre-proliferative diabetic retinopathy.
5. Central retinal vein occlusion.
6. Papilloedema.

After the examination

- Ask the patient if he has any questions or concerns.
- Thank the patient.
- Summarise your findings and offer a differential diagnosis.

Conditions most likely to come up in a vision and the eye examination
Cataract: • absent red reflex, on approaching ophthalmoscope the lens may look like cracked ice
Senile macular degeneration: • drusen (characteristic yellow deposits) in the macula, exudative changes resulting from blood and fluid under the macula
Hypertensive retinopathy: • stage I: arteriolar narrowing and tortuosity • stage II: AV nicking, silver-wiring • stage III: dot, blot, and flame haemorrhages, microaneurysms, soft exudates (cotton wool spots), hard exudates • stage IV: papilloedema
Diabetic retinopathy: • background: microaneurysms, macular oedema, hard exudates, haemorrhages • pre-proliferative: cotton-wool spots, venous beading • proliferative: neovascularisation, vitreous haemorrhage
Glaucoma: • increased cup to disk ratio (> 0.5), haemorrhages
Central retinal artery occlusion: • pale retina with swelling or oedema, markedly decreased vascularity, cherry red spot in the central fovea
Central retinal vein occlusion: • widespread haemorrhages throughout the retina with swelling and oedema, sometimes described as a 'stormy sunset'
Papilloedema: • blurring of disc margins, cupping and swelling of the disc, haemorrhages, exudates, distended veins

Station 48

Smell and the nose examination

Specifications: This station may involve a model of a nose in lieu of a patient.

Before starting

- Introduce yourself to the patient.
- Explain the examination and ask him for his consent to carry it out.
- Position him so that he is sitting in a chair facing you.
- Ensure that he is comfortable.

The history

- Briefly establish the nature of the problem.
- If there is obstruction of the nasal passages, determine its:
  - characteristics (nasal passage affected, onset, duration, timing, severity)
  - associated symptoms (facial pain, inflammation, itching, rhinorrhoea, sneezing, snoring, anosmia)
  - possible causes (asthma, hay fever, other allergies, trauma, surgery, other)
  - impact on everyday life

The examination

Inspection

- Observe the external appearance of the nose from the front, from the side, and from above. Look for evidence of deformity, inflammation, nasal discharge, skin disease, and scars.
- Examine the nasal vestibule, anterior end of the septum, and anterior ends of the inferior turbinates. Do this first by elevating the tip of the nose, and then with the help of a Thudicum speculum and torch.
- Look into the mouth.

Otoscopy

- Use an otoscope in conjunction with a Thudicum speculum to assess the nasal septum and the inferior and middle turbinates. Make sure that the otoscope has a very wide end-piece on it. Look for septal deviation, mucosal inflammation, bleeding, perforation, polyps, and foreign objects.

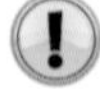

A more detailed view of the nasal cavities can be obtained using a flexible (fibre-optic) nasendoscope.

Nasal airflow

- Ask the patient to breathe out through his nose onto a mirror or cold tongue depressor positioned under the nose. If the nasal passages are not obstructed, there should be condensation under both nostrils.
- Assess inspiratory flow by occluding one nostril and asking the patient to sniff. Repeat for the other side.

Smell

- Assess sense of smell by asking the patient to identify fragrances from a series of bottles containing different odours.

Sinuses

- With your thumb, press over the supra- and infra-orbital areas to elicit tenderness. Tenderness in these areas is likely to indicate inflammation of the frontal and maxillary sinuses (sinusitis).

After examining the nose

- Ask the patient if he has any questions or concerns.
- Thank the patient.
- Offer to examine the throat and ears.
- Summarise your findings and offer a differential diagnosis.

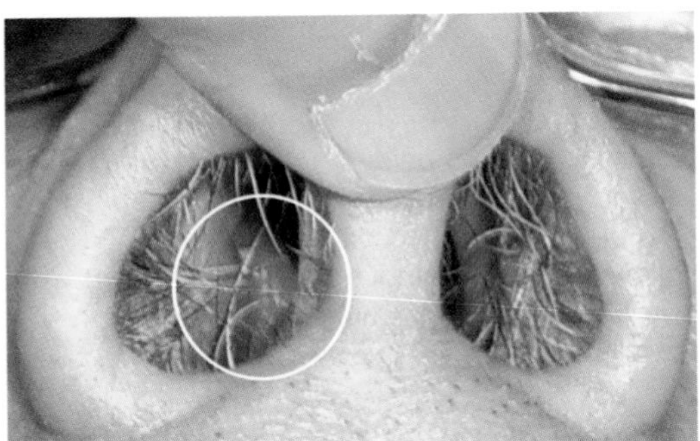

Figure 46. Nasal polyp. Swollen turbinates are often mistaken for polyps. However, swollen turbinates differ from polyps in that they tend to be pink rather than grey/yellow in colour, and in that they tend to be sensitive rather than insensitive to touch.

Reproduced from www.askdrshah.com with permission from Dr Rajesh Shah.

Conditions most likely to come up in a smell and nose examination station

- Congenital or trauma-induced deviated nasal septum
- Septum perforation secondary to cocaine use, nose picking, or granulomatous disease
- Chronic rhinitis
- Nasal polyps
- Anosmia secondary to viral infection or head injury

Lump in the neck examination

Before starting

- Introduce yourself to the patient.
- Explain the examination and ask for his consent to carry it out.
- Ask him to expose his neck and upper body.
- Sit him in a chair.

The examination

Inspection

- Inspect the patient generally, in particular looking for any signs of thyroid disease. The age and sex of the patient has an important bearing on the differential diagnosis of a goitre.
- Inspect the neck from the front and side, looking for goitre, other lumps, scars, and any other abnormalities.

A goitre, or enlarged thyroid gland, is seen as a swelling below the cricoid cartilage, on either side of the trachea.

- Ask the patient to take a sip of water. The following structures move upon swallowing: thyroid gland, thyroid cartilage, cricoid cartilage, thyroglossal cyst, lymph nodes.
- Ask him to stick his tongue out. A midline swelling which moves upwards when the tongue is protruded is a thyroglossal cyst.

Palpation

- Ask him if there is any tenderness in the neck area.
- Putting one hand on either side of his neck, examine the anterior and posterior triangles of the neck with your fingertips. For any lump, assess its site, size, shape, surface, consistency, and fixity. Is the lump tender to touch? Note that the normal thyroid gland is often not palpable.
- Palpate the cervical lymph nodes.
- Palpate for tracheal deviation in the suprasternal notch (see *Station 16: Respiratory system examination*).

Percussion

- Percuss for the dullness of a retrosternal goitre over the sternum and upper chest.

Auscultation

- Auscultate over the thyroid for bruits. Ask the patient to hold his breath as you listen; a soft bruit is sometimes heard in thyrotoxicosis.

Assessment of thyroid function

- Examine the patient for signs of hyper- and hypothyroidism, as appropriate (see below). Once you have examined the neck, this involves examining the hands (temperature, nails, skin, hair, tremor, pulse) and the eyes (chemosis, lid retraction, lid lag, periorbital oedema, proptosis, ophthalmoplegia and diplopia), and looking for evidence of congestive cardiac failure, pre-tibial myxoedema, and hyporeflexia. To look for exophthalmos, stand behind the patient and look at the eyes from above. To look for lid lag and ophthalmoplegia, test eye movements and ask the patient to tell you if he sees double at any time.

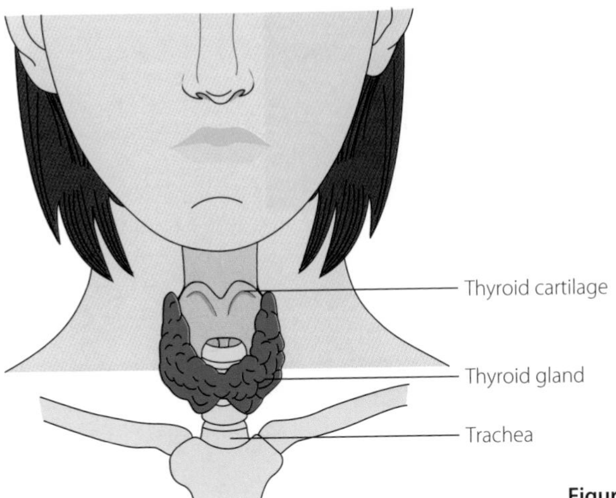

Figure 47. Anatomy of the normal thyroid gland.

After the examination

- Help the patient to put his clothes back on.
- Ensure that he is comfortable.
- Ask him if he has any questions or concerns.
- Thank him.
- Offer a diagnosis or differential diagnosis.
- Give suggestions for further management, e.g. thyroid function tests, thyroid antibodies, ultrasound examination of the thyroid, iodine thyroid scan, fine needle aspiration cytology.

Goitres and thyroid disease

Signs of **hyperthyroidism**: enlarged thyroid gland or thyroid nodules, thyroid bruit, hyperthermia, diaphoresis, dehydration, tremor, tachycardia, arrhythmia, congestive cardiac failure, onycholysis.

- Grave's disease (commonest cause of hyperthyroidism): uniformly enlarged smooth thyroid gland usually in a younger patient; lid retraction, lid lag, chemosis, periorbital oedema, proptosis, diplopia, pre-tibial myxoedema (non-pitting oedema and skin thickening, seen in <5% of cases), thyroid acropachy (finger clubbing, seen in <1% of cases).
- Toxic multinodular goitre: enlarged multinodular goitre in a middle-aged patient.
- Toxic nodule and de Quervain's thyroiditis are less common.

Signs of **hypothyrodism**: hypothermia and cold intolerance, weight gain, slowed speech and movements, hoarse voice, dry skin, hair loss, coarse facial features and facial puffiness, hypotension, bradycardia, and hyporeflexia.

- Hashimoto's thyroiditis (commonest cause of hypothyroidism): moderately enlarged rubbery thyroid gland, usually in a female patient aged 30–50 years; initial hyperthyroidism that progresses to hypothyroidism and, if untreated, to myxoedema.

[Note] Iodine deficiency can also cause a goitre but this is rarely seen in developed countries.

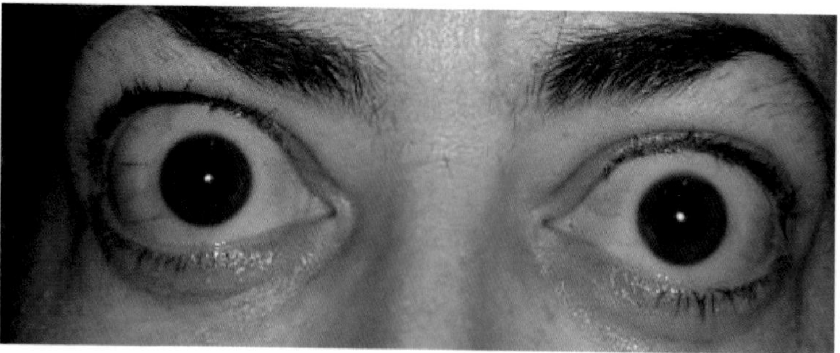

Figure 48. Eye signs in Graves' disease.
Reproduced from www.eyeplastics.net.

Conditions most likely to appear in a lump in the neck examination station
Toxic goitre: • diffuse (Graves' disease), multinodular, toxic nodule (see above)
Hashimoto's thyroiditis (see above)
Physiological goitre of puberty or pregnancy (or both)
Thyroglossal cyst: • fibrous cyst that forms from a persistent thyroglossal duct • midline lump in the region of the hyoid bone that is smooth and cystic and usually painless • moves upwards upon swallowing and upon tongue protrusion
Enlarged lymph nodes NB. Other, less likely, possibilities include thyroid carcinoma, branchial cyst, cystic hygroma (lymphangioma), carotid body tumour, and sternocleidomastoid tumour.

Dermatological history

Before starting

- Introduce yourself to the patient.
- Explain that you are going to ask him some questions to uncover the nature of his skin problem, and ask for his consent to do this.
- Ensure that he is comfortable; if not, make sure that he is.

The history

- Name and age.

Presenting complaint

- Use an open question to ask the patient to describe his skin problem.

History of presenting complaint

Ask about:

- When, where, and how the problem started.
- What the initial lesions looked like and how they have evolved. Are the hair and nails also involved?
- Symptoms: especially, pain, pruritus, blistering and bleeding.
- Aggravating factors such as sunlight, heat, soaps, etc.
- Relieving factors, including any treatments so far.
- Effect on everyday life.
- Details of previous episodes, if any.

Past medical history

- Previous skin disease.
- Atopy (asthma, allergic rhinitis, childhood eczema).
- Present and past medical illnesses.
- Surgery.

Drug history

- Prescribed and OTC/complementary medications, including topical applications such as gels and creams.
- Cosmetics and moisturising creams.
- Relationship of symptoms to use of medication.
- Allergies.

Family history

- Has anyone in the family had a similar problem?
- Medical history of parents, siblings, and children, focusing on skin problems.
- Sexual contacts.

Social history

- Occupation (in some detail). Has the patient's occupation exposed him to any allergens or irritants? Have colleagues been suffering from similar symptoms? Do the symptoms improve during holiday periods?
- Hobbies (in some detail). Have the patient's hobbies exposed him to any allergens or irritants? Has he been using sunbeds?
- Home circumstances.
- Alcohol use.
- Smoking.
- Recent travel, especially to the tropics.

Systems review

(If appropriate.)

After taking the history

- Ask the patient if there is anything that he might add that you have forgotten to ask about.
- Thank the patient.
- Summarise your findings and offer a differential diagnosis.
- State that you should next like to carry out a dermatological examination.

Station 51

Dermatological examination

Before starting

- Introduce yourself to the patient.
- Explain the examination and ask for his consent to carry it out.
- Ask him to undress to his undergarments.
- Ensure that he is comfortable.
- Ask him to report any pain or discomfort during the examination.
- Ensure that there is adequate lighting.

The examination

- Describe the distribution of the lesions: are they generalised or localised, symmetrical or asymmetrical, affecting only certain areas, e.g. flexor or extensor surfaces. Make a point of looking at all parts of the body.
- Describe the morphology of the individual lesions, commenting upon their colour, size, shape, borders, elevation, and spatial relationship. Use precise dermatological terms. A glossary of dermatological terms with accompanying images can be found at: www.dermnetnz.org/terminology.html.
- Note any secondary skin lesions such as scaling, lichenification, crusting, excoriation, erosion, ulceration, and scarring.
- Palpate the lesions (ask the patient if this is OK first). Assess their consistency. Do they blanch?
- Examine the finger nails and toe nails.
- Examine the hair and scalp.
- Examine the mucous membranes.
- Check for lymphadenopathy, if appropriate.
- Check the pedal pulses, if appropriate.

After the examination

- If appropriate, offer to help the patient to put his clothes back on.
- Thank the patient.
- Ensure that he is comfortable.
- Wash your hands.
- Summarise your findings and offer a differential diagnosis.

Examiner's questions

Differentiating skin cancers

BCC (75% of skin cancers) most often looks like a pearly bump or nodule on sun-exposed areas of skin. Bleeding or crusting may develop in the centre of the tumour, as in the photograph above. In contrast, squamous cell carcinoma (SCC, 20% of all skin cancers) most often looks a red, scaling, thickened patch, sometimes with bleeding, crusting, or ulceration. Although less common than either BCC or SCC, malignant melanoma is more commonly fatal. Pigmented lesions of the skin should be suspected to be malignant melanomas if they are **a**symmetrical, if they have irregular **b**orders, if their **c**olour varies from one area to another, or if their **d**iameter is larger than that of a pencil eraser (6 mm). This is easily remembered as A, B, C, D.

(A)

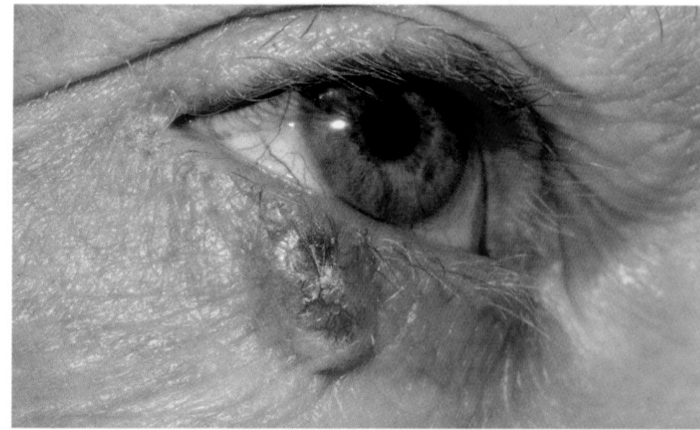

(B)

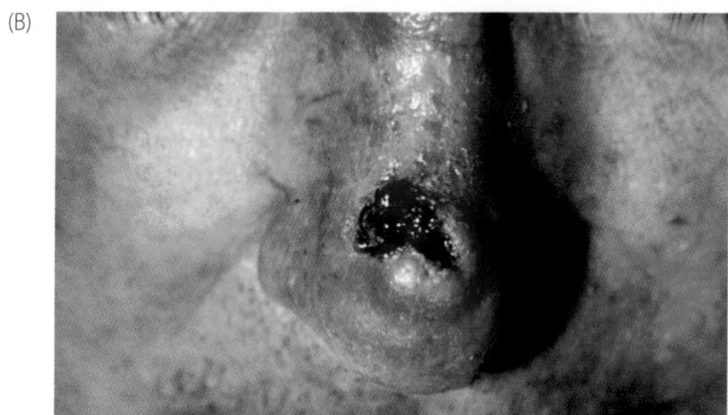

Figure 49. (A) Basal cell carcinoma (BCC). Reproduced from http://picasaweb.google.com/schalock. (B) Squamous cell carcinoma. Reproduced from http://commons.wikimedia.org/wiki/file:squamous_cell_carcinoma.jpg

Conditions most likely to come up in skin examination station

Psoriasis:

- chronic, autoimmune skin disease
- plaque psoriasis is most common type (c. 90%)
- red plaques with silvery scales due to inflammation and excessive skin production
- frequently on the elbows or knees, but can also affect any area including the scalp, palms, and soles
- may be accompanied by nail dystrophy
- may be accompanied by joint inflammation (psoriatic arthritis)
- may be aggravated by stress, alcohol, smoking, and certain drugs, e.g. lithium, beta blockers, chloroquinine

Eczema:

- most common types are atopic or flexural eczema and irritant-induced contact dermatitis
- recurrent dryness, itching, and skin rashes that may be accompanied by redness, inflammation, cracking, weeping, blistering, crusting, flaking, and skin discoloration
- frequently on the flexor aspects of joints (cf. psoriasis)

Acne vulgaris:

- changes in the pilosebaceous units as a result of increased androgen stimulation
- comedones (blackheads), inflammatory papules, pustules, and nodules that affect the face and neck and also the chest, back, and shoulders, and that can result in scarring
- usually appears during adolescence and may persist into early adulthood

Rosacea:

- chronic condition that primarily affects fair-skinned people and that is 2–3 times more common in women
- peak age of onset is 30–50
- typically begins as flushing and redness on the central face
- may be accompanied by telangiectasia, red domed papules and pustules, red gritty eyes, burning and stinging sensations, and, in some advanced cases, a red lobulated nose (rhinophyma)
- may be aggravated by stress, sunlight, cold weather, alcohol

Skin cancer (see *Examiner's questions* above)

Station 52

Advice on sun protection

Read in conjunction with Station 110: Explaining skills.

Before starting

- Introduce yourself to the patient.
- Tell him what you are going to explain, and determine how much he already knows.

The advice

Explain that there are three types of ultraviolet radiation from the sun: UVA, UVB, and UVC.

- UVA and UVB can cause skin cancer.
- UVC does not reach the surface of the earth and is therefore of no concern.

Explain that, other than causing skin cancer, UV radiation can also cause the skin to burn and (horror!) to age prematurely.

UV levels depend on a number of factors such as the time of day, time of year, latitude, altitude, cloud cover, and ozone cover.

Explain that there are four principal methods of protecting against the sun's rays:

1. Avoid the outdoors. The sun's rays are most direct around midday and so one should avoid being outdoors from around 11 am to 3 pm.
2. Seek shade.
3. Cover up (clothing should include a wide-brimmed hat and sunglasses that conform to British Standard 2724).
4. Use sunscreen.
    - A sunscreen's star rating is a measure of its level of protection against UVA.
    - A sunscreen's sun protection factor is a measure of its level of protection against UVB.
    - Use a sunscreen that has a star rating of at least three stars *** and an SPF of at least 15.
    - The sunscreen should be applied thickly over all sun-exposed areas, and re-applied regularly.

It is important that you explain that sunscreens should not simply be used as a means of spending more time in the sun.

Finally advise the patient to report any moles that change in size, shape, colour, or texture.

After giving the advice

- Summarise the information and ensure that the patient has understood it.
- Tell them that, if anything, they can remember 'Slip, slap, slop' – slip on some clothes, slap on a hat, and slop on sunscreen.
- Ask the patient if he has any questions or concerns.
- Give the patient a leaflet on sun protection.

Paediatric history

General points:

- As a rule of thumb, the older the child the more he should be involved in the history-taking process.
- Observe the child's behaviour as you take the history.
- The parent's concerns and the child's concerns are likely to differ: try as much as possible to address both.

Before starting

- Introduce yourself to the parent and child (in that order).
- Explain that you are going to ask some questions and obtain consent to do this.
- Ensure that the patient is comfortable; younger children may need some toys to keep them distracted.

The history

- Ask the age, sex, and preferred name of the child.
- Confirm the relationship of the accompanying adult.

Presenting complaint and history of presenting complaint

- Ask about the nature of the presenting complaint and how it has affected the child's daily routine. Start by using open questions and then explore the symptoms as you might in any other history. Ask about onset, duration, previous episodes, pain, associated symptoms (e.g. nausea, vomiting, diarrhoea, urinary frequency, constipation, altered consciousness), and treatments.

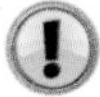 *Do not under any circumstances denigrate, or omit to address, the parent's concerns.*

Systems review

- The major systems should be covered briefly, placing the emphasis on areas of particular relevance.
  - *General health*: liveliness, change in behaviour, feeding, fever.
  - *ENT*: sore throat, earache, infections, deafness, nose bleeds.
  - *CVS and RS*: breathing problems (feeding problems in young infants), shortness of breath, exercise tolerance, colour changes (blue attacks, pallor), cough, croup, wheeze, stridor, chest infections, heart murmurs.
  - *GIS*: weight gain, feeding, vomiting, diarrhoea, constipation, jaundice, abdominal pain.
  - *GUS*: frequency, discharge, enuresis.
  - *NS*: headaches, fits, visual disturbances, balance and coordination, muscle problems.
  - *MSS*: limps, joint stiffness, pain, swelling, redness.
  - *Skin*: rash, eczema.

Past medical history

Similar problems in the past?

Ask about these topics if you think that they might be relevant to the child's presenting complaint.

- Medical problems (epilepsy, diabetes, asthma, etc.)

- Surgery.
- Birth history:
  - maternal obstetric history (illnesses or infections during pregnancy, blood pressure, foetal growth, drugs during pregnancy, e.g. anti-convulsants, narcotics, smoking, alcohol)
  - mode of delivery and any problems
  - gestation at delivery
  - birth weight
  - problems after birth and admission to Special Care Baby Unit
- Developmental milestones (smiling, sitting, walking and talking – see *Station 54: Developmental assessment*).
- Feeding (breast, bottle, how long, how much).
- Sleeping patterns.
- Childhood illnesses.
- Immunisations.

Drug history

- Prescribed and over-the-counter medications.
- Allergies.

Family history

- Health of parents and siblings.
- Congenital/genetic abnormalities. (*"Are there any illnesses that run in the family?"*)
- Cosanguinity.

Social history

- Parental occupation.
- Details of home life, siblings.
- Behaviour at home and at school.
- Pets and smokers in the home (if relevant).

After taking the history

- Ask the parent if there is anything that he/she might add that you have forgotten to ask about.
- Ask the parent and child if they have any specific questions or concerns.
- Thank the parent and child.
- Summarise your findings and offer a differential diagnosis.

Conditions most likely to come up in a paediatric history station

- Respiratory conditions, e.g. asthma, upper respiratory tract infection
- Headache
- Behavioural problems, e.g. enuresis
- Fits, e.g. febrile convulsions, epilepsy
- Childhood infections/rashes and immunisation compliance (see *Station 62: Child immunisation programme*).

Developmental assessment

Development in the early years of life is fairly consistent from child to child and any significant deviation from this pattern is thus a reliable marker of pathology.

The four parameters by which development is assessed

1. Gross motor skills
2. Vision and fine movement
3. Hearing and language
4. Social behaviour

Key ages for developmental assessment

1. Newborn
2. Supine infant (1.5–2 months)
3. Sitting infant (6–9 months)
4. Toddler (18–24 months)
5. Communicating child (3–4 years)

The developmental assessment

Specifications: This station may require you to carry out a developmental assessment or watch a short video and answer some questions about it.

The developmental assessment is usually performed alongside a general history, so many of the subject headings are the same as in *Station 53: Paediatric history*. Remember to tailor the assessment to the age of the child and that much of the assessment can and should be carried out by observation alone.

Before starting

- Introduce yourself to the parent and child.
- Explain that you are going to ask some questions and obtain consent to do this.
- Ensure that the child is comfortable; younger children may need toys to keep them distracted.
- Ask for the child's red book.

The assessment

- Ask for the age, sex, and preferred name of the child.

Presenting complaint and history of presenting complaint

- Ask about the nature of the presenting complaint and its effects on the child's daily routine. Use open questions.

Table 20. Average age for the acquisition of key milestones

	Motor skills	Vision and fine movement	Hearing and language	Social behaviour
Newborn	Symmetrical movements, limbs flexed, head lag on pulling up	Looks at light/ faces in direct line of vision	Startles to noises/ voices	Responds to parents
Supine infant (1.5–2 months)	Raises head in prone position	Tracks objects	Cries, coos, grunts	Smiles at faces
Sitting infant (6–9 months)	6/12: sits unsupported 8/12: crawls 9/12: stands supported	6/12: 'palmar grasp' 6–7/12: transfers objects	Babbles	Develops stranger and separation anxiety. Likes playing 'peek-a-boo'
Toddler (18–24 months)	12/12: stands unsupported and makes first steps 15/12: walks 24/12: climbs stairs	12/12: 'pincer grip' 16/12: uses spoon or fork	12/12: vocabulary of 1–3 words 24/12: vocabulary of >200 words; makes phrases	Is prone to temper tantrums
Communicating child (3–4 years)	Stands on one leg. Jumps. Pedals tricycle	Mature pencil grip. Draws a circle and a cross	Makes complete sentences	Plays co-operatively with other children. Imitates parents. Achieves urinary continence

Developmental/past medical history

- Birth history:
  - maternal obstetric history
  - mode of delivery and any problems
  - gestation at delivery
  - birth weight
  - problems after birth and admission to Special Care Baby Unit
  - initial feedings
  - medical problems, childhood illnesses, immunisations
- Key milestones:
  - smiling
  - sitting
  - walking
  - talking
- Current abilities:
  - motor skills
  - vision and fine movement
  - language and hearing
  - social behaviour

Systems review

Drug history

Family history

Social history

After the assessment

- Ask the parent if there is anything he/she might add that you have forgotten to ask about.
- Ask the parent if he/she has any specific questions or concerns.
- Thank the parent and child.
- Summarise your findings and offer a differential diagnosis.

Conditions most likely to come up in a developmental assessment station

- Late walker
- Developmental disorder, e.g. autism
- Mental retardation
- Emotional disorder, e.g. enuresis, elective mutism, sleep disorders
- Behavioural disorder, e.g. conduct disorder, ADHD

Neonatal examination

Specifications: A mannequin in lieu of a baby. The baby's 'mother' is also in the room.

Before starting

- Introduce yourself to the mother, explain the examination, and ask her for her consent to carry it out.
- Wash your hands.
- Ask the mother about:
  - complications of the pregnancy, if any
  - type of delivery and any complications
  - the baby's gestational age at the time of birth
  - the baby's birth weight
  - the baby's feeding, urination, and defaecation
  - any concerns that she might have

The examination

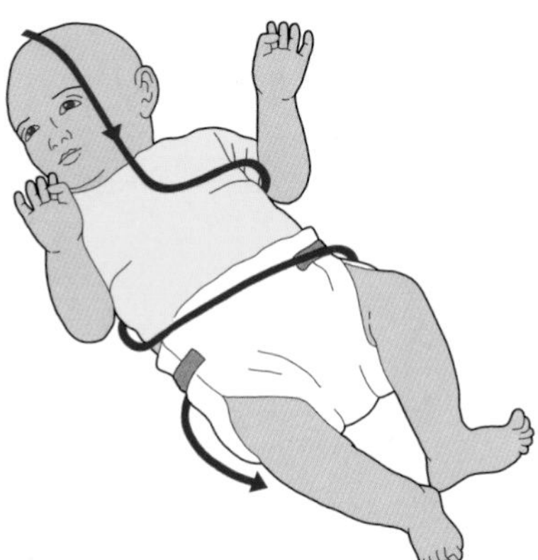

Figure 50. Neonatal examination, general order of the examination.

General inspection

Note size, colour (e.g. cyanosis, jaundice), posture, tone, movements, skin abnormalities (e.g. rash, petechiae, birth marks), and any other obvious abnormalities (e.g. dysmorphic features or birth trauma such as forceps marks or chignon). Are there any signs of respiratory distress?

Head

- Palpate the anterior and posterior fontanelles for bulging (raised intracranial pressure) or depression (dehydration).
- Measure the head circumference with the tape measure passing above the ears. Head circumference in the neonate should be 33–38 cm.

Face

- Inspect the face for dysmorphological features, e.g. dysplastic or folded ears, upward slanting palpebral fissures, and a flat nasal bridge (all may be seen in Down syndrome).
- Inspect the sclerae for redness (subconjunctival haemorrhage related to birth trauma) and the irises for Brushfield spots (Down syndrome).
- Using an ophthalmoscope, test the red reflex (congenital cataracts if the red reflex is absent, retinoblastoma if instead there is a white reflex) and pupillary reflexes.
- Test eye movements (squint).
- Check the patency of the ears and nostrils.
- Elicit the rooting reflex by lightly touching a corner of the baby's mouth.
- Introduce a finger into the baby's mouth to assess the sucking reflex and the soft palate (cleft palate).
- Also examine the soft palate using a torch and spatula.

Chest

- Inspect the chest for signs of laboured breathing and for deformities, e.g. *pectus carinatum, pectus excavatum*, shield-shaped chest with widely-spaced nipples (Turner syndrome).
- Take the brachial and femoral pulses, one after the other and then both at the same time (brachio-femoral delay). Pulse rate in the neonate should be 100–160.
- Palpate the precordium and locate the apex beat.
- Auscultate the heart using the bell of your stethoscope (congenital heart defects).
- Auscultate the lungs using the diaphragm of your stethoscope. Turn the infant over and listen over the back. The respiratory rate should be less than 60 breaths per minute.

Back

- Examine the spine, focusing on the sacral pit (neural tube defects).
- Check the position and patency of the anus (anal atresia).

Abdomen

- Inspect the abdomen and the umbilical stump.
- Palpate the abdomen.
- Palpate specifically for the spleen, liver, and kidneys (thumb in front, finger in the loin), and for any masses.
- Auscultate for bowel sounds.
- Feel in the inguinoscrotal region for inguinal hernias.
- Examine the genitalia, in male infants note the position of the urethral meatus (hypospadias) and feel for the testicles (undescended testes).
- Feel for the femoral pulses.

Hips

- *Ortolani test*. With your thumbs on the inner aspects of the thighs and your index and middle fingers over the greater trochanters, flex the hips and knees to 90 degrees and then abduct the hips (an audible and palpable clunk indicates relocation of a dislocated hip).
- *Barlow test*. Next, adduct them whilst applying downward pressure with your thumbs (an audible and palpable clunk indicates an unstable hip that can be dislocated).

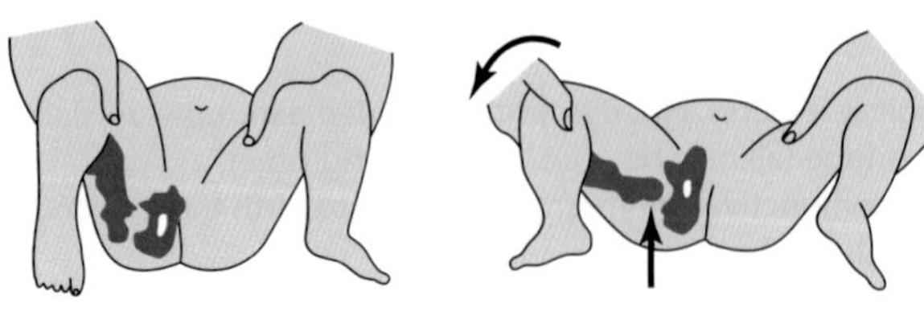

Ortolani test

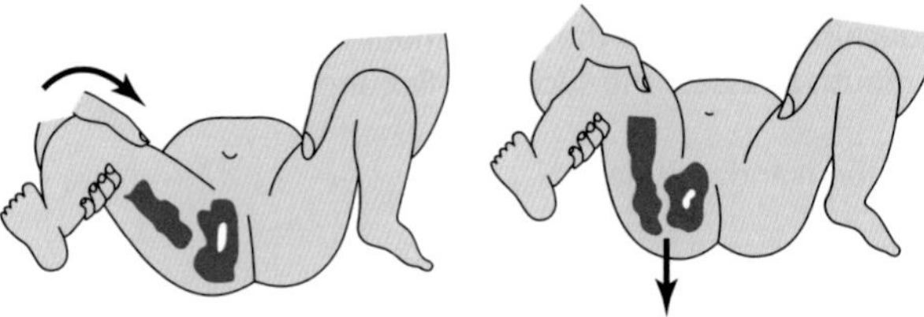

Barlow test

Figure 51. The Ortolani and Barlow tests.

Arms and hands

- Inspect the arms and hands, paying particular attention to the palmar creases (Simian crease – Down syndrome).
- Count the number of digits on each hand.

Feet

- Inspect the feet for deformities and test their range of movement.
- Count the number of digits on each foot.

Posture and reflexes

- *Head lag.* Lay the baby supine and pull up the upper body by the arms – the head should first 'lag' back, then straighten and fall forward.
- *Ventral suspension.* Hold the baby prone – the head should lie above the midline.
- *Moro or startle reflex.* Lift the head and shoulders and then suddenly drop them back – the arms and legs should abduct and extend symmetrically, and then adduct and flex (NB. some examiners may prefer that you did not test the Moro reflex).
- *Grasp reflex.* Place a finger in the baby's hand – the hand should close around your finger.

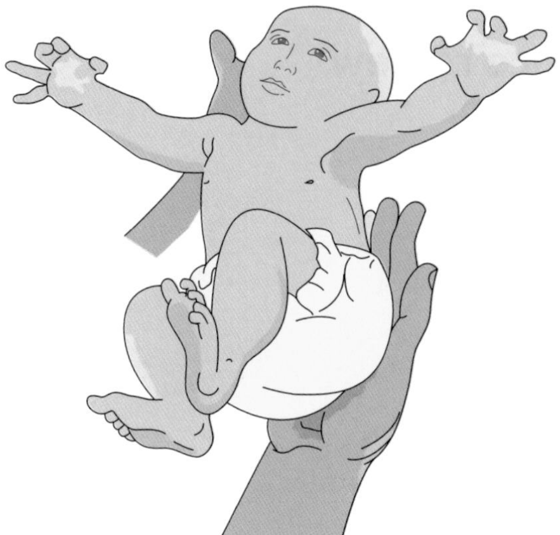

Figure 52. Eliciting the Moro reflex.

After the neonatal examination

- State that you would also measure and weigh the baby and record your findings on a growth centile chart.
- Summarise your findings.
- Reassure the mother, and tell her that you are going to have the baby examined by a senior colleague.

The six-week surveillance review

Specifications: A mannequin in lieu of a baby.

Before starting

- Introduce yourself to the parent.
- Explain the nature of the examination and obtain consent.
- Ask for the parent-held record.

The history

- Ask for the exact age, sex, and preferred name of the child.

Main concerns

- Ask if the parent has any specific concerns.

Past medical history

- Birth history:
  - pregnancy
  - gestation
  - delivery
  - birth weight
  - neonatal history
- Present health:
  - current health status
  - medication
  - social history

The examination

PART 1 – DEVELOPMENTAL ASSESSMENT

Motor skills

- Symmetrical limb movements.
- Head lag.

Vision and fine movement

- Looks at light/faces.
- Follows an object.

Hearing and language

- Responds to noises/voices.
- Normal cry.
- Ask parent if he/she is concerned about the baby's hearing.

Social behaviour

- Smiles responsively.

PART 2 – PHYSICAL EXAMINATION

Growth

- Weight.
- Length.
- Head circumference.
- Plot findings on a centile chart.

Head

- Palpate the fontanelles.

Face

- Eyes: red reflex, papillary reflexes, and eye movements (squints).
- Ears.
- Mouth – use a pen torch.

Chest

- Feel for the radial and femoral pulses.
- Auscultate the heart.
- Auscultate the lungs.

Back

- Examine the spine, particularly the sacral pit.

Abdomen

- Inspect and palpate the abdomen.
- Examine the external genitalia.

Hips

- Abduct the hips (Ortolani test, see *Figure 51*).
- Next, adduct them whilst applying downward pressure with your thumbs (Barlow test, see *Figure 51*).

After the surveillance review

- Discuss your findings with the parent.
- Use the opportunity for health promotion, e.g. immunisations, accident prevention, services available for the parents of young children.
- Elicit any remaining concerns that the parent may have.
- Thank the parent.

Station 57

Paediatric examination: cardiovascular system

[Note] This station should be read in conjunction with *Station 12*.

If you are asked to examine the cardiovascular system of a younger child (an unlikely event), be prepared to change the order of your examination and to modify your technique as appropriate. For example, you may need to examine the child on his parent's knees or auscultate his heart as soon as he stops crying. As in all paediatric stations, the quality of your rapport with the child will be of considerable importance.

Before starting

- Introduce yourself to the child and the parent.
- Explain the examination and ask for consent to carry it out.
- Position the child at 45 degrees, and ask him to remove his top(s).
- Ensure that he is comfortable.

The examination

General inspection

- From the end of the couch, inspect the child carefully, looking for any obvious abnormalities in his general appearance and in particular for any dysmorphic features suggestive of Down syndrome (e.g. oblique eye fissures, epicanthic folds, Brushfield spots, flat nasal bridge, Simian crease), Turner syndrome (e.g. short stature, low-set ears, webbed neck, shield chest), or Marfan syndrome (e.g. tall stature, elongated limbs, *pectus carinatum* or *pectus excavatum*).
- Does the child look his age? Ask to look at the growth chart.
- Is he breathless or cyanosed?
- Look around the child for clues such as a oxygen, PEFR meter, inhalers, etc.
- Inspect the precordium and the chest for any scars and pulsations. A median sternotomy or thoracotomy scar under the axillae may indicate the repair of a congenital heart defect such as a patent ductus arteriosus or a ventricular septal defect.

Inspection and examination of the hands

- Take both hands and assess them for:
  - colour and temperature
  - clubbing
  - nail signs
- Determine the rate, rhythm, and character of both radial pulses (in younger infants, the brachial pulses). Take both femoral pulses at the same time to exclude a radiofemoral delay (coarctation of the aorta).
- Indicate that you would record the blood pressure in both arms. If you are asked to record the blood pressure, remember to use a cuff of appropriate size.

Table 21. Normal pulse rates in children

Age in years	Pulse (beats per minute)
< 1	100–160
2–4	90–140
4–10	80–140
> 10	65–100

Inspection and examination of the head and neck

- Inspect the conjunctiva for signs of anaemia or jaundice.
- Inspect the mouth and tongue for signs of central cyanosis and a high arched palate (Marfan syndrome).
- Assess the jugular venous pressure (difficult in very young infants).
- Locate the carotid pulse and assess its character.

Palpation of the heart

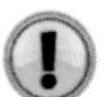 *Ask the child if he has any pain in the chest.*

- Determine the location and character of the apex beat. In children (up to 8 years), this is found in the fourth intercostal space in the mid-clavicular line.
- Palpate the precordium for thrills and heaves.

Auscultation of the heart

 *Warm up the diaphragm of your stethoscope.*

- Listen for heart sounds, additional sounds, and murmurs. Using the stethoscope's diaphragm, listen in:
  - the *aortic* area
  - the *pulmonary* area
  - the *tricuspid* area
  - the *mitral* area

(See *Station 12, Figure 9.*)

- Any murmur heard must be classified according to:
  - timing
  - grading
  - site
  - radiation

Innocent murmurs are common in childhood

Innocent murmurs are:

- Systolic.
- Low-grade.
- Heard over only a relatively small area.
- Asymptomatic.

Chest examination

Auscultate the bases of the lungs and check for sacral oedema.

Abdominal examination

Palpate the abdomen to exclude ascities and/or an enlarged liver. Note that the liver edge can usually be palpated in younger infants.

Peripheral pulses

Feel the temperature of the feet, palpate the femoral pulses, and check for pedal oedema.

After the examination

- Cover the child.
- Ask the child and parent if they have any questions or concerns.
- Thank the child and parent.
- Indicate that you would test the urine, examine the retina with an ophthalmoscope and, if appropriate, order some key investigations, e.g. a CXR, ECG, echocardiogram.
- Summarise your findings and offer a differential diagnosis.

Conditions most likely to come up in a paediatric cardiovascular examination station
Ventricular septal defect (VSD) • Pansystolic murmur best heard over the left lower sternal edge and possibly accompanied by a palpable thrill, parasternal heave, and displaced apex beat. Most VSDs are small and asymptomatic and may close spontaneously within the first year of life. However, a large VSD may progressively lead to higher pulmonary resistance and, finally, to irreversible pulmonary vascular changes, producing the so-called Eisenmenger syndrome (reversal of shunt to right-to-left shunt). Eisenmenger syndrome can also result from atrial septal defect and patent ductus arteriosus.
Patent ductus arteriosus (PDA) • Continuous machine-like murmur best heard over the pulmonary area and possibly accompanied by a left subclavicular thrill, displaced apex beat, and collapsing pulse. The first heart sound is normal but the second is often obscured by the murmur. The ductus arteriosus is a shunt that runs from the pulmonary artery to the descending aorta and which enables blood to bypass the closed lungs *in utero*. A small PDA may cause no signs or symptoms and may go undetected into adulthood, but a large one can cause signs and symptoms of heart failure soon after birth.
Atrial septal defect • Ejection systolic murmur best heard in the pulmonary area due to increased blood flow across the pulmonic valve with an associated mid-diastolic murmur best heard in the tricuspid area due to increased blood flow across the tricuspid valve. These murmurs, neither of which is particularly loud, are accompanied by a wide fixed splitting of the second heart sound and a displaced apex beat. The patient is often asymptomatic.

Pulmonary stenosis

- Loud ejection systolic murmur with an ejection click that is best heard in the pulmonary area. This murmur may be accompanied by a widely split second heart sound, and by a systolic thrill and parasternal heave. The patient is often asymptomatic.

Aortic stenosis

- Ejection systolic murmur with an ejection click best heard in the aortic area and radiating to the carotids. The murmur may be accompanied by a slow-rising pulse and a heaving cardiac apex. The patient is often asymptomatic.

Coarctation of the aorta

- Arterial hypertension in the right arm with normal to low blood pressure in the legs. There is radio-femoral delay between the right arm and the femoral artery and, in severe cases, a weak or absent femoral artery pulse. In contrast, mild cases may go undetected into adulthood.

Tetralogy of Fallot

- The tetralogy refers to VSD, pulmonary stenosis, overriding aorta, and right ventricular hypertrophy, and there may also be other anatomical abnormalities. There is cyanosis from birth or developing in the first year of life.

Paediatric examination: respiratory system

[Note] This station should be read in conjunction with *Station 16*.

If you are asked to examine the respiratory system of a younger child (an unlikely event), be prepared to change the order of your examination and to modify your technique as appropriate. For example, you may need to examine the child on his parent's knees or auscultate his chest as soon as he stops crying. As in all paediatric stations, the quality of your rapport with the child will be of considerable importance.

Before starting

- Introduce yourself to the child and parent.
- Explain the examination and ask for consent to carry it out.
- Position the child at 45 degrees, and ask him to remove his top(s).
- Ensure that he is comfortable.

The examination

General inspection

- From the end of the couch inspect the child carefully, looking for any obvious abnormalities in his general appearance.
- Does the child look his age? Ask to look at the growth chart.
- Is he breathless or cyanosed?
- Is his breathing audible?
- Note the rate, depth, and regularity of his breathing.
- Look around the child for clues such as a PEFR meter, inhalers, etc.

Table 22. Normal respiratory rates in children

Age in years	Respiratory rate (breaths per minute)
Premature infant	40–60
Term infant	30–50
6 years	19–24
12 years	16–21

Look for:

- Deformities of the chest (barrel chest, *pectus excavatum*, *pectus carinatum*) and spine.
- Asymmetry of chest expansion.
- Signs of respiratory distress such as the use of accessory muscles of respiration, suprasternal, intercostal, and/or subcostal recession, nasal flaring, and difficulty speaking.
- Added sounds such as cough, croup, wheeze, stridor.
- Harrison's sulci.
- Operative scars.

Inspection and examination of the hands

- Take both hands and assess them for colour and temperature.
- Look for clubbing.

- Determine the rate, rhythm, and character of the radial pulse (in younger infants, the brachial pulse).
- State that you would record the blood pressure.

Inspection and examination of the head and neck

- Inspect the conjunctivae for signs of anaemia.
- Inspect the mouth for signs of central cyanosis.
- Assess the jugular venous pressure and jugular venous pulse form.
- Palpate the cervical, supraclavicular, infraclavicular, and axillary lymph nodes.

Palpation of the chest

 *Ask the child if he has any pain in the chest.*

- Palpate for tracheal deviation by placing the index and middle fingers of one hand on either side of the trachea in the suprasternal notch. (As this may be uncomfortable, it is probably best omitted in younger children.)
- Palpate for the position of the cardiac apex.

[Note] Carry out all subsequent steps on the front of the chest and, once this is done, repeat them on the back of the chest.

- Palpate for equal chest expansion, comparing one side to the other.
- Palpate for tactile fremitus.

Percussion of the chest

- Percuss the chest. Start at the apex of one lung and compare one side to the other. Do not forget to percuss over the clavicles and on the sides of the chest. Note that percussion of the chest is not useful in young infants.

Auscultation of the chest

 *Warm up the diaphragm of your stethoscope.*

- If old enough, ask the child to take deep breaths through the mouth and, using the diaphragm of the stethoscope, auscultate the chest. Start at the apex of one lung, and compare one side to the other. Are the breath sounds vesicular or bronchial? Are there any added sounds?

Oedema

- Assess for sacral and pedal oedema.

After the examination

- Cover the child.
- Ask the child and parent if they have any questions or concerns.
- Thank the child and parent.
- Indicate that you would like to look at the sputum pot, measure the PEFR and, if appropriate, order some key investigations, e.g. a CXR, FBC, etc.
- Summarise your findings and offer a differential diagnosis.

Conditions most likely to come up in a paediatric respiratory examination station
Cystic fibrosis • Autosomal recessive progressive multisystem disease that is related to a mutation in the *CFTR* gene and that leads to viscous secretions. • In terms of the respiratory system, findings on physical examination may include delayed growth and development, finger clubbing, nasal polyps, recurrent chest infections, shortness of breath, coughing with copious phlegm production, haemoptysis, hyper-inflated chest, *cor pulmonale*.
Broncho-pulmonary dysplasia (BPD) • Chronic lung disorder that involves inflammation and scarring in the lungs and which is most common among children who were born prematurely and who received prolonged mechanical ventilation for respiratory distress syndrome. • Findings on physical examination may include delayed growth and development, shortness of breath, crackles, wheezes, and decreased breath sounds, hyper-inflated chest, *cor pulmonale*.
Pneumonia • Findings on physical examination may include signs of consolidation accompanied by fever, lethargy, poor feeding, shortness of breath, productive cough, and, in some cases, haemoptysis and pleuritic chest pain.
Asthma • Findings on physical examination may include shortness of breath, chest tightness, wheezing and coughing, signs of respiratory distress such as the use of accessory muscles of respiration and intercostal recession, hyper-inflated chest.

Paediatric examination: abdomen

[Note] This station should be read in conjunction with *Station 21*.

Before starting

- Introduce yourself to the child and parent.
- Explain the examination and ask for consent to carry it out.
- Position the child so that he is lying flat and expose his abdomen as much as possible (customarily 'nipples to knees', although this is not appropriate in an OSCE setting).
- Ensure that he is comfortable.

The examination

General inspection

- From the end of the couch, observe the child's general appearance:
  - does the child look his age? Ask to look at the growth chart
  - nutritional status
  - state of health/other obvious signs
- Inspect the abdomen noting any:
  - distension
  - localised masses
  - scars and skin changes
- Look around the child for clues such as oxygen, tubes, drains, etc.

 *A distended abdomen is often a normal finding in younger infants.*

Inspection and examination of the hands

- Take both hands looking for:
  - temperature and colour
  - clubbing
  - nail signs
- Take the pulse.

Inspection and examination of the head, neck, and upper body

- Inspect the sclera and conjunctivae for signs of jaundice or anaemia.
- Inspect the mouth, looking for ulcers (Crohn's disease), angular stomatitis (nutritional deficiency), atrophic glossitis (iron deficiency, vitamin B12 deficiency, folate deficiency), furring of the tongue (loss of appetite), and the state of the dentition.
- Examine the neck for lymphadenopathy.

Palpation of the abdomen

- Abdominal palpation can be difficult in children if they do not relax the abdominal muscles. Attempt to distract the child by handing him a toy or try to make him relax by coaxing him into palpating his abdomen and then copying his actions.

Ask the child if he has any tummy pain and keep your eyes on his face as you begin palpating his abdomen.

- *Light palpation* – begin by palpating furthest from the area of pain or discomfort and systematically palpate in the four quadrants and the umbilical area. Look for tenderness, guarding, and any masses.
- *Deep palpation* – for greater precision. Describe and localise any masses.

Palpation of the organs

- *Liver* – starting in the right lower quadrant, feel for the liver edge using the flat of your hand. Note that in younger infants the liver edge is normally palpable.
- *Spleen* – palpate for the spleen as for the liver, starting in the right lower quadrant.
- *Kidneys* – position the child close to the edge of the bed and ballot each kidney using the technique of deep bimanual palpation. Beyond the neonatal period, it is unlikely that you should be able to feel a normal kidney.

Percussion

- Percuss the liver area, also remembering to detect its upper border.
- Percuss the suprapubic area for dullness (bladder distension).
- If the abdomen is distended, test for shifting dullness (ascites).

Auscultation

- Auscultate in the mid-abdomen for abdominal sounds. Listen for 30 seconds at least before concluding that they are hyperactive, hypoactive, or absent.

Examination of the groins and genitalia

- Inspect the groins for hernias and, in boys, examine the testes (this is particularly important in younger infants).
- Note that examination of the groins and genitalia may only need to be mentioned, as it is not usually carried out in the OSCE setting.

Rectal examination

- PR is not routine practice in paediatrics and should be avoided unless specifically indicated.

After the examination

- Ask to test the urine.
- Cover the child.
- Ask the child and parent if they have any questions or concerns.
- Indicate that you would test the urine and order some key investigations, e.g. ultrasound scan, FBC, LFTs, U&Es, and clotting screen.
- Thank the child and parent.
- Summarise your findings and offer a differential diagnosis.

Conditions most likely to come up in a paediatric abdomen station

Constipation

- The majority of children with constipation do not have a medical disorder causing the constipation. Many things can contribute to constipation such as avoidance of the toilet (for various reasons), changes in diet or poor diet, and dehydration.
- Medical disorders that can cause chronic constipation include hypothyroidism, diabetes, cystic fibrosis, and disorders of the nervous system such as cerebral palsy and mental retardation. Constipation since birth may be from Hirschprung disease (a.k.a. congenital aganglionic megacolon).
- Other causes of chronic constipation include depression, drug side-effects, coercive toilet training, and sexual abuse.

Coeliac disease

- An autoimmune disorder of the small intestine that occurs in genetically predisposed people of all ages, but often from infancy. It is caused by a reaction to gliadin, a prolamin (gluten protein) found in wheat, barley, and rye, and results in villous atrophy.
- Symptoms include abdominal pain and cramping, diarrhoea, steatorrhoea, failure to thrive, and fatigue. Signs include short stature, a distended abdomen, wasted buttocks, mouth ulcers, and signs of anaemia.

Kidney transplant

- A kidney transplant has been required as a consequence of end-stage renal failure, which may itself have been a consequence of a birth defect, a structural malformation, a hereditary disease such as polycystic kidney disease or Alport syndrome, a glomerular disease, or a systemic disease such as diabetes or lupus.

Paediatric examination: gait and neurological function

Before starting

- Introduce yourself to the child and parent.
- Tell the child that you are going to examine him.
- Ensure that he is comfortable.

Examination of neurological function in children is principally a matter of observation. If the child is old enough to obey commands, a more formal assessment of gait and neurological function can be carried out, as in adults.

The examination

Neurological overview

- A brief developmental assessment should be performed to enable you to gauge the child's subsequent performance. Ask the parent the child's age and if there are any concerns about the child's vision and/or hearing.

Gait and movement

- If the child is too young to walk, observe him crawling or playing. Is he using all his limbs equally?
- If possible, observe the child walking and running. Common abnormalities of gait in children include:
  - scissoring or tiptoeing gait – suggestive of cerebral palsy or of Duchenne muscular dystrophy
  - broad-based gait: suggestive of a cerebellar disorder
  - limp – limps have many causes including dislocated hip, trauma, sepsis, and arthritis
- If possible, observe the child rising from the floor. The Gower sign (the child rising from the floor by 'climbing' up his legs) is suggestive of Duchenne muscular dystrophy.

Inspection

- Inspect all four limbs, in particular looking for muscle wasting or hypertrophy. Hypertrophy of the calves is suggestive of Duchenne muscular dystrophy.

Tone

- Assess tone and range of movement in all four limbs.
- In younger children also assess truncal tone by trying to get the child to sit unsupported.
- In young infants test head lag by lying the infant supine and pulling up his upper body by the arms.

Power

- Observe the child playing, and look for appropriate anti-gravity movement. A more formal assessment can be carried out if the child is old enough to carry out instructions.

Reflexes

- Check all reflexes as in the adult. Practice is the key!

- Note that eliciting the Babinsky sign (extensor plantar reflex) is not very discriminative in children.

Co-ordination

- If the child is old enough to carry out instructions, assess co-ordination by the finger-to-nose test or just by asking the child to jump or hop. If the child cannot carry out instructions, give him toys or some bricks and assess his co-ordination by observing him at play.

Sensation

- Indicate that you would test sensation.

Cranial nerves

- Indicate that you would test the cranial nerves – where possible this is done as in the adult.

After the examination

- Thank the parent and child.
- If appropriate, indicate that you would order some key investigations, e.g. CT, MRI, nerve conduction studies, electromyography, etc.
- Summarise your findings and offer a differential diagnosis.

Conditions most likely to appear in a paediatric gait and neurological function station
Cerebral palsy • In most cases of cerebral palsy there is a spastic, scissoring gait. The hips, knees, and ankles are flexed, producing a crouching and tiptoeing demeanour. In addition, the hips are adducted and internally rotated, such that the knees cross or hit each other in a scissor-like movement. There is a similar pattern of flexion and adduction in the upper limbs.
Duchenne muscular dystrophy • Severe recessive X-linked form of muscular dystrophy. • There is rapid progression of muscle degeneration leading to generalised and symmetrical weakness of the proximal muscles. • Symptoms and signs include muscle wasting, pseudohypertrophy of the calves, waddling gait, toe walking, frequent falls, poor endurance, difficulties running, jumping, or climbing stairs, difficulties standing unaided, and positive Gower's sign, with the child 'walking' his hands up his legs to stand upright.
Myotonic dystrophy • Autosomal dominant progressive and highly variable multisystemic disease characterised by muscle wasting, myotonia (delayed relaxation of the muscles after voluntary contraction), cataracts, heart conduction defects, endocrine defects, and cognitive abnormalities, amongst others. • The first muscles to be affected by wasting and weakness are typically those of the face and neck (leading to a 'fish face' and 'swan neck' appearance), hands, forearms, and feet. • The disease commonly affects adults but it has several forms and can also present as early as birth.
Ex-premature infant

Infant and child Basic Life Support

Specifications: A mannequin in lieu of an infant or child.

[Note] For the purposes of Basic Life Support, an infant is defined as being under 1 year, and a child as being between 1 year and puberty.

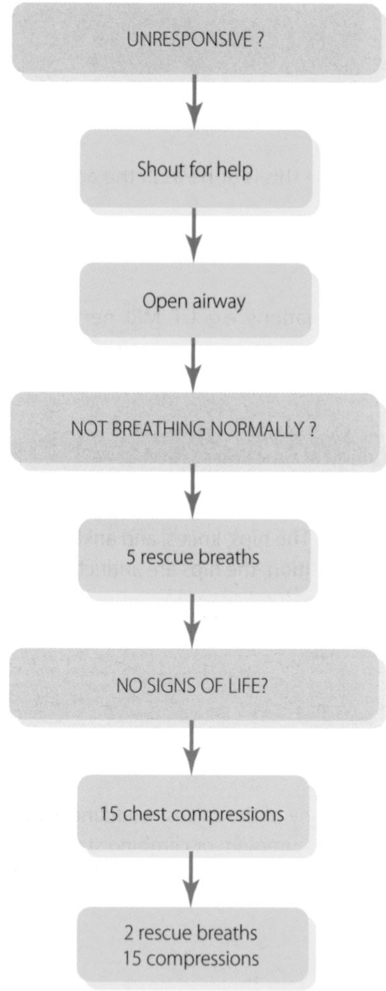

Figure 53. Paediatric Basic Life Support algorithm. Resuscitation Guidelines 2010.

- Ensure the safety of the rescuer and child
- Check the child's responsiveness by gently stimulating the child and asking loudly, 'Are you all right?'

 *Do not shake infants or children with suspected cervical spine injuries.*

- If the child responds by answering or moving:
  - leave the child in the position in which you find him (provided he is not in further danger)
  - check his condition and get help if needed
  - reassess him regularly
- If the child does not respond:
  - shout for help
  - turn the child onto his back and open his airway by using the head-tilt, chin-lift technique (see *Station 86*); if you have difficulty opening the airway using the head-tilt, chin-lift technique, try the jaw-thrust technique (see *Station 87*)

If you suspect that there may have been injury to the neck, try to open the airway using chin lift or jaw thrust alone. If this is unsuccessful, add head tilt a small amount at a time until the airway is open.

- Holding the child's airway open, put your face close to his mouth and look along his chest. Listen, feel, and look for breathing for no more than 10 seconds.
- If the child is breathing normally:
  - turn him into the recovery position
  - send for help
  - check for continued breathing
- If he is not breathing normally or is making agonal gasps (infrequent, irregular breaths):
  - carefully remove any obvious airway obstruction
  - give 5 initial rescue breaths
- While performing the rescue breaths, note any gag or cough response to your action.
- To deliver rescue breaths to a child over 1 year:
  - ensure head tilt and chin lift
  - pinch the soft part of his nose closed with the index finger and thumb of the hand on his forehead
  - allow his mouth to open, but maintain chin lift
  - take a breath and place your lips around his mouth, making sure that you have a good seal
  - blow steadily into his mouth over 1–1.5 seconds, watching for his chest to rise
  - maintaining head tilt and chin lift, take your mouth away from the victim and watch for his chest to fall
  - take another breath and repeat this sequence 4 more times
- To deliver rescue breaths to an infant:
  - ensure a neutral position of the head and apply chin lift
  - take a breath and cover the mouth and nasal apertures of the infant with your mouth, making sure you have a good seal
  - blow steadily into the infant's mouth and nose over 1–1.5 seconds so that the chest rises visibly
  - maintaining head tilt and chin lift, take your mouth away from the victim and watch for his chest to fall
  - take another breath and repeat this sequence 4 more times
- If you have difficulty achieving an effective breath, the airway may be obstructed.
  - Open the child's mouth and remove any visible obstruction.
  - Ensure that there is adequate head tilt and chin lift, but also that the neck is not over extended.
  - If the head-tilt, chin-lift method has not opened the airway, try the jaw thrust method.
  - Make up to 5 attempts to achieve effective rescue breaths. If still unsuccessful, move on to chest compression.
- Check for signs of a circulation (signs of life).
  - Take no more than 10 seconds to check for signs of circulation such as movement, coughing, or normal breathing (but not agonal gasps).

- Check the pulse but take no longer than 10 seconds to do this. In a child check the carotid pulse, in an infant check the brachial pulse.

- If you are confident that you have detected signs of circulation:
  - continue rescue breathing, if necessary, until the child starts breathing effectively on his own
  - turn the child into the recovery position if he remains unconscious
  - reassess the child frequently
- If there are no signs of life, unless you are CERTAIN that you can feel a definite pulse of greater than 60 beats per minute within 10 seconds, start chest compression. To deliver chest compressions to all children, compress the lower third of the sternum.
  - Locate the xiphisternum and compress the sternum one finger's breadth above this.
  - Compress the sternum by one-third of the depth of the chest or more. In infants, use the tips of two fingers or, if there are two or more rescuers, use the encircling technique with two thumbs. In children, use the heel of one hand or, in larger children, the heels of both hands, as in adults.
  - Aim for a rate of 100–120 compressions per minute.
- After 15 compressions, tilt the head, lift the chin, and give two effective breaths.
- Continue compressions and breaths in a ratio of 15:2.
- Continue resuscitation until the child shows signs of life (spontaneous respiration, pulse, movement) or further help arrives or you become exhausted.

When to go for assistance

- If more than one rescuer is present, one rescuer begins resuscitation whilst another goes for assistance.
- If only one rescuer is present, he should undertake resuscitation for 1 minute before going for assistance. It may be possible for him to carry the infant or child whilst going for assistance.
- The exception to this rule is in the case of a child with a witnessed, sudden collapse when the rescuer is alone. In this case the cause is likely to be an arrhythmia and the child may need defibrillation. Go for assistance immediately if there is no one to go for you.

Adapted from Resuscitation Council (UK), 2010 Guidelines.

Child immunisation programme

The instructions for this station may involve explaining the immunisation programme to a parent, or talking to an anxious parent about the pros and cons of the MMR vaccine. This station covers the facts, see *Station 110: Explaining skills* for the method.

Table 23. The UK Immunisation schedule

Age	Vaccine	Specifications
2 months	DTP triple vaccine (diphtheria, tetanus and pertussis) Hib (*Haemophilus influenzae* type b) Polio PCV (pneumococcal conjugate vaccine)	One injection (DTP, Hib and polio) One injection (PCV)
3 months	DTP + Hib + polio (2nd dose) MenC (meningitis C)	One injection One injection
4 months	DTP + Hib + polio (3rd dose) MenC (2nd dose) PCV (2nd dose)	One injection One injection One injection
Around 12 months	Hib/MenC (4th dose of Hib and 3rd dose of MenC)	One injection
Around 13 months	MMR (measles, mumps and rubella) PCV (3rd dose)	One injection One injection
Around 3 years and four months (pre-school age booster)	DTP + polio (booster) MMR (2nd dose)	One injection One injection
Around 12–13 years (girls)	HPV (human papillomavirus)	Three injections • 2nd injection 1–2 months after the first • 3rd injection 6 months after the 1st
Around 13–18 years	Diphtheria (low dose) + tetanus + polio	One injection as a booster
Adults	*H. influenzae* and PCV Diphtheria + tetanus + polio	If aged 65 or over or in a high-risk group At any age if not fully immunised as a child

A vaccine is a small sample of an attenuated pathogen, the function of which is to prime the body's immune system to recognise the pathogen and to mount a successful defence against it. Vaccines are very effective both at the individual and at the population level. As a result of the UK immunisation programme, a number of potentially deadly infectious diseases have become uncommon in the UK. That having been said, they are still very common in some other countries, from where they may be reintroduced to unvaccinated children in the UK. Vaccines can and often do have side-effects, but these are usually very mild. They include redness and swelling at the injection site, flu-like symptoms, and a fever. Some vaccines are given together in a single injection so as to minimise the number of injections required and to prevent delayed or missed vaccinations. There is no added benefit to giving them separately.

The MMR controversy

- Measles can cause pneumonia, fits, encephalitis, sub-acute sclerosing panencephalitis, and death.
- Mumps can cause meningitis, encephalitis, deafness, and sterility.
- Rubella in pregnancy can cause severe damage to the foetus.
- The MMR vaccine is safe and effective, and more than 500 million doses of the vaccine have been given since 1972.
- Common side-effects of the MMR vaccine are a sore injection site and flu-like symptoms. Very rarely, an allergic reaction can occur.
- There is no evidence to support a distinct syndrome of MMR-induced autism or inflammatory bowel disease.
- Separate administration of the measles, mumps, and rubella vaccines provides no added benefit over administration of the combined MMR vaccine, but means three injections and potentially delayed or missed vaccinations.

Geriatric history

Before starting

- Introduce yourself to the patient.
- Explain that you are going to ask him some questions to determine the nature of his problems, and ask for his consent to do this.
- Ensure that he is comfortable; if not, make sure that he is.
- Ask if you can take a collateral history from a caretaker.

The history

- Name, age, and past occupation if this information has not already been provided.

Presenting complaint

- Enquire about the patient's presenting complaint, if any. Use open questions and active listening.
- Explore any symptoms, e.g. onset, duration, previous episodes, pain, associated symptoms.
- Enquire about the effects that his symptoms are having on his everyday life.
- Elicit his ideas, concerns, and expectations.

Then aim to cover:

- Physical independence, e.g. describe a typical day.
- Functional assessment: can he stand up and walk, climb the stairs, get on and off the toilet, get in and out of the bathtub, dress, cook/clean/shop, and manage his finances and administration?
- Living arrangements: housing, heating, lighting, stairs, toileting, cooker and smoke alarm, slippery bathtubs, loose rugs, adaptive or home safety aids, e.g. grab bars in the bathroom, stair lift, raised toilet seat, shower stool, bedside commode.
- Carers and support services.
- Social interaction: family, friends, clubs, etc. If appropriate, ask *"Who will help you if you become ill? Who should make decisions for you if you become too ill to speak for yourself?"*
- Daily diet, including nausea, vomiting, and change in appetite or weight.
- Urinary and faecal incontinence.
- Mood (e.g. *"How are you keeping in your spirits?"*). Also ask about sleep and appetite.
- Memory and cognitive impairment.
- Dizziness/falls (see *Station 30: History of 'funny turns'*).
- Vision (corrective aids, accidents, difficulty reading, feeding, dressing, grooming, driving, and recognising pills or items).

Past medical history

- Current, past, and childhood illnesses. Ask about rheumatic fever and polio.
- Surgery.

Drug history

- Prescribed medication and *compliance*.
- Over-the-counter drugs.
- Smoking and alcohol use.
- Allergies.

Family history

- Parents, siblings, and children. Ask specifically about diabetes, Alzheimer's disease, and cancer.

After taking the history

- Ask the patient if there is anything that he might add that you have forgotten to ask about.
- Ask if he has any questions or concerns.
- Thank him.
- Indicate that you would like to examine the patient and order some investigations.
- Formulate a problem list and suggest treatment options.

Geriatric physical examination

Examining a patient in old age (>65 years old) is very similar to examining a patient at any other age. If asked to examine a patient in old age, important features to look out for or aspects to consider are:

Vital signs

Temperature, pulse, blood pressure (lying and standing), respiratory rate, height, weight.

General inspection

Nutritional status, posture, tremor, gait, aids

Skin

Pressure sores, senile keratoses, senile purpura, bruises, pre-malignant or malignant lesions.

Eyes, ears, nose and throat

Vision (including fundoscopy), hearing, mouth, throat.

Musculoskeletal system

Arthritis, muscle wasting, contractures, range of motion in different joints.

Cardiovascular system

Arrhythmias, added sounds, murmurs, carotid bruits, pedal oedema, absent peripheral pulses, gangrene.

Respiratory system

Chest expansion, basal crackles (may be difficult to hear because of basilar rales).

Abdomen

Organomegaly, bladder distension, abdominal aortic aneurysm, frequency and quality of abdominal sounds, rectal examination.

Breast and genitourinary

Malignancy.

Neurological examination

Tone, power, sensation, reflexes, gait, co-ordination.

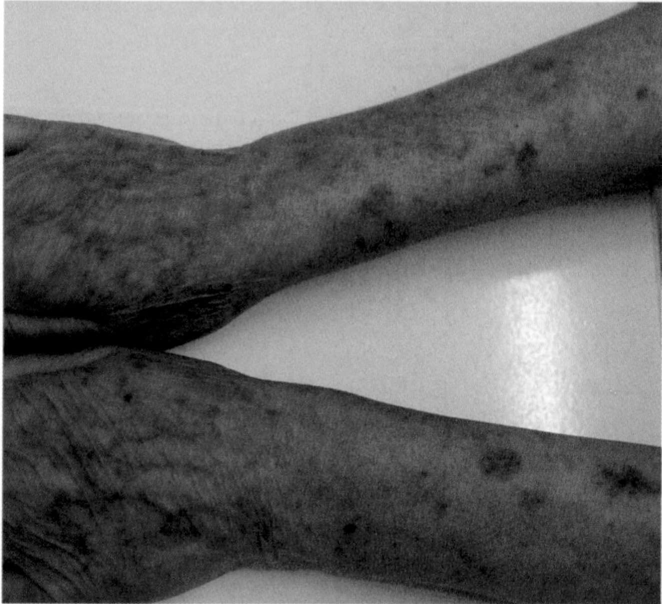

Figure 54. Senile purpura.

Obstetric history

Specifications: You may be asked to focus on only a certain aspect or certain aspects of the obstetric history.

Before starting

- Introduce yourself to the patient.
- Explain that you are going to ask her some questions to uncover the nature and background of her obstetric complaint, and ask for consent to do this.
- Ensure that she is comfortable.

The history

- Name, age, and occupation.

Presenting problem (presenting complaint)

Ask about the presenting problem (if any) in some detail, e.g. onset, duration, pain, bleeding, associated symptoms, previous occurrences.

History of the present pregnancy

- Determine the duration of gestation and calculate the expected due date (EDD).
  - Ask about the date of the patient's last menstrual period (LMP).
  - Ask if her periods had been regular prior to her LMP.
  - Ask if she had been on the oral contraceptive pill (OCP). If yes, determine when she stopped taking it and the number of periods she had before becoming pregnant.
  - Determine the duration of gestation and calculate the EDD. To calculate the EDD add 9 months and 7 days to the date of the LMP. Alternatively, add 1 year, subtract 3 months, and add 7 days.
- Ask about foetal movements and, if present, about any changes in their frequency.
- Take a detailed history of the pregnancy, enquiring about:

First trimester:

- date and method of pregnancy confirmation
- was the pregnancy planned or unplanned? If it was unplanned, is it desired?
- symptoms of pregnancy (e.g. sickness, indigestion, headaches, dizziness…)
- bleeding during pregnancy
- ultrasound scan (10–12/52)
- chorionic villus sampling (10–13/52)
- type of antenatal care (e.g. shared care, midwife-led care, domino scheme, consultant-led scheme)

Second trimester:

- amniocentesis (16–18/52)
- anomaly scan (18–20/52)
- quickening (16–18/52)

Third trimester:

- antenatal clinic findings – you *must* ask about blood pressure and proteinuria
- vaginal bleeding
- hospital admissions

History of previous pregnancies (past reproductive history)

Ask her if she has any children.

For each previous pregnancy, ask about:

The pregnancy, including:

- the date (year) of birth
- the duration of the pregnancy and any problems
- the mode of delivery and any problems
- the outcome

The child, including:

- the child's birth weight
- problems after birth
- the child's present condition

Do not forget to also ask about miscarriages, stillbirths, and terminations.

Gynaecological history

Take a focussed gynaecological history, and ask about the date and result of the last cervical smear test.

Past medical history

- Current, past, and childhood illnesses. Ask specifically about hypertension, epilepsy, diabetes and DVT.
- Surgery.
- Recent visits to the doctor.

Drug history

- Prescribed medication.
- Over-the-counter drugs.
- Folic acid supplements (should be taken from 3 months prior to conception to 3 months into pregnancy).
- Rhesus antibody injections (if required).
- Smoking.
- Alcohol use.
- Recreational drug use.
- Allergies.

Family history

- Parents, siblings, and children. Has anyone in the family ever had a similar problem?
- Is there a family history of hypertension, heart disease, or diabetes?
- *Is there a history of twins or triplets in your family or in your partner's family?*

Social history

- Support from the partner and/or family.
- Employment.
- Income and financial support.
- Housing.

After taking the history

- Ask the patient if there is anything she might add that you have forgotten to ask about.
- Thank the patient.
- If asked, summarise your findings and offer a differential diagnosis.

Conditions most likely to come up in an obstetric history station
Ectopic pregnancy • In about 1% of pregnancies the fertilised egg implants outside the uterine cavity, most often in the Fallopian tube, but also in the cervix, ovaries, and abdomen. Clinical presentation occurs at a mean of about 7 weeks after the LMP, with a range of 5–8 weeks. Symptoms principally involve lower abdominal pain which may be worse upon moving and straining, and vaginal and internal bleeding which can be life-threatening. The principal differential is from normal pregnancy and miscarriage.
Miscarriage • In about 15–20% of all recognised pregnancies, the pregnancy ends spontaneously at a stage when the embryo or foetus is incapable of surviving (before approximately 20–22 weeks of gestation, although most miscarriages occur prior to 13 weeks of gestation). The most common symptoms, which can range from very mild to severe, are cramping and vaginal bleeding with blood clots. The principal differential is from ectopic pregnancy.
Placenta praevia • In about 0.5% of pregnancies, usually during the second or third trimester, the placenta attaches to the uterine wall close to or covering the cervix. This classically leads to painless, bright red vaginal bleeding that increases in frequency and intensity over a period of weeks.
Placental abruption • In about 1% of pregnancies the placenta partially or completely separates from the uterus, depriving the baby of oxygen and nutrients and causing heavy bleeding in the mother. Placental abruption can begin at any time after 20 weeks of gestation, classically with variable amounts of vaginal bleeding, abdominal pain, back pain, uterine tenderness and contraction, and rapid and repetitive uterine contractions.
False labour
Normal pregnancy

Examination of the pregnant woman

Specifications: Most likely an anatomical model in lieu of a patient.

Before examining the patient

- Introduce yourself to the patient.
- Explain the examination and ensure consent.
- Indicate that you would weigh the patient, take her blood pressure (pre-eclampsia), dipstick her urine (pre-eclampsia, gestational diabetes) and ask her to empty her bladder.
- Position the patient so that she is lying supine (she can sit up if she finds lying supine uncomfortable).
- Ask her to expose her abdomen.
- Ensure that she is comfortable.

The examination

General inspection

Carry out a general inspection from the end of the couch.

Inspection of the abdomen

- Abdominal distension and symmetry. Is the umbilicus everted?
- Foetal movements (after 24 weeks).
- *Linea nigra* (brownish streak running vertically along the midline from the umbilicus to the pubis).
- *Striae gravidarum* (purplish stretch marks from the current pregnancy).
- *Striae albicans* (silvery stretch marks from previous pregnancies).
- Scars.

Palpation of the abdomen

- Enquire about pain before palpating the abdomen.
- Then, facing the mother, determine the:
  - size of the uterus
  - liquor volume (normal, polyhydramnios, oligohydramnios)
  - number of foetuses
  - size of the foetus(es)
  - lie
  - presenting part
- Turning to face the mother's feet, determine the:
  - engagement

Table 24. Some important obstetric definitions

Lie. The relationship of the long axis of the foetus to that of the uterus, described as longitudinal, transverse, or oblique.

Presenting part. The part of the foetus that is in relation with the pelvic inlet, e.g. cephalic/breech for a longitudinal lie or shoulder/arm for a transverse/oblique lie.

Engagement. During engagement, the presenting part descends into the pelvic inlet in readiness for labour. Engagement is usually described in fifths of head palpable above the pelvic inlet, although sometimes the presenting part may not be the head. Engagement usually occurs after 37 weeks of gestation, before which the foetus is said to be 'floating' or 'ballotable'.

Although not usually performed, indicate that you could also determine the position, station, and attitude of the foetus. Position refers to the relationship of a point of reference on the foetus to the quadranted pelvis; station (see *Figure 55*) refers to the depth of the presenting part in relation to the ischial spines (from −5 to +5); attitude refers to the degree of flexion of the foetus' body parts.

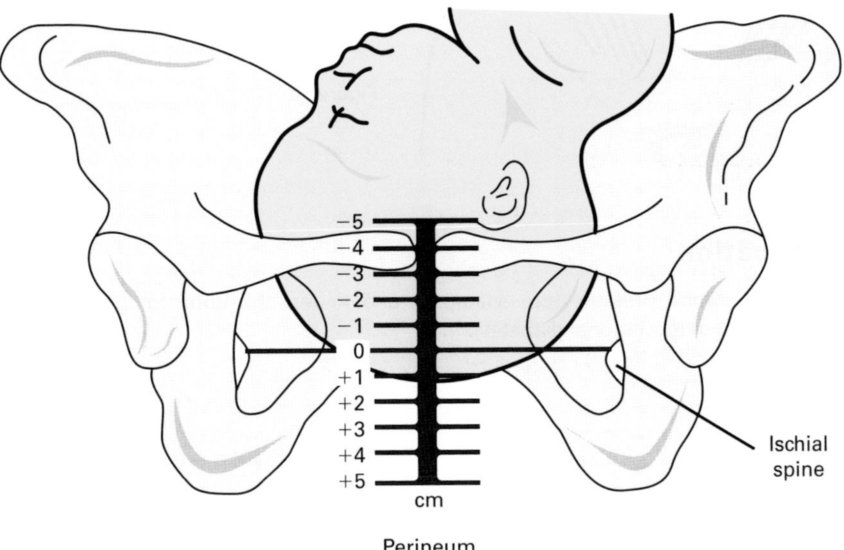

Figure 55. Measurement of station.

Symphyseal–fundal height (SFH)

Using a tape measure, measure from the mid-point of the symphysis pubis to the top of the uterus. From 20 to 38 weeks of gestation, the SFH in centimetres approximates to the number of weeks of gestation ± 2 (see *Figure 56*).

Auscultation

Listen to the foetal heart by placing a Pinard stethoscope over the foetus' anterior shoulder and estimate the heart rate (usually 110–160 bpm). Ensure that your hands are free from the abdomen.

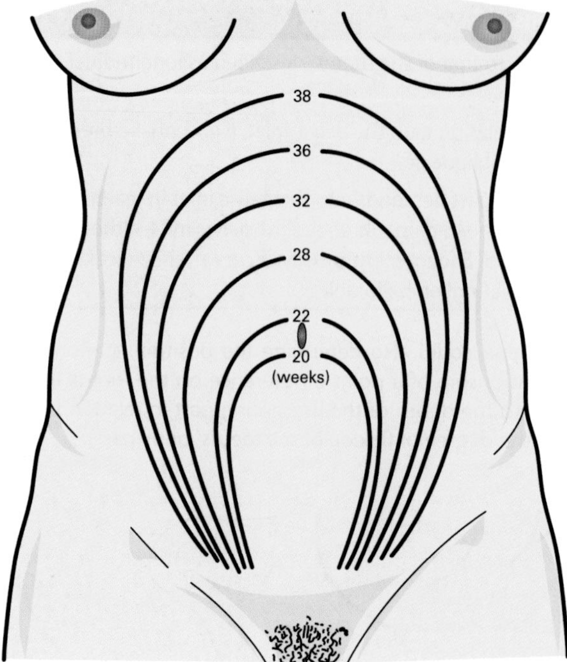

Figure 56. Expansion of the uterus during pregnancy.

After the examination

- Ask to record the blood pressure (pre-eclampsia) and to test the urine for protein (pre-eclampsia) and glucose (gestational diabetes).
- Cover the patient up.
- Thank the patient.
- Summarise your findings.

Gynaecological history

Specifications: You may be asked to circumscribe your questioning to certain aspects of the gynaecological history only.

Before starting

- Introduce yourself to the patient.
- Explain that you are going to ask her some questions to uncover the nature and background of her gynaecological complaint, and ask for her consent to do this.
- Ensure that she is comfortable.

The history

- Name, age, and occupation.

Presenting complaint and history of presenting complaint

- Ask about the presenting problems (if any) in some detail, e.g. onset, duration, pain, bleeding, associated symptoms, previous occurrences. Explore the patient's ideas, concerns and expectations. Then ask about:
  - age at menarche
  - regularity of the menses
  - dysmenorrhoea
  - date of LMP – did the LMP seem normal?
  - inter-menstrual (or post-menopausal) bleeding
  - post-coital bleeding
  - vaginal discharge – if there is a vaginal discharge, ask about its amount, colour, and smell. Is it causing the patient to itch?
  - date and result of the last cervical smear test
  - vaginal prolapse
  - urinary incontinence
  - coitus, present or past (*"Are you sexually active?"*)
  - dyspareunia
  - use of contraception

Past medical history

- Past gynaecological history.
- Past reproductive history: previous pregnancies in chronological order, including terminations and miscarriages.
- Past medical history:
  - current, past, and childhood illnesses
  - surgery
  - recent visits to the doctor

Drug history

- Prescribed medication, including, if appropriate oral contraceptives and HRT.
- Over-the-counter medication.
- Recreational drug use.
- Allergies.

Family history

- Ask about parents, siblings, children. Has anyone in the family had a similar problem? In the case of a suspected STD, don't forget to ask about the partner.

Social history

- Employment.
- Housing and home-help.
- Travel.
- Smoking.
- Alcohol use.

After taking the history

- Ask the patient if there is anything she might add that you have forgotten to ask about.
- Thank the patient.
- Summarise your findings and offer a differential diagnosis.

Conditions most likely to come up in a gynaecological history station

Menopause

- The permanent cessation of the primary functions of the ovaries, namely, the ripening and release of ova and the release of hormones that cause both the creation and the subsequent shedding of the uterine lining. It normally occurs gradually over a period of years during the late 40s or early 50s.
- Signs and symptoms may include irregular menses, hot flushes and night sweats, increased stress, mood changes, sleep disturbances, atrophy of genitourinary tissue, vaginal dryness, and breast tenderness.

Amenorrhoea

- The absence of a menstrual period in a pre-menopausal woman for a period of 3 months (or 9 months in women with a history of oligomenorrhoea). It is a sign with many causes including normal pregnancy, lactation, and oral contraceptives.
- Primary amenorrhoea (menstruation has not started by age 16 or age 14 if there is a lack of secondary sexual characteristics) is often related to chromosomal or developmental abnormalities.
- Secondary amenorrhoea (menstruation has started but then stops) is often related to disturbances in the hypothalamo–pituitary axis due to, for example, stress, excessive dieting or exercising, PCOS, or a prolactin-secreting pituitary tumour; hypothyroidism; certain drugs such as antipsychotics and corticosteroids; intrauterine scar formation; premature menopause.

Dysmenorrhoea

- Severe uterine pain possibly radiating to the back and thighs either preceding menstruation by several days or accompanying it. Associated symptoms might include menorrhagia, nausea and vomiting, diarrhoea, headache, dizziness, fainting, and fatigue.
- Secondary dysmenorrhoea is diagnosed in the presence of an underlying cause, commonly endometriosis or uterine fibroids.

Menorrhagia

- Abnormally heavy (>80 ml) and/or prolonged (>7 days) menstrual period at regular intervals possibly associated with dysmenorrhoea and signs and symptoms of anaemia. In many cases, no cause can be found. However, common causes include hormonal imbalance, pelvic inflammatory disease, endometriosis, uterine polyps or fibroids, adenomyosis, intrauterine device, coagulopathy, and certain drugs such as NSAIDs and anticoagulants.

Inter-menstrual bleeding

- Bleeding between periods may be associated with sexual intercourse or may occur spontaneously. Causes of spontaneous inter-menstrual bleeding include physiological hormone fluctuations, oral contraceptives, cervical smear test, certain drugs such as anticoagulants and corticosteroids, vaginitis, infection (e.g. chlamydia), cervicitis, cervical polyps, uterine polyps or fibroids, and adenomyosis. It is particular important to consider cervical cancer, endometrial adenocarcinoma, threatened miscarriage, and ectopic pregnancy.

Vaginal discharge (see *Station 72*)

Dyspareunia (see *Station 72*)

Gynaecological (bimanual) examination

Specifications: A pelvic model in lieu of a patient.

Before starting

- Introduce yourself to the patient.
- Explain the examination, reassuring the patient that, although it may feel uncomfortable, it should not cause any pain.
- Obtain consent.
- Ask for a chaperone.
- Confirm that the patient has emptied her bladder.
- Indicate that you would normally carry out an abdominal examination prior to a gynaecological examination.
- Once undressed, ask the patient to lie flat on the couch, bringing her heels to her buttocks and then letting her knees flop out.
- Ensure that she is comfortable, and cover her up with a drape.

The examination

Always tell the patient what you are about to do.

- Don a pair of non-sterile gloves and adjust the light source to ensure maximum visibility.
- Inspect the vulva, paying close attention to the pattern of hair distribution, the labia majora, and the clitoris. Note any redness, ulceration, masses, or prolapse.
- Palpate the labia majora for any masses.
- Try to palpate Bartholin's gland (the structure is not normally palpable).
- Lubricate the index and middle fingers of your gloved right hand.
- Use the thumb and index finger of your left hand to separate the labia minora.
- Insert the index and middle fingers of your right hand into the vagina at an angle of 45 degrees.
- Palpate the vaginal walls for any masses and for tenderness.
- Use your fingertips to palpate the cervix. Assess the cervix for size, shape, consistency, and mobility. Is the cervix tender? Is it open?
- Palpate the uterus: place the palmar surface of your left hand about 5 cm above the symphysis pubis and the internal fingers of your right hand behind the cervix and gently try to appose your fingers in an attempt to 'catch' the uterus. Assess the uterus for size, position, consistency, mobility, and tenderness. Can you feel any masses?

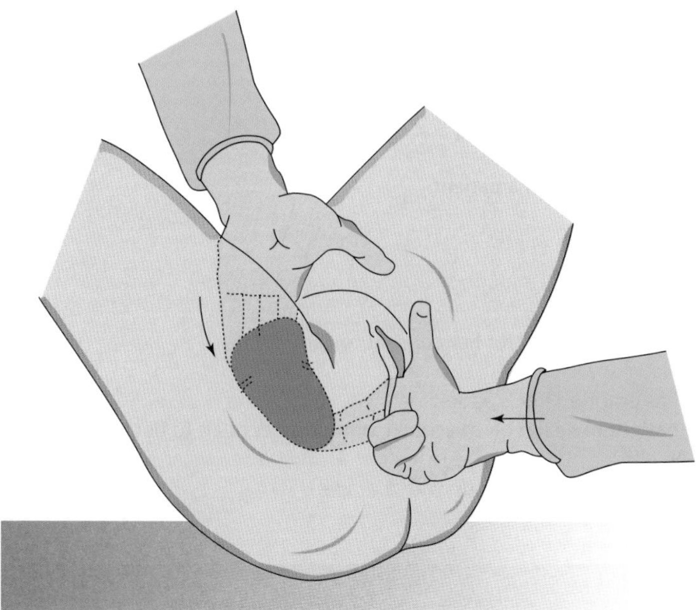

Figure 57. Technique for bimanual examination

- Palpate the right adnexae: place the palmar surface of your left hand in the right iliac fossa and the internal fingers of your right hand in the right fornix and gently try to appose your fingers in an attempt to 'catch' the ovary. Assess the ovary for any masses and for excitation tenderness (look at the patient's face).
- Use a similar technique for palpating the left adnexae.
- Once you have removed your internal fingers, inspect the glove for any blood or discharge.

After the examination

- Dispose of the gloves and wash your hands.
- Offer the patient a box of tissues and give her the opportunity to dress.
- Thank the patient.
- Ensure that she is comfortable.
- Indicate that you could also have carried out a speculum examination and taken a cervical smear (see *Station 69: Cervical smear test*).
- Summarise your findings and offer a differential diagnosis.

Conditions most likely to come up in gynaecological examination station
Uterine fibroids • Common and often multiple benign tumour of the smooth muscle (myometrium) of the uterus, typically found during the middle and later reproductive years. In most cases uterine fibroids are asymptomatic, but in some cases they can cause menorrhagia, dysmenorrhoea, inter-menstrual bleeding, dyspareunia, urinary frequency and urgency, and fertility problems.
Ovarian cyst • Functional fluid-filled sacs within or on the surface of an ovary. Ovarian cysts are very common, particularly in women of reproductive age, and are generally benign and asymptomatic. Symptoms can include pelvic pain, pain during urination, defecation, or sexual intercourse, urinary frequency, nausea and vomiting, abdominal fullness, breast tenderness, and menstrual irregularities.

Cervical smear test and liquid based cytology test

Specifications: An anatomical model in lieu of a patient.

Before starting

- Introduce yourself to the patient.
- Explain the procedure to her, and ask her for her consent to carry it out.
- Request a chaperone.
- Confirm that the patient has emptied her bladder.
- Once undressed, ask the patient to lie flat on the couch, bringing her heels to her buttocks and then letting her knees flop out.
- Ensure that she is comfortable, and cover her up with a drape.
- Gather the appropriate equipment.

The equipment

On a trolley, gather:

- non-sterile gloves
- Ayres spatula
- fixative spray (or 95% alcohol)
- bivalve speculum
- brush, if post-menopausal
- labelled slides (name, date of birth, hospital number)

The procedure

- Indicate that you would record the patient's name, date of birth, and hospital number on the slide.
- Adjust the light source to ensure maximum visibility.
- Don the pair of gloves.
- Inspect the vulva, paying close attention to the pattern of hair distribution, the labia majora, and the clitoris. Note any redness, ulceration, masses or prolapse.
- Warm the speculum's blades in your palm.
- Place a small amount of K-Y jelly on either side of the speculum near the tip.
- With your non-dominant hand, part the labia to ensure all hair and skin are out of the way.
- With your other hand, slowly but gently, insert the speculum with the screw facing sideways, rotating it into position (screw upwards) and then opening it.
- Place the back of your non-dominant hand against her pubic area and gently open the speculum to identify the cervix.
- Fix the speculum in the open position by tightening the screw.

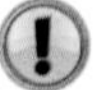

A smear should not be taken if there is any bleeding or vaginal discharge.

- Place the tip of the Ayres spatula in the external os and rotate the spatula by 360 degrees in either direction, all the while keeping it firmly applied to the cervix.
- Spread the material thus obtained evenly onto the labelled slides.
- Immediately spray fixative onto the slides.
- Carefully remove the speculum. Hold the speculum in the open position and completely unscrew it. Then remove the speculum slowly rotating it sideways and allowing it to close naturally as you withdraw it.

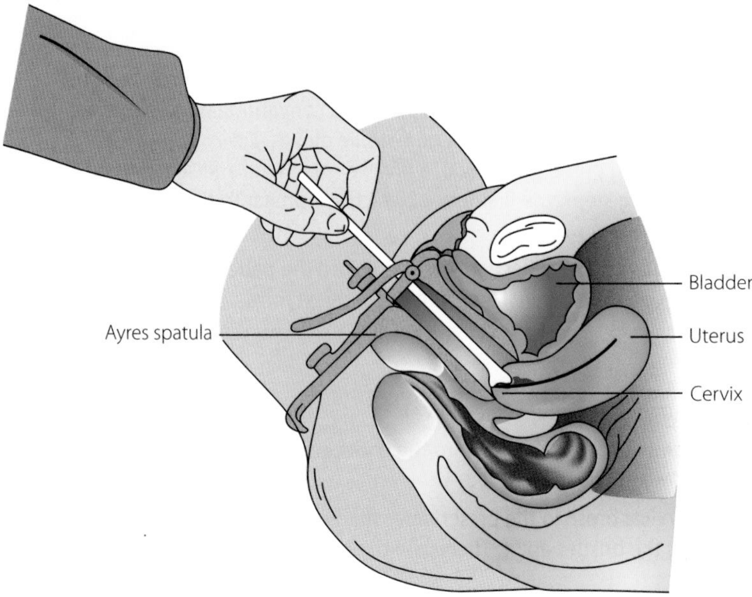

Figure 58. The cervical smear test.

After the procedure

- Dispose of the speculum and of the gloves.
- Offer the patient a box of tissues and give her the opportunity to dress.
- Meanwhile, complete an investigation form and send it off together with the labelled slide.
- Warn the patient about the possibility of spotting/bleeding after the test.
- Explain to her when and how she will receive the test results and the possible outcomes:
  - normal test – do nothing;
  - inadequate or unsatisfactory test – repeat the test;
  - borderline or mild dyskaryosis – repeat the test in 6 months;
  - moderate or severe dyskaryosis – refer for colposcopy
- Also explain when her next screening test is (the test is carried out 3-yearly if between 25 and 49 years of age, or 5 yearly if between 50 and 64 years of age).
- Ask her if she has any questions or concerns.
- Thank her.

Liquid based cytology test

Liquid based cytology (LBC) is a new method of preparing cervical samples for examination in the laboratory. It is currently being introduced and is soon to replace the conventional cervical smear test. If asked to perform an LBC test you must gather a pair of non-sterile gloves, a cervical examination brush (Cervex-Brush®), a vial containing preservative fluid, a bivalve speculum, and some K-Y jelly. Then you must carry out the following steps, the first four of which are similar to those outlined above:

- Check the expiry date on the sample collection vial and record the patient's name, date of birth and hospital number on both the vial and cytology request form.
- Adjust the light source.
- Don the pair of gloves.
- Warm, lubricate, and insert the speculum (see above).
- Insert the central bristles of the cervical brush into the endocervical canal and rotate it by 360 degrees in a clockwise direction five times.
- Immediately rinse the cervical brush in the preservative fluid by pushing it into the bottom of the vial ten times, forcing the bristles apart. Then swirl the brush vigorously to further release material.
- Inspect the cervical brush to ensure that it is free of material.
- Discard the brush.
- Carefully remove the speculum (see above).
- Tighten the cap on the vial and place it in a specimen bag, along with the request form.

Examiner's questions

Staging of cervical cancer

Stages are described in terms of the International Federation of Gynecology and Obstetrics (FIGO) system, which is based on clinical rather than surgical findings.

Stage 0	Carcinoma *in situ*. Tumour is present only in epithelium.
Stage I	Invasive cancer with tumour strictly confined to cervix.
Stage II	Invasive cancer with tumour extending beyond cervix or upper two-thirds of vagina, but not onto pelvic wall.
Stage III	Invasive cancer with tumour spreading to lower third of vagina or onto pelvic wall.
Stage IV	Invasive cancer with tumour spreading to other parts of the body.

NB: Various sub-stages are also described.

Breast history

Before starting

- Introduce yourself to the patient.
- Explain that you are going to ask her some questions to uncover the nature of her complaint, and ask for her consent to do this.
- Ensure that she comfortable; if not, ensure that she is.

The history

- Name, age, and occupation, if this information has not already been provided. Is the patient pregnant or lactating?

Presenting complaint and history of presenting complaint

- Use open questions to ask about the presenting complaint. Explore the patient's ideas, concerns and expectations.
- Ask specifically about pain, a lump in the breast, and nipple discharge.

For pain, determine:

- Site.
- Severity.
- Nature.
- Onset.
- Duration.
- Aggravating and alleviating factors.
- Associated signs and symptoms:
  - locally, e.g. lump, discharge, bleeding, skin changes, nipple retraction/inversion
  - systemically, e.g. tiredness, fever, night sweats, weight loss, chest or back pain
- Cyclicity.
- If the patient has had it before.
- Any other changes in the breast.

For a lump in the breast, determine:

- Site.
- Size.
- Onset.
- Duration.
- Cyclicity.
- Associated symptoms:
  - locally, e.g. pain, discharge, bleeding, skin changes, nipple retraction/inversion
  - systemically, e.g. tiredness, fever, night sweats, weight loss, chest or back pain
- If the patient has had it before.

For nipple discharge, determine:

- Amount.
- Colour.
- If it is unilateral or bilateral.
- If it is from one duct or several.
- If it is spontaneous.

- Associated symptoms:
  - locally, e.g. pain, lump, bleeding, skin changes, nipple retraction/inversion
  - systemically, e.g. tiredness, fever, night sweats, weight loss, chest or back pain
- If the patient has been breast-feeding.
- If the patient has had it before.

Past medical history

- Age at menarche and (if applicable) menopause.
- Regularity of menses and date and character of LMP.
- Does the patient have any children? How old are they? Did she breast-feed them?
- Current, past, and childhood illnesses.
- Surgery.
- Previous breast investigations.
- Recent visits to the doctor.

Drug history

- Prescribed medication, especially oral contraceptives and HRT. Note that certain drugs, e.g. antipsychotics, can cause hyperprolactinaemia and galactorrhoea.
- Over-the-counter medications.
- Recreational drug use.
- Allergies.

Family history

- Parents, siblings, and children. Ask specifically about breast problems and cancers.

Social history

- Smoking.
- Alcohol use.
- Employment, past and present.
- Housing.
- Hobbies.

Systems enquiry

(If appropriate.)

After taking the history

- Ask the patient if there is anything that she might add that you have forgotten to ask about.
- Thank the patient.
- Summarise your findings and offer a differential diagnosis.
- State that you would like to examine the patient and possibly order some investigations, e.g. mammogram, ultrasound scan, fine-needle aspiration cytology (FNAC), to confirm your diagnosis.

Conditions most likely to come up in a breast history station

Fibroadenoma

- Noncancerous mass of fibrous and glandular breast tissue most commonly affecting young women and presenting as a painless, smooth, solitary, firm ('rubbery hard'), and highly mobile lump.
- Fibroadenomas can be multiple and bilateral.

Fibrocystic disease

- Common condition characterised by noncancerous lumps in the breast which can sometimes cause persistent or cyclical discomfort that peaks just before the menses. The lumps are smooth with defined edges, usually free-moving, and most often found in the upper, outer section of the breast. They may be associated with a nipple discharge that is clear, white, or green in colour. The condition usually subsides after the menopause.

Mastitis

- Bacterial infection of the breast tissue, sometimes in connection with pregnancy or breastfeeding (puerperal mastitis). Signs and symptoms include fever, malaise, breast swelling and tenderness, skin redness (often in a wedge-shaped pattern), and pain or a burning sensation either persistently or only while breast-feeding. The most serious complication is breast abscess.

Breast abscess

- The lump and nearby area are red, hot, tender, and painful. Other signs and symptoms can include fever, purulent nipple discharge, and axillary lymphadenopathy. Principal complications are gangrene and septicaemia.

Mammary duct ectasia

- Refers to dilatation and inflammation of a milk duct. It is most common in women in their 40s and 50s and is often asymptomatic. However, some women may have nipple discharge and breast tenderness or inflammation in the area near the nipple.

Carcinoma

- Cancer originating from breast tissue, most commonly from the inner lining of milk ducts (ductal carcinoma) or the lobules (lobular carcinoma). Signs and symptoms include an irregular breast lump or thickening, a change in the size or shape of the breast, changes to the skin over the breast such as dimpling, inverted nipple, bloody nipple discharge, and lymphadenopathy.

Intraductal papilloma

- A benign proliferation of duct epithelial cells that may present as a small painful lump in the area of the nipple. It is the most common cause of a bloody nipple discharge in young women.

Breast examination

Specifications: In this station you may be asked to examine a patient wearing synthetic breasts. You may also be asked to take a brief history beforehand.

A full breast examination involves inspection, palpation of the breast tissue, palpation of the nipple, and palpation of the lymph nodes.

Before starting

- Introduce yourself to the patient.
- Explain the examination, and ask her for consent to carry it out.
- Request a chaperone.
- Ask her to undress from the waist up and hand her a drape or blanket to cover herself up with.
- Ask her to sit on the edge of the couch, and ensure that she is comfortable.

The examination

General inspection

- From a distance, observe the patient's general appearance (age, state of health, any obvious signs).

Inspection of the breasts

- Note the size, symmetry, contour, and colour of the breast; also note the pattern of venous drainage. In particular, look for the important signs of nipple inversion or retraction and *peau d'orange* (breast carcinoma). Is there a visible discharge? Are there any scars? Also remember to look under the breasts (ask the patient to lift up her breasts for you).
- Now ask the patient to put her hands atop her head and then to press them against her hips. Look for tethering and asymmetrical changes in the breast contour.

Palpation of the breasts

- Ask the patient to sit back on the couch, reclining at 45 degrees.
- Warm up your hands.
- Before palpating the breasts, ask if there is any breast or chest pain.
- Starting with the normal breast, palpate the breast tissue with the palmar surface of the middle three fingers, using an even rotary movement to compress the breast tissue gently towards the chest wall. If the breasts are large, use one hand to steady the breast on its lower border.
- Examine each breast following a circular, concentric trail (*Figure 59*). Alternatively, use the vertical strip or wedge palpation techniques.

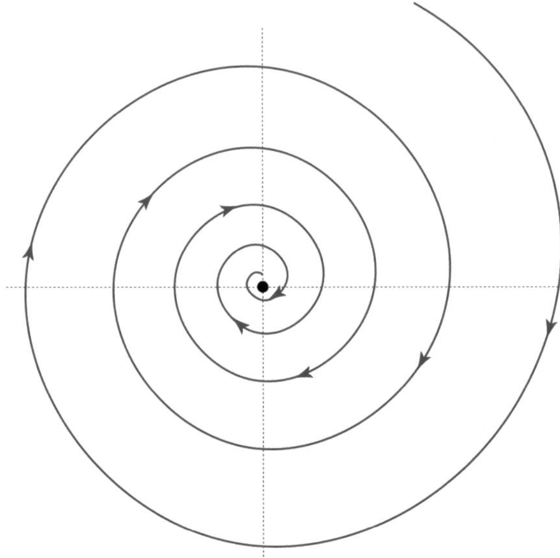

Figure 59. The circular palpation technique. Other palpation techniques include the vertical strip and wedge techniques.

- Ask the patient to put her hands atop her head and palpate the tail of Spence between thumb and forefinger.

Assess any lump for size, shape, consistency, mobility, surface, temperature, and tenderness.

Don't forget that there are two breasts that need examining, a common enough oversight in the artificial and anxiety-provoking OSCE situation.

Palpation of the nipple

- Hold the nipple between thumb and forefinger and gently compress it in an attempt to express a discharge (or ask the patient to do this). A discharge could signify normal lactation, galactorrhoea, duct ectasia, a carcinoma, or an intraductal papilloma. Any fluid expressed should be smeared for cytology and swabbed for microbiology.

Palpation of the lymph nodes

- Expose the right axilla by lifting and abducting the arm and supporting it at the wrist with your right hand.
- With your left hand, palpate the following lymph node groups (See *Figure 4* in *Station 8*):
  - apical
  - anterior
  - posterior
  - infraclavicular and supraclavicular
  - nodes of the medial aspect of the humerus
- Now expose the left axilla by lifting and abducting the left arm and supporting at the wrist with your left hand.
- With your right hand, palpate the lymph node groups, as listed above.

Assess any nodes for size, shape, consistency, mobility, and tenderness.

After the examination

Indicate that you could also:

- palpate the liver edge for an enlarged liver (liver metastases)
- palpate the spine for tenderness (spinal metastases)
- auscultate the lung bases (pleural effusions)

- Cover up the patient.
- Thank the patient.
- Ensure that she is comfortable.
- Summarise your findings and offer a differential diagnosis.
- Offer further investigations if appropriate, e.g. mammogram, USS, or FNAC

Conditions most likely to come up in a breast examination station	
• Fibroadenoma	• Mammary duct ectasia
• Fibrocystic disease	• Carcinoma
• Mastitis	• Interductal papilloma
• Breast abscess	• See *Station 70* for a description of these conditions

Sexual history

This is a history that students often find difficult because of the highly personal nature of the questions involved. The trick is to remain formal and professional throughout, yet to exert tact and, if the patient becomes uncomfortable, a measure of restraint. The OSCE may ask you to focus on either risk assessment or sexual function. If the latter, do not forget that sexual dysfunction often results from medical and psychiatric disorders and/or their treatments, e.g. antihypertensives, antidepressants.

Before starting

- Introduce yourself to the patient.
- Set the scene: *"I'd like to ask you a few questions about your sex life. I don't mean to embarrass you, and it's alright if you prefer not to answer some of my questions. May I begin?"*
- Reassure the patient about confidentiality.
- Explore the patient's ideas, concerns and expectations.

The history

Would you describe yourself as heterosexual, homosexual, or bisexual?

Who

- *"Who did you last have sex with, and when was this?"*
- *"Who else have you had sex with in the last three months?"*
- *"Were they regular or casual partners?"*
- *"Were they male or female (or both)?"*

How

- *"Did you have vaginal/oral/anal sex?"*
- *"If oral or anal sex, did you give it or receive it?"*
- *"Did you use protection on each occasion?"*
- If yes, *"did you have any problems with it?"*
- *"Have you ever been hurt or abused by your partner?"*

Where

- *"Have you had sex whilst abroad? Whom with?"*
- *"Where are your partners from?"*
- *"Is it possible that they have had sex whilst abroad?"*

Sexually transmitted diseases

Ask about:

- Any sores, discharge, itching, dysuria, and abdominal pain (in females). Explore any positive findings.
- History of sexually transmitted diseases (including HIV) in both the patient and his partner(s).
- In females, date and result of the last cervical smear test.

Sexual function

- *"Do you have any problems with, or concerns about, having sex?"* You may ask specifically about erectile dysfunction and ejaculatory dysfunction in males, and about hypoactive sexual desire, anorgasmia, vaginismus, and dyspareunia in females.
- Determine the onset, course, and duration of the problem. Is the problem primary or secondary?
- Determine the frequency and timing of the problem. Is the problem partial or situational? In situational erectile dysfunction, the patient is still able to have morning erections.
- Assess the effect that the problem is having on the patient's life.

Table 25. Types of sexual dysfunction (common types are in bold)

Type of sexual dysfunction	Male	Female
Sexual desire disorders	Hypoactive sexual desire Sexual aversion (rare)	**Hypoactive sexual desire** (F > M) Sexual aversion (rare)
Sexual arousal disorders	**Erectile dysfunction***	Failure of genital response
Sexual pain disorders	Dyspareunia	Dyspareunia (F > M) Vaginismus§
Orgasm disorders	Ejaculatory impotence **Premature ejaculation****	**Anorgasmia** (F > M)

*Erectile dysfunction or impotence is more common in elderly males.

**Premature ejaculation is more common in young males engaging in their first sexual relationships.

§Vaginismus describes involuntary vaginal contractions in response to attempts at penetration.

Past medical history

- History of sexually transmitted diseases.
- History of sexual problems.
- Menstrual history: regularity of menses and date and character of LMP.
- Medical conditions and previous hospital admissions.

Drug history

Social history

After taking the history

- Ask if there is anything that the patient would like to add which you may have forgotten to ask about.
- Thank the patient.
- Summarise your findings and offer a further course of action, e.g. physical examination, microbiological testing, contact tracing.

Conditions most likely to come up in a sexual history station

Candidiasis

- Common fungal infection involving any of the *Candida* species. Infection of the vagina or vulva is often asymptomatic but may cause severe itching, burning, soreness, irritation, and a whitish or whitish-grey 'cottage cheese' discharge.
- In men, there may be red and itchy or painful sores on the penile head or foreskin. Candidiasis is not classified as an STD.

Bacterial vaginosis (BV)

- Common bacterial infection involving, amongst others, *Gardnerella vaginalis*. Although BV is not classified as an STD, it is more common in women who are sexually active and increases their susceptibility to STDs. It may be asymptomatic or there may be a thin, homogeneous, off-white, and malodorous vaginal discharge, usually in the absence of redness, itchiness, or pain.

Chlamydia

- One of the most common STDs involving the bacterium *Chlamydia trachomatis*. In women it may be asymptomatic or it might present with a yellow and odourless mucopurulent cervical discharge, dysuria, and frequency.
- In men, it is usually symptomatic, presenting with a white penile discharge with or without dysuria.
- Major complications are pelvic inflammatory disease in women, epididymitis in men, and Reiter's syndrome in both.

Gonorrhoea

- A common STD caused by *Neisseria gonorrhoeae*. In women it may be asymptomatic or it might present with a greenish–yellow malodorous vaginal discharge, dysuria, and frequency.
- In men, it presents with a yellow–white penile discharge and dysuria. Symptoms typically occur 4–6 days after being infected.
- Major complications are pelvic inflammatory disease in women and epididymitis in men, or systemic spread to affect the joints and heart valves.

Trichomoniasis

- STD caused by the protozoan parasite *Trichomonas vaginalis*. Typically, only women experience symptoms but even they may be asymptomatic. Symptoms include copious amounts of a frothy, foul-smelling greenish–yellow mucopurulent discharge, itchiness, dysuria, and frequency. Discomfort may Increase during intercourse and upon urination. Symptoms typically occur 5–28 days after being infected.

Syphilis

- STD caused by the bacteria *Treponema pallidum*. The disease can also be transmitted from mother to foetus, resulting in congenital syphilis. The signs and symptoms depend on which of the four stages it presents in:
  - primary stage presents at an average of 21 days after initial exposure, typically with a single chancre or
  - secondary stage presents with a diffuse rash and other symptoms
  - latent stage with little to no symptoms
  - tertiary stage with gummas, neurological, and cardiac symptoms.

Genital herpes

- Genital infection by herpes simplex virus (HSV) that may lead to clusters of inflamed papules and vesicles on the outer surface of the genitals or on surrounding skin. These usually appear 4–7 days after sexual exposure to HSV. Other common symptoms include pain, itching, discharge, fever, and myalgia. After 2–3 weeks, the lesions progress into ulcers and then crust and heal.

Genital warts

- Highly contagious STD caused by some sub-types of human papillomavirus (HPV), and spread through direct skin-to-skin contact during oral, genital, or anal sex. Approximately 70% of those who have sexual contact with a partner with an active infection develop genital warts, and while less than 1% of those become symptomatic, those infected can still transmit the virus.

Sexual dysfunction

- Sexual dysfunction can occur at any stage of sexual intercourse: initiation, arousal, penetration, and orgasm (see *Table 25*). It can result from organic causes (such as diabetes, angina, prostate surgery, antihypertensives, antidepressants, antipsychotics) or from psychological causes (such as depression, anxiety, sexual inexperience, traumatic sexual experience, relationship difficulties, stress), or from a combination of either.
- In secondary dysfunction there is a history of normal function, but in primary dysfunction such a history is lacking. The epidemiology of sexual dysfunction is difficult to establish, but erectile dysfunction and premature ejaculation are common in males, and anorgasmia and hypoactive sexual desire are common in females.

HIV risk assessment

Before starting

- Introduce yourself to the patient.
- Explain that you are going to ask him some questions to determine his risk of having contracted HIV, and ask him for his consent to do this.
- Remember to be especially sensitive, tactful, and empathetic.

The risk assessment

- Explore the patient's reason for attendance.

Sexual behaviour

Establish:

- Whether the patient has sex with men, women, or both.
- Whether he has had unprotected anal, vaginal, or oral sex. If so, when, where, how often, and with how many different partners? Receptive anal intercourse is especially high risk.
- Whether he has recently contracted any sexually transmitted diseases.
- The HIV status and sexual practices of the patient's partners.

Illicit drug use

Establish:

- Whether the patient has been injecting himself. If so, has he been sharing needles?
- Whether any of his partners inject themselves.

Blood products and transfusions

Establish:

- Whether the patient is a haemophiliac.
- Whether he has received blood products or transfusions prior to about 1985.

Occupational risk

- Ask about the patient's occupation to determine if he poses an occupational risk.

After the risk assessment

- Ask the patient if there is anything that he might add that you have forgotten to ask about.
- Give him feedback on his HIV risk and, if appropriate, indicate a further course of action, e.g. an HIV test.
- Address his concerns.
- Thank him.

Condom explanation

Male and female condoms are barrier methods of contraception and prevent sperm from reaching the egg. They are very effective at preventing sexually transmitted infections but less effective than methods such as the pill in preventing pregnancy.

There are many different types of male condoms available on the market. These include plain-end or teat-end, shaped/ribbed or straight-sided, and lubricated (e.g. with inert silicone or nonoxynol-9 spermicide) condoms. Femidom is the only female condom available in the UK.

Spermicidal condoms are no longer recommended as evidence suggests that nanoxynol-9 may increase the risk of HIV and other sexually transmitted infections such as chlamydia and gonorrhoea.

Before starting

- Introduce yourself to the patient.
- Establish how much he already knows about using condoms. If correctly used, the male condom is 98% effective, and the female condom is 95% effective. Condoms also protect against STDs.

The equipment

- Two condoms.
- A model of a penis.
- An information booklet on condom use.

Explain the use of a condom

Explain that condom use should be discussed with the partner(s) and that the condom should be put on before any genital contact has taken place.

Explain/demonstrate to:

- check for the British Kite mark (*Figure 60*) or equivalent symbol, a guarantee of quality
- check the expiry date
- carefully tear open the pack and remove the condom – do not use teeth or sharp nails
- position the condom on the tip of the erect penis
- squeeze out the air from the tip of the condom and gently roll it out to the base of the penis
- hold the condom at the base of the penis during penetration
- after intercourse, remove the condom ensuring that semen is not spilt
- dispose of the condom in the bin – condoms must never be re-used

Ask the patient to repeat the procedure.

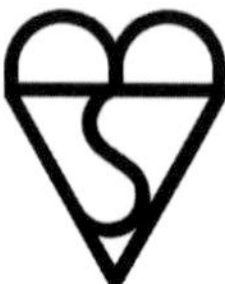

Figure 60. British kite mark.

Explain that condoms can occasionally tear and that, in this event, the patient and his partner should consult a GP or family planning clinic.

Principal side-effects are due to latex allergy and spermicide sensitivity.

Principal contraindications are oil-based lubricants such as Vaseline, hormonal vaginal creams, and antifungal preparations (Canesten is safe to use).

After the explanation

- Ask if the patient has any questions or concerns. (He may ask you about other methods of contraception.)
- Tell him to return should he have any further questions.
- Give him an information booklet on condom use.

Combined oral contraceptive pill (COCP) explanation

Before starting

- Introduce yourself to the patient.
- Ask for her name and age.
- Confirm the reason for her attendance.
- Has she considered other methods of contraception?

Explaining the COCP – items to cover

Efficacy

99.9% if used correctly, 97% in practice.

It is important to emphasise that the pill does not protect against STDs.

Principal benefits

- More regular periods, less blood loss, fewer period pains.
- Decreased risk of ovarian cancer and endometrial cancer.
- Acne often improves.

Principal risks

- Increased risk of deep vein thrombosis and pulmonary embolism.
- Increased risk of myocardial infarction.
- Increased risk of breast cancer and adenoma of the cervix.

Principal adverse effects

- Headache.
- Nausea.
- Dizziness.
- Hypertension.
- Breast tenderness.
- Weight gain.
- Depression.

Principal contraindications

Absolute

- Thrombophlebitis, thromboembolitic disorder, or history of thromboembolism.
- Stroke.
- Ischaemic heart disease.
- Liver disease.
- Kidney disease.
- History of breast cancer or other oestrogen-dependent cancers of the reproductive organs.
- Pregnancy.

Relative

- Uncontrolled hypertension.
- Migraine.
- Smoking (> 15 cigarettes a day and over the age of 35).
- Abnormal vaginal bleeding.
- Sickle cell disease.
- Breast-feeding.
- Family history of hyperlipidaemia, heart disease, or kidney disease.

Remember to take a quick drug history, as many common drugs such as ampicillin or carbamazepine can alter the effectiveness of the pill.

How to take the pills

- Start taking the pill on the first Sunday after periods begin.
- Take one pill a day at the same time every day for either 21 or 28 days, depending on the number of pills in the pack.
- After finishing the 28-day pack, start another one immediately (the last seven pills in the 28-day pack are 'dummy pills').
- After finishing the 21-day pack, stop taking the pill for 7 days and then start another pack.
- Use barrier contraception during the first month on the pill.
- If you develop vomiting or diarrhoea, use barrier contraception until your next period.

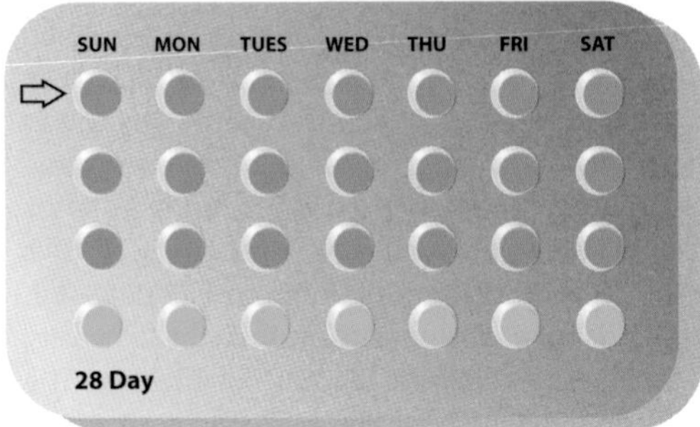

Figure 61. A 28-day pack.

What if pills are missed

If one pill is missed:

- take a pill as soon as you can remember to do so
- take the next pill at the regular time
- use barrier contraception for 7 days

If two pills are missed:

- take two pills a day for 2 days
- use barrier contraception for 7 days

If three pills are missed:

- stop taking the pill and start on another pack in 7 days' time

Before finishing

- Summarise and check understanding.
- Hand out a leaflet on the COCP.
- Tell the patient to report any severe or unexpected symptoms.

Examiner's questions

Other forms of contraception

Combined hormonal contraceptives are also available as a skin patch, worn for 3 out of every 4 weeks.

Low-dose progestogen-only contraceptives such as the traditional progestogen-only pill (POP, 'mini-pill'), subdermal implants (e.g. Norplant), and intrauterine systems (e.g. Mirena) inconsistently inhibit ovulation but thicken the cervical mucus and reduce sperm penetration, and also make the endometrium unsuitable for implantation. Intermediate-dose progestogen-only contraceptives such as the Cerazette pill are much more reliable at inhibiting ovulation, and high-dose progestogen-only contraceptives such as the injectable Depo-Provera inhibit ovulation completely (in the case of Depo-Provera, for up to 3 months).

The POP is taken continuously without any breaks. Whereas the COCP can be taken within a window of 12 hours, the mini-pill has a much shorter window of 3 hours. Thus, whilst the efficacy of the mini-pill is similar to that of the COCP, it is more dependent on user compliance. The POP is not affected by broad-spectrum antibiotics, and can often be used when the COCP is contraindicated, e.g. in smokers above the age of 35. It is contraindicated in cardiovascular disease, liver disease, breast cancer, ovarian cysts, and migraine. Side-effects, if any, are generally mild and transient. There is a small increased risk of ectopic pregnancy and breast cancer. Unlike the COCP, the POP does not regulate menstruation and can lead to either irregular menstruation or amenorrhoea.

Emergency post-coital contraception comes either in the form of an intrauterine device (IUD) or an emergency contraceptive pill (ECP, 'morning-after pill') that, in contrast to medical abortion methods, act before implantation, either by postponing ovulation or by preventing implantation. The Levonelle brand contains levonorgestrel which is a progestogen hormone, and is licensed for use up to 72 hours after intercourse. There is an approximate 80% reduction in the risk of pregnancy, to about 1–2% (this compares to virtually 0% for the IUD). Generally speaking, the advantages of using the ECP outweigh any theoretical or proven risks, and harm to a foetus that has already implanted is thought to be very unlikely. Side-effects include nausea, vomiting, abdominal pain, fatigue, headache, and dizziness. The ECP should not be confused with the 'abortion pill' (high dose mifepristone, RU 486).

Pessaries and suppositories explanation

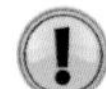 *Read in conjunction with* Station 110: Explaining skills.

Like tablets, pessaries and suppositories are medication. Suppositories are for rectal use, common examples being pain-killers and steroids, whereas pessaries are for vaginal use, common examples being antibiotics and progesterone.

They are used if oral drugs cannot be given, for example, in the post-operative period or if the patient is vomiting, and if the site of action of the drug is the rectum or vagina, or near enough, for example, the colon or cervix.

In this station you may be asked to explain the use of a pessary and/or a suppository to a patient. Both scenarios have been described here.

Before starting

- Introduce yourself to the patient.
- Confirm her/his reason for attendance.
- Ask her/him if she/he has ever used a pessary or suppository before.

The explanation: items to cover

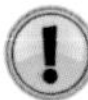 *Be sensitive to the psychological and sociocultural issues involved in placing a finger into the vagina or rectum, and be sympathetic and understanding.*

Pessaries

- Pessaries are bullet-shaped medicines designed for easy insertion into the vagina using your fingers or an applicator. Your body temperature will slowly dissolve the pessary and release the medicine into your vagina.
- Wash and dry your hands.
- Remove the pessary and applicator (if supplied) from its foil or wrapper.
- If an applicator is supplied, push the pessary into the hole at its end.
- Lie down with your knees bent and legs apart.
- Carefully push the pessary high up into your vagina, pointed end first, using either your fingers or the applicator.
- If using an applicator, push the plunger to release the pessary and then remove the applicator.
- Wash your hands afterwards.
- The pessary may leak from your vagina, so it may be best to insert it before bedtime and to use a sanitary towel to avoid staining of the clothes.
- If you miss a dose, insert the pessary as soon as you remember, and then carry on as normal.
- Check the expiry date before using your pessary.
- Store in a cool, dry place and out of children's reach.
- Continue using your pessaries until the course is completed, even if this means inserting them during your monthly period.

Suppositories

- Suppositories are bullet-shaped medicines designed for easy insertion into the lower bowel (rectum) using your fingers. Your body temperature will slowly dissolve the suppository and release the medicine across your rectum and into the bloodstream.
- Empty your bowels if necessary.
- Wash and dry your hands.
- Remove the suppository from its foil or wrapper.
- Lie down on your side with one leg bent and the other straight.
- Carefully push the suppository 2–3 cm up your bottom, pointed end first, using your finger. Some people may prefer to wear a glove, but this is not necessary.
- Close your legs and lie still for a few minutes.
- Wash your hands afterwards.
- If you open your bowels within 2 hours after inserting the suppository, you need to insert another.
- The suppository may leak from your rectum, so it may be best to insert it before bedtime and (if female) to use a sanitary towel to avoid staining of the clothes.
- If you miss a dose, insert the suppository as soon as you remember, and then carry on as normal.
- Check the expiry date before using your suppository.
- Store in a cool, dark place and out of children's reach.
- Continue using your suppositories until the course is completed.

After the explanation

- Summarise and check the patient's understanding.
- Ask if she/he has any questions or concerns.
- Offer her/him a leaflet.

Rheumatological history

Before starting

- Introduce yourself to the patient.
- Explain that you are going to ask him some questions to uncover the nature of his complaint, and ask him for his consent to do this.
- Ensure that he is comfortable.

The history

Name, age, and occupation, if this information has not already been supplied.

Presenting complaint

Ask the patient about the nature of his complaint. Use open questions.

Pain

Ask specifically about any pain and determine its site (i.e. which joints are affected), severity, and timing.

Stiffness

Ask specifically about stiffness and determine its site, severity and timing.

History of presenting complaint

Ask about:

- The onset and any provoking factors such as trauma or infection.
- The progression.
- Any associated features:
  - local: swelling or inflammation, deformity, cracking, clicking, locking, loss of movement
  - systemic: skin problems, eye problems, GI disturbances, urethral discharge
  - general: fever, night sweats, weight loss
- Any aggravating or relieving factors such as activity, rest, NSAIDs, steroids

Social history

Ask about:

- Difficulty in completing everyday tasks and the effect that this is having on his life. If need be, you can get him to describe a typical day: getting out of bed, toileting, dressing, etc. What did he used to do that he can no longer do?
- Housing and home-help.
- Mood. Screen for the core features of depression: low mood, fatiguability, and loss of interest.
- Recent travel.

Past medical history

- Current, past, and childhood illnesses.
- Surgery.
- Recent visits to the doctor.

Drug history

- Prescribed medication, e.g. NSAIDs, steroids, immunosuppressants.
- Over-the-counter medications.
- Allergies.
- Smoking, alcohol use, and recreational drug use.

Family history

- Parents, siblings, children. Has anyone in the family ever had similar problems?

After taking the history

- Ask the patient if there is anything he might add that you have forgotten to ask about.
- Thank the patient.

Conditions most likely to come up in rheumatological history station

Rheumatoid arthritis:

- chronic, systemic inflammatory disorder that may affect many tissues and organs, but principally the synovial joints, leading to destruction of articular cartilage and ankylosis of the joints
- women are three times more commonly affected than men
- onset is often at age 40–50, but can be at any age
- affects multiple joints, often in a symmetrical fashion, and most commonly the small joints of the hands, feet, and cervical spine
- affected joints are swollen, warm, painful, and stiff, particularly early in the morning, on waking, or following prolonged activity
- in time, there is decreased range of movement and deformity, e.g. ulnar deviation, boutonnière deformity, swan neck deformity, Z-thumb

Osteoarthritis:

- 'wear and tear' arthritis
- commonly affects the hands, feet, spine, and the large weight-bearing joints
- affected joints are painful, tender, and stiff, with symptoms worsening throughout the day and after exercise
- there may be hard bony enlargements called Heberden's nodes on the distal interphalangeal joints and Bouchard's nodes on the proximal interphalangeal joints
- there may be crepitus upon movement, restricted range of movement, joint mal-alignment, and effusions

Psoriatic arthritis:

- systemic inflammatory disorder associated with psoriasis
- asymmetrical or relatively asymmetrical arthritis most commonly affecting the distal joints in the hands and feet
- symptoms of inflammation, pain, and stiffness typically wax and wane
- there may be swelling of an entire finger or toe (dactylitis) as well as fingernail and toenail involvement

Gout:

- caused by elevated levels of urate in the blood
- more common in men
- presents as recurrent attacks of acute inflammatory arthritis
- commonly (but not exclusively) affects the metatarsal–phalangeal joint at the base of the big toe
- the joint is red, tender, hot, and swollen
- may be associated with hard, painless deposits of uric acid called tophi
- pseudogout can be difficult to distinguish from gout; it involves calcium pyrophosphate dihydrate rather than urate deposition, and it normally affects the knee and larger joints rather than the foot

Ankylosing spondylitis:

- chronic, inflammatory disorder principally affecting the axial skeleton and sacroiliac joints and potentially leading to fusion of the spine ('bamboo spine') and to damage of the spinal cord, roots, and nerves
- there is a strong genetic component
- it is more common and tends to be more severe in males
- commonly presents at ages 20–40
- morning stiffness is characteristic, and pain improves with physical activity
- may be associated with systemic features such as fever and weight loss and extra-articular manifestations such as uveitis

Septic arthritis:

- results from direct invasion of one or several joint spaces by various microorganisms, with the knee being the joint that is most commonly affected
- acute onset of joint pain with possible systemic symptoms and possible history of underlying joint disease or trauma or unprotected sexual intercourse or intravenous drug abuse
- the joint itself is red, tender, hot, and swollen, and there is often an effusion
- septic arthritis is a medical emergency

Polymyositis and dermatomyositis:

- polymyositis is an inflammatory myopathy related to dermatomyositis
- it commonly presents in early adulthood with bilateral and progressive proximal muscle weakness
- the muscles may be painful and tender and there may be systemic symptoms such as fatigue and fever
- in dermatomyositis there is also a skin rash
- the cause or causes of polymyositis and dermatomyositis is unknown

Polymyalgia rheumatica: • muscle pain and stiffness in the neck, shoulders, and hips, especially in the morning or after inactivity • the disorder may develop either rapidly or gradually • systemic symptoms may include fatigue, fever, and anorexia • there is an association with temporal arteritis • usually affects older adults, more commonly females • the cause of polymyalgia rheumatica is unknown • prognosis is good, especially with corticosteroid treatment
Tendon rupture
Complications of steroid treatment

The GALS screening examination

GALS: 'Gait, arms, legs, and spine'. Remember that GALS is a screening test and that a detailed examination should therefore not be required.

Before starting

- Introduce yourself to the patient.
- Explain the examination and ask for his consent to carry it out.
- Ask him to undress to his undergarments.
- Ensure that he is comfortable.

The GALS screening examination

Brief history

- Name, age, and occupation, if this information has not already been supplied.
- *"Do you have any pain or stiffness in your muscles, back, or joints?"*
- *"Do you have any difficulty in climbing stairs?"*
- *"Do you have any difficulty washing or dressing?"*

The examination

General inspection

Inspect the patient standing. Note any obvious scars, swellings, deformities, and/or unusual posturing.

Spine

Look

- From the front.
- From behind, looking in particular for list, scoliosis and lumbar lordosis.
- From the side, looking in particular for kyphos, kyphosis and fixed flexion deformity.

Feel

- Press on each vertebral body in turn, trying to elicit tenderness.

Move

- Ask the patient to bend forwards and touch his toes. Look for lumbar lordosis and for scoliosis, which should become more pronounced.

Ask him to sit down on the couch.

- Lateral flexion of the neck. Ask him to put his ear on his shoulder and then do the same on the other side.
- Flexion and extension of the neck. Ask him to put his chin on his chest and then look up towards the ceiling.
- Spinal rotation. Ask him to turn his upper body to either side.

Demonstrate each of these movements to the patient. In particular, look for restricted range of movement and pain on movement.

Arms

Look

- Skin: rashes, nodules, nail signs
- Muscles: wasting, fasciculation
- Joints: swelling, asymmetry, deformity

Do not forget to inspect both surfaces of the hands.

Feel

- Skin: temperature
- Muscles: general muscle bulk
- Joints: tenderness and warmth; squeeze each hand at the level of the carpal and metacarpal joints, and try to localise any tenderness by squeezing each individual joint in turn

Move

- Hands: ask the patient to squeeze your finger (grip strength); then ask him to make a pinch and attempt to 'break' his pinch (precision pinch)
- Wrists: ask him to put his hands in the prayer position and then in the reverse prayer position
- Elbows: ask him to bring up his forearms as if he were lifting weights and then to straighten out his arms alongside his body
- Shoulders: ask him to raise his arms above his head (abduction) and to then to put his hands behind his head (internal rotation); coming from below, ask him to touch his back between the shoulder blades (external rotation).

Demonstrate these movements to the patient. Look for restricted range of movement and pain on movement.

Legs

Now ask the patient to lie on the couch.

Look

- Skin: rashes, nodules, callosities on the soles of the feet
- Muscles: wasting, fasciculation
- Joints: swelling, asymmetry, deformity

Feel

- Skin: temperature
- Joints: tenderness, warmth, and swelling; palpate each knee along the joint margin; squeeze each foot, and try to localise any tenderness by squeezing each individual joint in turn

Move

- Ask the patient to bring his heels to his bottom.
- Hold the knee and hip at 90 degrees of flexion and internally and externally rotate the hip. Keep an eye on the patient's face as you do this and ensure that you do not cause the patient unnecessary pain.
- Next, place one hand on the knee joint and extend it, feeling for any crepitus as you do so.
- Repeat on the other side.

Gait

Ask the patient to walk, observing:

- general features: rhythm, speed, stride length, limp
- the phases of gait: heel-strike, stance, push-off, and swing
- arm swing
- turning
- transfer ability: sitting and standing from a chair (note that you should already have had a chance to observe this)

After the examination

- Thank the patient.
- Offer to help the patient dress.
- Ensure that he is comfortable.
- Summarise your findings.
- If appropriate, indicate that you would perform a more detailed physical examination.

Hand and wrist examination

Before starting

- Introduce yourself to the patient.
- Explain the examination and ask for his consent to carry it out.
- Ask him to expose his arms.
- Ensure that he is comfortable.

The examination

Look

First inspect the dorsum and then the palmar surfaces of the hands.

- Skin: colour, rheumatoid nodules, scars, nail changes.
- Joints: swelling, Heberden's nodes, Bouchard's nodes.
- Shape and position: normal resting position of the hand, ulnar deviation, boutonnière and swan neck deformity of the fingers, mallet finger, finger droop, Z-deformity of the thumb, muscle wasting, Dupuytren's contracture.
- Elbows: psoriatic plaques, gouty tophi, rheumatoid nodules.

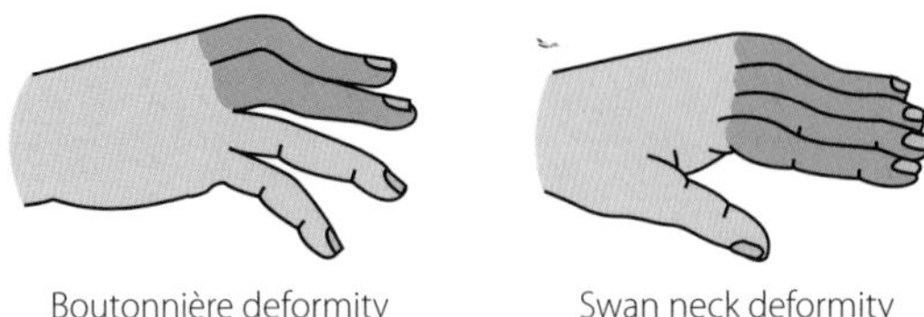

Figure 62. The arthritic hand. Boutonnière and swan neck deformity of the fingers.

Feel

Ask if the hands are painful.

- Skin: temperature.
- Finger and wrist joints: swelling, synovial thickening, tenderness.
- Anatomical snuff box (fractured scaphoid).
- Tip of the radial styloid (de Quervain's disease) and head of the ulna (extensor carpi ulnaris tendinitis).

Move

Test active and passive movements, looking for limitation in the normal range of movement. Ask the patient to report any pain.

Wrist

- Flexion and extension.
- Ulnar and radial deviation.
- Pronation and supination.

Thumb

- Extension. *"Stick your thumb out to the side."*
- Abduction. *"Point your thumb up to the ceiling."*
- Adduction. *"Collect your thumb in your palm."*
- Opposition. *"Appose the tip of your thumb to the tip of your little finger."*

Fingers

Each finger should be fully extended and flexed. Look at the movements of the metacarpophalangeal and interphalangeal joints. Test the grip strength by asking the patient to make a fist and try to squeeze your fingers. Try to open the fist. Test the pincer strength by trying to break the pinch between his thumb and first finger.

Special tests

- Carpal tunnel tests:
  - try to elicit Tinnel's sign by extending the hand and tapping on the median nerve in the carpal tunnel
  - try to elicit Phalen's sign by holding the hand in forced flexion for 30–60 seconds

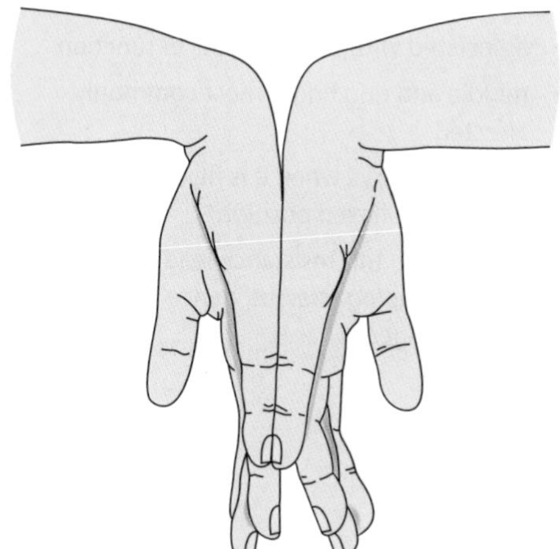

Figure 63. An alternative and quicker method for eliciting Phalen's sign.

- *Flexor profundus*: hold a finger extended at the proximal interphalangeal joint and ask the patient to flex the distal interphalangeal joint of that same finger.
- *Flexor superficialis*: ask the patient to flex a finger whilst holding all the other fingers on the same hand extended.
- Assess function by asking the patient to make use of an everyday object such as a pen or cup.

After the examination

- State that you would also like to examine the vascular and neurological systems of the upper limb.
- If appropriate, indicate that you would order some tests, e.g. X-ray, FBC, ESR, rheumatoid factor, etc.
- Thank the patient.
- Ensure that he is comfortable.
- Offer to help the patient put his clothes back on.
- Offer a differential diagnosis.

Conditions most likely to come up in a hand and wrist examination station	
Osteoarthritis (see *Station 77*) **Rheumatoid arthritis** (see *Station 77*) **Psoriatic arthritis** (see *Station 77*)	**De Quervain's tenosynovitis:** • idiopathic inflammation of the tendons of *extensor pollicis brevis* and *abductor pollicis longus* muscles concerned with radial abduction of the thumb • accompanied by difficulty gripping and pain, tenderness, and swelling over the radial styloid • the diagnosis is verified by holding the thumb inside a clenched fist and ulnar deviating the wrist; this stretches the inflamed tendons over the radial styloid, thereby exacerbating the patient's pain (Finkelstein's test)
Lesions of the median, radial, or ulnar nerves (see *Station 32*) **Gout** (see *Station 77*)	
Carpal tunnel syndrome: • compression of the median nerve in the carpal tunnel • more common in females • burning pain, tingling, and numbness in the distribution of the median nerve • possible wasting of the thenar eminence and weakness of the *abductor pollicis brevis* • Tinnel's sign and Phalen's sign are positive	**Trigger finger:** • idiopathic catching, snapping, or locking of the involved finger flexor tendon • associated with pain and loss of function • middle and ring finger most commonly affected • the finger clicks when it is flexed and gets stuck in the flexed position • overcoming this resistance leads to the finger snapping straight, hence the name 'trigger finger'
Dupuytren's disease: • fixed flexion contracture of the hand with the ring and little fingers most commonly affected • scar tissue palpable beneath the skin of the palm with dimpling and puckering of the skin over that area	

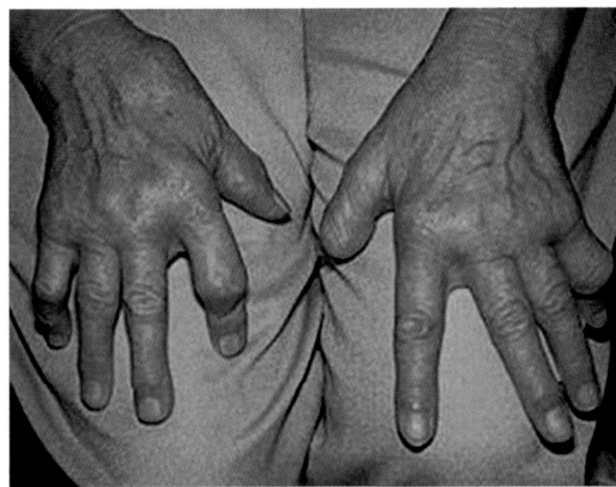

Figure 64. Rheumatoid arthritis of the hands.

Reproduced from www.mrcophth.com.

Elbow examination

This station is unlikely to come up on its own but may be asked as part of a hand and wrist examination, and is included here for completeness.

Before starting

- Introduce yourself to the patient.
- Explain the examination and ask for his consent to carry it out.
- Ask him to expose his arms.
- Ensure that he is comfortable.

The examination

Look

Ask the patient to hold his arms by his side.

- Overall impression: varus or valgus deformities (look from behind), effusions, inflammation of the olecranon bursa
- Skin: rheumatoid nodules, gouty tophi, scars
- Muscle wasting: biceps, triceps, forearm

Feel

Ask if the arms are painful.

- Skin: temperature, psoriatic plaques, rheumatoid nodules, gouty tophi
- Joints: tenderness, effusions, synovial thickening
- Bones: tenderness of the lateral and medial epicondyles

Move

- Flexion and extension:
  - tennis elbow: ask about pain at the *lateral* epicondyle on elbow *extension* and forced wrist *extension*
  - golfer's elbow: ask about pain at the *medial* epicondyle on elbow *flexion* and forced wrist *flexion*
- Pronation and supination. Show the patient how to tuck his elbows into his sides and to turn his arms so that the palm of his hands face up and down (a bit like the gesture for 'I don't know').

After the examination

- State that you would also like to examine the wrist and hand.
- State that you would also like to examine the vascular and neurological systems of the upper limb.
- If appropriate, indicate that you would order some tests, e.g. X-ray, FBC, ESR, rheumatoid factor, etc.
- Thank the patient.
- Offer to help the patient put his clothes back on.
- Ensure that he is comfortable.
- Summarise your findings and offer a differential diagnosis.

Conditions most likely to come up in an elbow examination station		
• Osteoarthritis	• Rheumatoid arthritis	• Olecranon bursitis

Shoulder examination

Before starting

- Introduce yourself to the patient.
- Explain the examination and ask for his consent to carry it out.
- Ask him to undress from the waist upward.
- Ensure that he is comfortable.

The examination

Look

Inspect from front and back.

- Overall impression: alignment, position of the arms, axillae, prominence of the acromioclavicular and sternoclavicular joints
- Skin: colour, sinuses, scars
- Muscle wasting: deltoid, periscapular muscles (supraspinatus and infraspinatus)

Feel

Ask if the shoulders are painful.

- Skin: temperature – compare both sides
- Bones and joints: palpate the bony landmarks of the shoulder, starting at the sternoclavicular joint and moving laterally along the clavicle. Try to localise any tenderness. Can you feel any effusions?
- Biceps tendon: ask the patient to flex his arms and palpate the biceps tendon in the bicipital groove. Tenderness suggests biceps tendinitis.

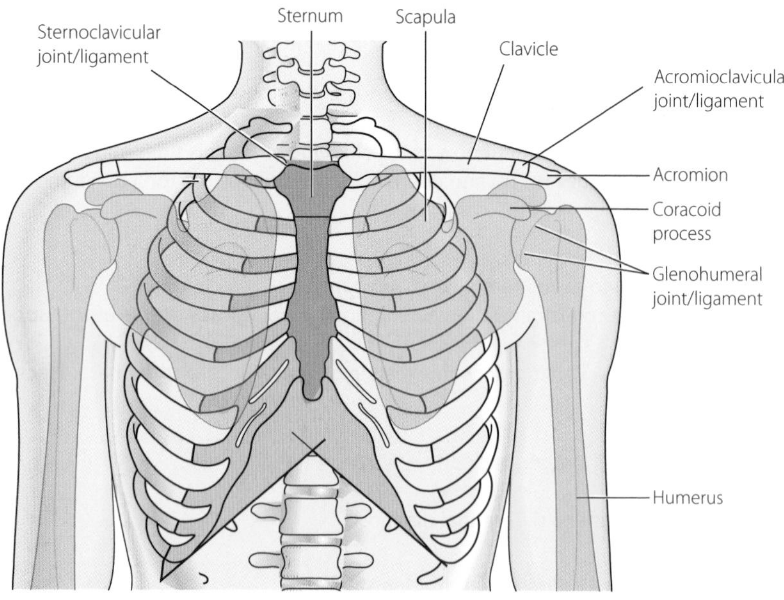

Figure 65. Anatomy of the shoulder joint.

Move

Demonstrate these movements to the patient. Note if there is a restricted range of movement and/or any pain on movement.

- Abduction: *Raise your arms above your head, making the palms of your hands touch.*
- Adduction: *Cross your arms across the front of your body.*
- Flexion: *Raise your arms forwards.*
- Extension: *Pull your arms backwards.*
- External rotation: *With your arms bent and your elbows tucked into your sides separate your hands.*
- Internal rotation: *With your arms bent and your elbows tucked into your sides bring your hands together.*
- Internal rotation in adduction: *Reach up your back and touch your scapulae.*
- External rotation in abduction: *Hold your hands behind your neck, like you do at the end of the day.*

If any one movement is limited, also test the passive range of movement.

Serratus anterior function

Ask the patient to put his hands against a wall and to push against it. Observe the scapulae from behind, looking for asymmetry or winging.

After the examination

- State that you would also like to examine the vascular and neurological systems of the upper limb.
- If appropriate, indicate that you would order some tests, e.g. X-ray, FBC, ESR, rheumatoid factor, etc.
- Thank the patient.
- Offer to help the patient put his clothes back on.
- Ensure that he is comfortable.
- Summarise your findings and offer a differential diagnosis.

Conditions most likely to come up in a shoulder examination station
Frozen shoulder (adhesive capsulitis): • the shoulder capsule becomes inflamed, resulting in pain and stiffness • range of active movements is almost the same as that of passive movements • the movement that is most severely restricted is external rotation • often idiopathic • more common in females • rarely presents under the age of 40
Calcific tendonitis: • pain and restricted movement results from deposits of hydroxyapatite in any tendon of the body, but most commonly in those of the rotator cuff • pain is aggravated by elevation of the arm • calcific deposits are visible on X-ray • calcific tendonitis predisposes to frozen shoulder
Rotator cuff tear: • tears of one or more of the four tendons of the rotator cuff muscles, particularly that of supraspinatus • often asymptomatic, but may cause tenderness and pain that may radiate along the arm • the movement that is most severely restricted is abduction; however, if the arm is passively abducted beyond 90°, the patient can abduct his arm further using the deltoid muscle
Impingement syndrome: • impingement of the supraspinatus tendon between the acromion and the humeral head • there is pain, weakness, and restricted movement with a painful arc of movement from 60 to 120° of abduction • impingement syndrome predisposes to rotator cuff tear
Shoulder dislocation: • separation of the humerus from the scapula at the glenohumeral joint • partial separation is referred to as subluxation • 95% of shoulder dislocations are anterior • anterior dislocations are usually caused by the arm being forced into abduction and external rotation • apart from a visibly displaced shoulder, there is severe pain that may radiate along the arm and a severely restricted range of movement
Bicipital tendinitis: • inflammation of the long head of the biceps tendon, often associated with trauma or overuse • there is shoulder pain that is exacerbated by overhead activity and by lifting • there is tenderness over the bicipital groove • in cases of rupture of the long head of the biceps tendon, the retracted muscle belly bulges over the anterior upper arm (Popeye sign)
Osteoarthritis (see *Station 77*)
Winging of the scapula
Referred pain from the cervical spine or the heart

Spinal examination

Before starting

- Introduce yourself to the patient.
- Explain the examination and ask for his consent to carry it out.
- Ask him to undress to his undergarments.
- Ensure that he is comfortable.

The examination

Look

Inspect from front and back.

- General inspection: ask the patient to stand and assess posture. Are there any obvious malformations?
- Skin: scars, pigmentation, abnormal hair, unusual skin creases.
- Shape and posture.
- Spine:
  - lateral curvature of the spine – *scoliosis* (observe from the back)
  - abnormal increase in the kyphotic curvature of the thoracic spine – *kyphosis* (observe from the side)
  - sharp, angular bend in the spine – a *kyphos* (observe from the side)
  - loss or exaggeration of lumbar lordosis
- Asymmetry or malformation of the chest.
- Asymmetry of the pelvis.

Feel

Ask if there is any pain.

- Palpate and percuss the spinous processes, the interspinous ligaments, and the paravertebral muscles.

Move

Ask the patient to copy your movements, looking for any limitation of range of movement. Ask the patient to indicate if any of the movements are painful.

Gait

Cervical spine

- Flexion: *Put your chin on your chest.*
- Extension: *Look at the ceiling.*
- Lateral flexion: *Put your ear onto your shoulder.*
- Rotation: *Look back over each shoulder.*

Thoracic spine

- Rotation. Please sit down (to stabilise the pelvis) and twist from side to side.

Measure chest expansion. It should be at least 5 cm.

Lumbar spine

- Flexion. *Touch your toes, keep your knees straight.*
- Extension. *Lean back, keep your knees straight.*
- Lateral flexion. *Slide your hand alongside the outside of your leg.*

Schober's test. Measure lumbar excursion by drawing a line from 10 cm above L5 to 5 cm below it and asking the patient to bend fully forwards. Extension of the line by <5 cm indicates movement restriction. (Rather than drawing a line, you can just use two fingers or a measuring tape.)

Special tests

Ask the patient to lie prone.

- Palpate the sacroiliac joints for tenderness.
- Press on the mid-line of the sacrum to test if movement of the sacroiliac joints is painful.
- Femoral stretch test (L2–L4):
  - with the patient lying prone, raise the leg so as to flex the knee
  - if this does not trigger any pain, raise the leg further so as to extend the hip – pain suggests irritation of the second, third, or fourth lumbar root of that side

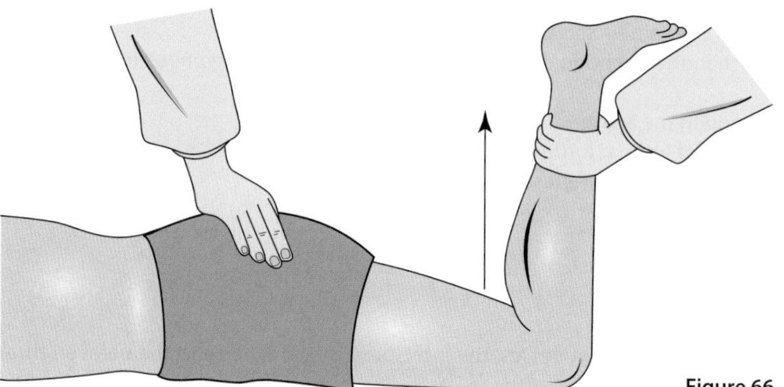

Figure 66. The femoral stretch test.

Ask the patient to lie supine.

- Straight leg raise (L5–S2):
  - with the patient lying supine, flex the hip while maintaining the knee in extension
  - pain in the thigh, buttock, and back suggests sciatica
  - the response can be amplified by concomitant dorsiflexion of the foot (Bragard's test)
  - perform Lasègue's test if you're after a gold medal! Flex the knee and then flex the hip to 90 degrees. With your left hand on the knee, gradually extend the knee with your right hand until the pain is reproduced.

After the examination

- State that you would also like to carry out neurological and vascular examinations.
- If appropriate, indicate that you would order some tests, e.g. X-ray, MRI, DEXA, FBC, ESR, bone profile, etc.
- Thank the patient.
- Offer to help the patient put his clothes back on.
- Ensure that he is comfortable.
- Summarise your findings and offer a differential diagnosis.

Conditions most likely to come up in a spinal examination station
Osteoarthritis (see *Station 77*)
Ankylosing spondylitis (see *Station 77*)
Prolapsed disc: • part of the nucleus pulposus herniates through the outer part of the disc with attending inflammation and nerve root compression • most cases occur in the lumbar spine, most commonly at L4/L5 and L5/S1 • symptoms may include back pain that is aggravated by coughing, sneezing, or straining and relieved by lying flat; nerve root pain (often involving the sciatic nerve, 'sciatica'); other nerve root symptoms such as numbness and paraesthesiae; cauda equina syndrome • the distribution of the symptoms helps to identify the level of the lesion • straight leg raise, Bragard's test, and Lasègue's test are positive • commonest in men and in middle age
Muscular back pain
Scoliosis

Hip examination

Before starting

- Introduce yourself to the patient.
- Explain the examination and ask for his consent to carry it out.
- Ask him to undress to his undergarments.
- Ensure that he is comfortable.

The examination

Look

Inspect from front and back.

- General inspection: posture, symmetry of legs and pelvis, deformity, muscle wasting, scars.
- Gait (observe from the front and back). Note any limp – antalgic, short leg, or Trendelenberg (see *Station 36*).
- Trendelenberg's test: ask the patient to stand on each leg in turn, lifting the other one off the ground by bending it at the knee. Face the patient and support him by the index fingers of his outstretched hands. The sign is positive if the pelvis drops on the non-weight bearing side.

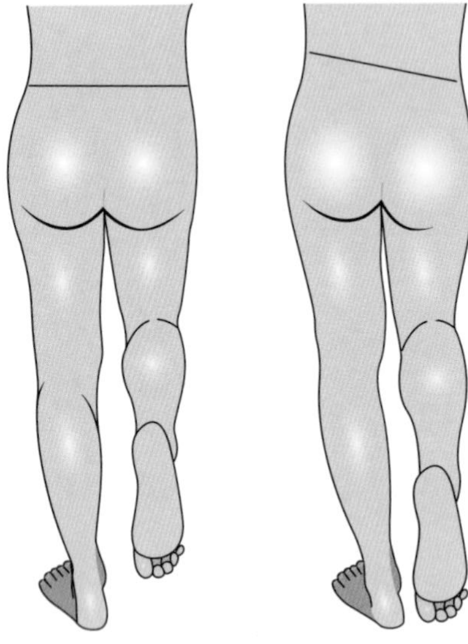

Figure 67. Negative (left) and positive Trendelenberg's test. A positive Trendelenberg's test suggests weakness of the abduction of the weight-bearing hip, and hence a problem in that hip.

Ask the patient to lie supine.

- Skin: colour, sinuses, scars.
- Position: limb shortening, limb rotation, abduction or adduction deformity, flexion deformity.
- Limb length.
  - To measure *true* leg length, position the pelvis so that the iliac crests lie in the same horizontal plane, at right angles to the trunk (this is not possible if there is a fixed abduction or adduction deformity) and then measure the distance from the anterior superior iliac spine (ASIS) to the medial malleolus. True leg shortening suggests pathology of the hip joint.

  - To measure *apparent* leg length, measure the distance from the xiphisternum to the medial malleolus. Apparent leg shortening suggests pelvic tilt, most often due to an adduction deformity of the hip.
- Circumference of the quadriceps muscles at a fixed point.

Feel

Ask if there is any pain.

- Skin: temperature, effusions (difficult to feel).
- Bones and joints: bony landmarks of the hip joint, inguinal ligament.

Move

Look for limitation of the normal range of movement, and ask the patient to report any pain.

- Flexion and Thomas' test:
  - flex both hips and place your hand in the small of the back to ensure that the lumbar lordosis has been eliminated
  - hold one hip flexed and straighten the other leg, maintaining your hand in the small of the back – if the leg cannot be straightened and the knee is unable to rest on the couch, a fixed flexion deformity is present
  - repeat for the other leg
- Abduction and adduction:
  - drop one leg over the edge of the couch to fix the pelvis
  - place one hand on the anterior superior iliac spine of the other leg and carry it through abduction and adduction
  - repeat for the other leg
- Rotation:
  - flex the hip and knee to 90 degrees
  - hold the knee in the left hand and the ankle in the right hand
  - using your right hand, rotate the hip internally and externally
  - repeat for the other leg

Ask the patient to lie prone.

- Look for scars, etc.
- Feel for tenderness.
- Extend each hip in turn. Keep a hand under a bent knee and extend the hip by pulling the leg up at the ankle.

After the examination

- State that you would also like to examine the vascular and neurological systems of the lower limbs.
- If appropriate, indicate that you would order some tests, e.g. hip and knee X-ray, DEXA, FBC, ESR, bone profile, etc.
- Thank the patient.
- Offer to help the patient put his clothes back on.
- Ensure that he is comfortable.
- Summarise your findings and offer a differential diagnosis.

Conditions most likely to come up in a hip examination station
Osteoarthritis: • the hip is held in flexion, external rotation, and adduction accompanied by pain and limited movement • there is apparent limb shortening • there are other signs of osteoarthritis, e.g. Heberden's nodes on the distal interphalangeal joints
Slipped upper femoral epiphysis: • fracture through the physis resulting in slippage of the overlying epiphysis, producing a 'melting ice-cream cone' on X-ray • limited movement of the hip, particularly internal rotation and abduction, and pain in the hip, groin, or knee • external rotation and shortening of the affected leg • often presents in obese prepubescent males
Trendelenburg gait (see *Station 36*)
Antalgic gait (see *Station 36*)
Hip replacement
Hip arthrodesis
Trochanteric bursitis

Knee examination

Before starting

- Introduce yourself to the patient.
- Explain the examination and ask for his consent to carry it out.
- Ask him to undress from the waist downwards.
- Ensure that he is comfortable.

The examination

Ask the patient to stand.

Look

- Gait: observe from in front and behind, looking for instability, limp, and limited range of movement.
- Position: neutral, varus, valgus, fixed flexion, hyperextension (recurvatum).
- Squat test (avoid in elderly patients).

Ask the patient to lie supine.

- Skin: colour, sinuses, scars (including arthroscopic scars).
- Shape: alignment, effusion, patellar alignment.
- Position: hyperextension, varus, valgus.

Measure quadriceps circumference a hand breadth above the patella.

Feel

Ask if there is any pain.

- Skin: temperature (compare both sides).
- Effusions: cross fluctuation, patellar tap test, and bulge test.
  - cross fluctuation: place the thumb and index finger of one hand on the joint line just below the patella and with the other hand empty the suprapatellar pouch. If an impulse is transmitted across the joint line, this indicates a large effusion.
  - patellar tap test: empty the suprapatellar pouch with one hand and dip the patella with the thumb, index finger, and middle finger of the other hand. If the patella is felt to tap the underlying bone and to bounce back up, this indicates a medium sized effusion.
  - bulge test: empty the medial parapatellar fossa by stroking the medial aspect of the joint; then empty either the suprapatellar pouch or the lateral parapatellar fossa. If the medial parapatellar fossa is seen to bulge out, this indicates a small effusion.
- Joint line at 90 degrees of flexion. Feel for any synovial thickening.
- Surrounding structures: ligaments, tibial tuberosity, femoral condyles.
- Patella: note size and height of patella and carry out patellar apprehension tests. Displace the patella laterally while flexing the knee. If the patella is unstable, the patient will either contract the quadriceps muscle or discontinue the test.

Move

- Active:
  - flexion
  - extension

- Passive:
  - flexion (to 140 degrees), feeling for crepitus and clicks
  - extension (to 0 to –10 degrees)

Special tests

- Collateral ligament tears.
  - Apply varus and valgus stresses at 0 degrees and 20 degrees of flexion. Hold the leg under one arm and apply pressure on the medial/lateral side of the knee joint.
- Cruciate ligament tears.
  - Posterior sag test: flex the knee to 90 degrees and look for a sag across the knee. The presence of a sag indicates a posterior cruciate ligament tear.
  - Anterior and posterior drawer tests: flex the knee to 90 degrees, sit on the foot (ask the patient first!), and pull the tibia back and forth. Exaggerated anterior displacement indicates that the anterior cruciate ligament is probably torn, whereas exaggerated posterior displacement indicates that the posterior cruciate ligament is probably torn.
  - Lachman's test (*Figure 68*): flex the knee to 30 degrees and, holding the thigh in one hand and the proximal tibia in the other, attempt to make the joint surfaces slide upon one another. Exaggerated anterior displacement of the tibia indicates that the anterior cruciate ligament is probably torn.

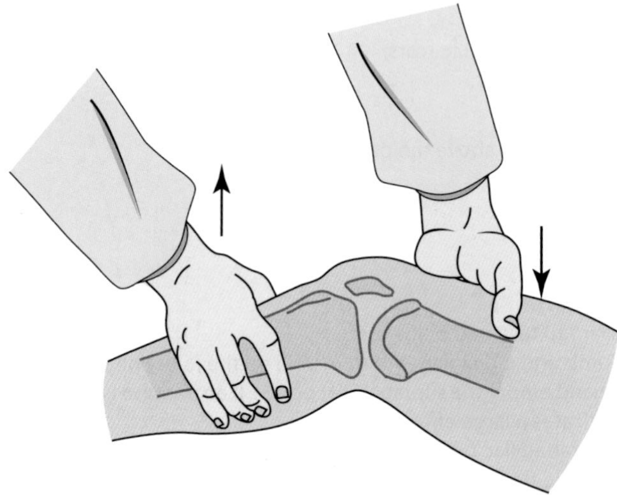

Figure 68. Lachman's test.

- Meniscal tears.
  - McMurray's test (*Figure 69*): place one hand on the knee and the other on the ankle. Flex the hip and knee. To test the medial meniscus, palpate the posteromedial margin of the joint. Then hold the leg in external rotation and extend the knee. To test the lateral meniscus, palpate the posterolateral margin of the joint. Then hold the leg in internal rotation and extend the knee. A positive test is one that elicits pain, resistance, or a reproducible click.
  - Apley's grinding test (not usually performed).

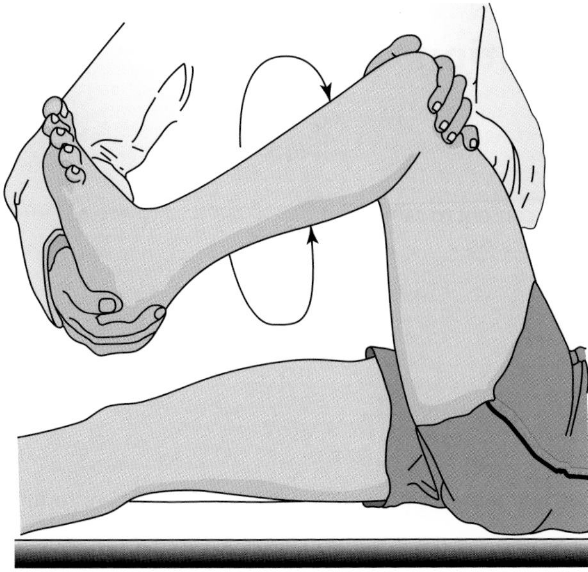

Figure 69. McMurray's test.

Lie the patient prone.

- Popliteal fossa:
  - inspect the popliteal fossa
  - palpate the popliteal fossa for a Baker's (popliteal) cyst

After the examination

- State that you would also like to examine the vascular and neurological systems of the lower limbs.
- If appropriate, indicate that you would order some tests, e.g. knee X-ray, FBC, ESR, bone profile, rheumatoid factor, etc.
- Thank the patient.
- Offer to help the patient put his clothes back on.
- Ensure that he is comfortable.
- Summarise your findings and offer a differential diagnosis.

 *The age and sex of the patient have a strong bearing on the differential diagnosis.*

Conditions most likely to come up in a knee examination station	
• Recurrent subluxation of the patella	• Osteoarthritis
• Chrondromalacia patellae	• Rheumatoid arthritis
• Collateral ligament tears	• Prepatellar and infrapatellar bursitis
• Cruciate ligament tears	• Baker's (popliteal) cyst
• Meniscal tears	• Tibial apophysitis (Osgood–Schlätter's disease)

Ankle and foot examination

Before starting

- Introduce yourself to the patient.
- Explain the examination and ask for his consent to carry it out.
- Ask him to undress from the waist downwards.
- Ensure that he is comfortable.

The examination

The patient is standing.

Look

- General inspection: posture, symmetry, and any obvious deformities. Ask the patient to turn around.
- Gait: observe from front and back. Ask the patient to stand on his tiptoes and then on his heels.

Ask the patient to lie on the couch.

- Skin: colour, sinuses, scars, corns, calluses, ulcers.
- Shape: alignment, *pes planus* (flat foot), *pes cavus* (arched foot), deformities of the toes (*hallux valgus*, claw, hammer, and mallet toes).
- Position: varus or valgus hindfoot deformity.

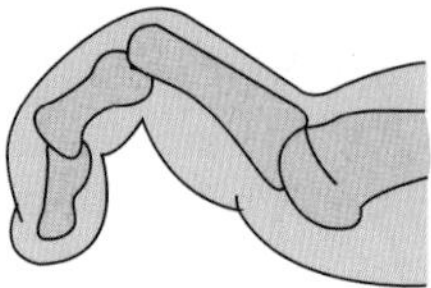
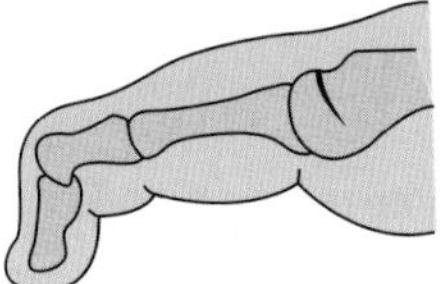
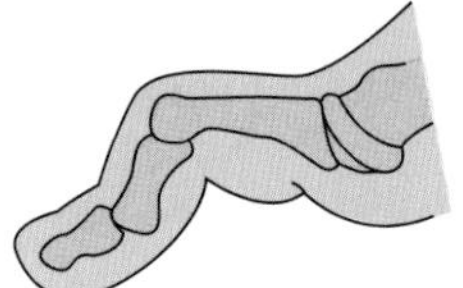

Figure 70. Claw, mallet, and hammer toes.

Feel

Ask about any pain.

- Skin: temperature (compare both sides), abnormal thickening on the soles of the feet.
- Pulses: dorsalis pedis, posterior tibial.
- Bone and joints: palpate the joint margin, forefoot (metatarsals and metatarsophalangeal joints) and hindfoot, and localise any tenderness. Remember to keep looking at the patient's face.

Move

Look for restriction of the normal range of movement. Ask the patient to report any pain.

Ankle joint

- Hold the heel in the left hand and the forefoot in the right hand.
- Plantarflex the foot (normal range 40 degrees).

- Dorsiflex the foot (normal range 25 degrees).
- Compare range of movement to that in the other foot.

Subtalar joint

- Hold the heel in the left hand and the forefoot in the right hand, as above, with the ankle fixed at 90 degrees.
- Invert the foot (normal range 30 degrees).
- Evert the foot (normal range 30 degrees).
- Compare the range of movement to that in the other foot.

Midtarsal joint

- Hold the heel in the left hand and the forefoot in the right hand.
- Flex, extend, invert, and evert the forefoot.

Toes

- Flex and extend each toe in turn. If there is any tenderness, try to localise it to a particular joint.

Ask the patient to lie prone.

- Look for any scars and for wasting of the calves.
- Palpate the calf muscle and the Achilles' tendon.
- Simmond's test: squeeze the calf – if the foot plantarflexes, the Achilles' tendon is intact.

After the examination

- State that you would also like to examine the vascular and neurological systems of the lower limbs.
- If appropriate, indicate that you would order some tests, e.g. foot and ankle X-ray, FBC, ESR, bone profile, rheumatoid factor, etc.
- Thank the patient.
- Offer to help the patient put his socks and shoes back on.
- Ensure that he is comfortable.
- Summarise your findings and offer a differential diagnosis.

Conditions most likely to come up in an ankle and foot examination station	
• Osteoarthritis • Rheumatoid arthritis • Ankle injuries	• Deformities of the foot • Plantar fasciitis

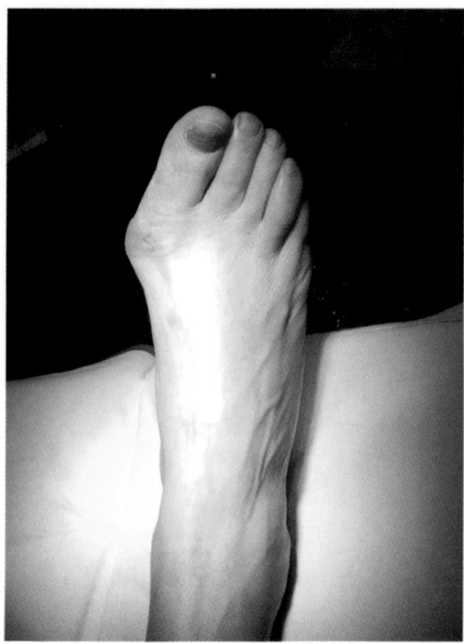

Figure 71. Hallux (abducto) valgus.

Reproduced from http://commons.wikimedia.org – photograph by Dr Henri Lelièvre.

Adult Basic Life Support

- Make sure the victim, any bystanders, and you are safe.
- Check the victim for a response. Gently shake his shoulders and ask loudly, *Are you all right?*

Adult Basic Life Support

UNRESPONSIVE ?
↓
Shout for help
↓
Open airway
↓
NOT BREATHING NORMALLY ?
↓
Call 999
↓
30 chest compressions
↓
2 rescue breaths 30 compressions

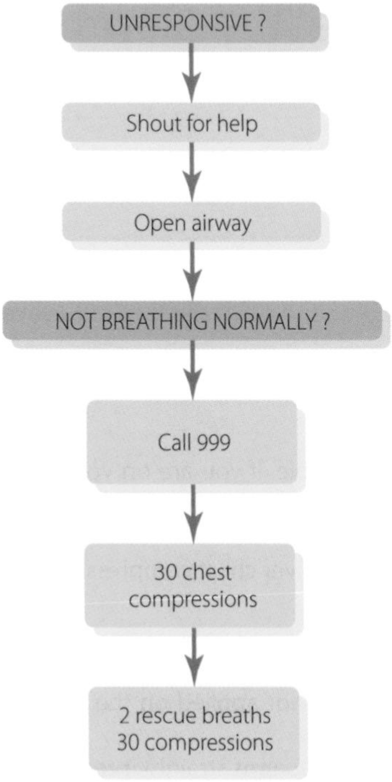

Figure 72. Basic Life Support algorithm.

If he responds:

- Leave him in the position in which you find him provided there is no further danger.
- Try to find out what is wrong with him and get help if needed.
- Reassess him regularly.

If he does not respond:

- Shout for help.
- Turn him onto his back and open the airway using the head-tilt, chin-lift technique.
  - Place your hand on his forehead and gently tilt his head back.
  - With your fingertips under the point of his chin, lift the chin to open the airway.
  - Holding his airway open, put your ear to his mouth. *Listen, feel*, and *look* for breathing for no more than 10 seconds. If you have any doubt about whether breathing is normal, assume that it is not.

Agonal breathing (occasional gasps, slow, laboured, or noisy breathing) is common in the early stages of cardiac arrest and should not be mistaken for a sign of life.

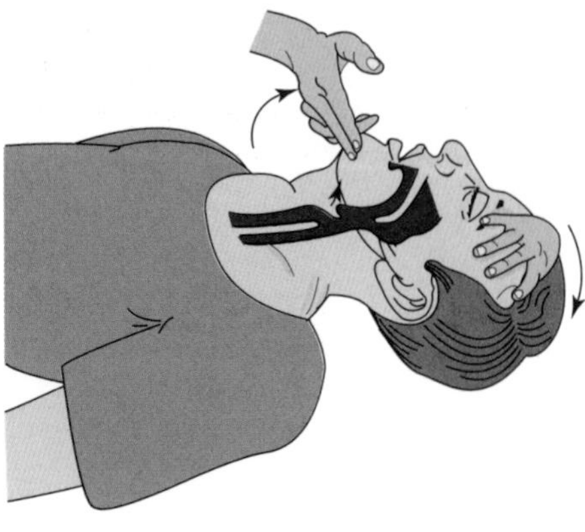

Figure 73. The head-tilt, chin-lift technique.

If he is breathing normally:

- Turn him into the recovery position.
- Call for an ambulance by mobile phone or, if this is not possible, send a bystander to call. Leave the victim only if there is no other way of obtaining help.
- Check for continued breathing.

If he is not breathing normally:

- Ask someone to call for an ambulance and bring an AED if available. If you are on your own, use your mobile phone to call for an ambulance. Leave the victim only if there is no other way of obtaining help.
- Deliver 30 chest compressions followed by 2 rescue breaths. To deliver chest compressions:
  - kneel by the side of the victim
  - place the heel of one hand in the centre of the victim's chest
  - place the heel of the other hand on top of the first hand
  - interlock the fingers of your hands and ensure that pressure is not applied on the victim's ribs, bottom end of his chest bone, or upper abdomen
  - position yourself vertically above the victim's chest and, with your arms straight, press down on the sternum 5–6 cm
  - after each compression, release all the pressure on the chest without losing contact between your hands and the sternum – repeat at a rate of about 100–120 per minute
  - compression and release should take an equal amount of time

  To deliver rescue breaths:
  - after 30 compressions, again open the airway using head tilt and chin lift
  - pinch the soft part of the victim's nose closed using the index finger and thumb of the hand on his forehead
  - allow his mouth to open, but maintain chin lift
  - take a normal breath and place your lips around his mouth, making sure that you have a good seal
  - blow steadily into his mouth whilst watching for his chest to rise – take about 1 second to make his chest rise
  - maintaining head tilt and chin lift, take your mouth away from him and watch for his chest to fall
  - deliver a second rescue breath and return to chest compressions without delay
- Continue with chest compressions and rescue breaths at a ratio of 30:2.
- Stop to re-check the victim only if he starts to show signs of regaining consciousness, such as coughing, opening his eyes, speaking or moving purposefully AND starts to breathe normally; otherwise do not interrupt resuscitation.

- If your rescue breaths do not make the chest rise as in normal breathing, check the victim's mouth and remove any obstruction and re-check that there is adequate head tilt and chin lift. Do not attempt more than 2 rescue breaths each time before returning to chest compressions.
- If there is more than one person present, the person providing chest compressions should change every 1–2 minutes with only minimal interruption to the chest compressions.

If the rescuer is unable or unwilling to give rescue breaths, he can give chest compressions at a rate of 100–120 compressions per minute, stopping only to recheck the victim if he shows signs of regaining consciousness AND starts to breathe normally.

Continue resuscitation until qualified help arrives or until the victim shows signs of regaining consciousness AND starts to breathe normally or until exhaustion.

The recovery position

- Remove the victim's spectacles, if any.
- Kneel beside the victim and make sure that both his legs are straight.
- Place the arm nearest to you out at right angles to his body, elbow bent, with the hand palm uppermost.
- Bring the far arm across the chest, and hold the back of the hand against the victim's cheek nearest to you.
- With your other hand, grasp the far leg just above the knee and pull it up, keeping the foot on the ground.
- Keeping his hand pressed against his cheek, pull on the far leg to roll the victim towards you and onto his side.
- Adjust the upper leg so that both the hip and knee are bent at right angles.
- Tilt the head back to ensure that the airway remains open.
- Adjust the hand under the cheek, if necessary, to keep the head tilted.

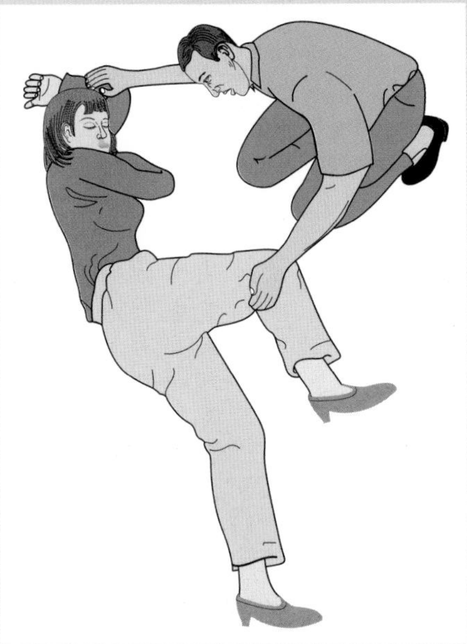

Figure 74. The recovery position.

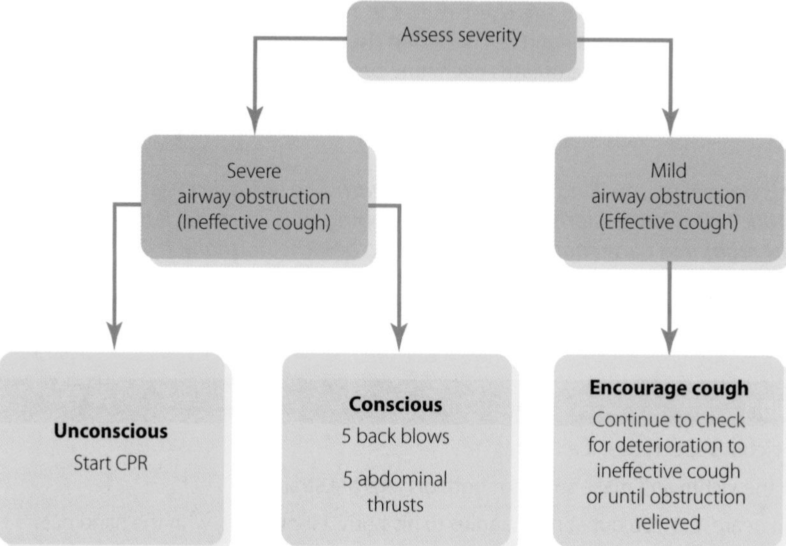

Figure 75. Adult choking algorithm.

Adapted from Resuscitation Council (UK) 2010 Guidelines.

In-hospital resuscitation

This sequence should be followed for a collapsed patient in hospital.

- Ensure personal safety.
- Shout for help.
- Check the patient for a response – gently shake his shoulders and loudly ask *"Are you all right?"*

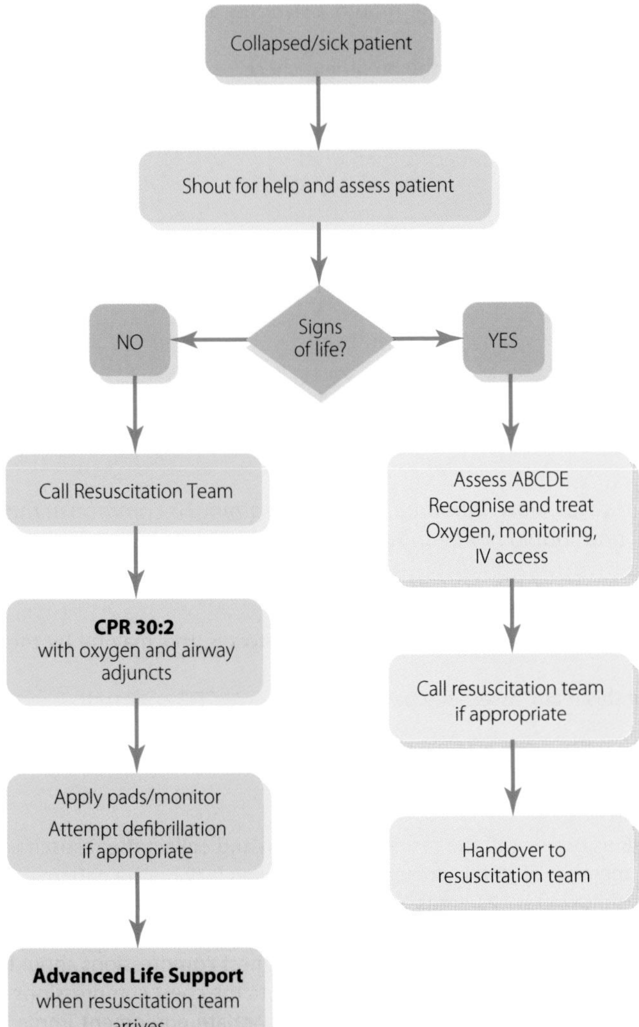

Figure 76. In-hospital resuscitation algorithm.

- If the patient responds:
  - urgent medical assessment is required – depending on local protocols, this may be by the resuscitation team
  - while awaiting the arrival of this team, assess the patient using the ABCDE approach
  - give the patient oxygen
  - attach monitoring

  - obtain venous access
- If the patient does not respond:
  - turn the patient onto his back
  - open the airway using the head-tilt, chin-lift technique
  - if there is a risk of C-spine injury, use the jaw-thrust or chin-lift technique with manual in-line stabilisation (MILS) of the head and neck by an assistant (if sufficient staff are available). If airway obstruction persists despite jaw thrust or chin lift, add head tilt a small amount at a time. Establishing an airway should take priority over concerns about a potential C-spine injury.
- Holding the patient's airway open, put your ear to his mouth. *Listen, feel*, and *look* for breathing for no more than 10 seconds.
- Assess the carotid pulse at the same time or after the breathing check.

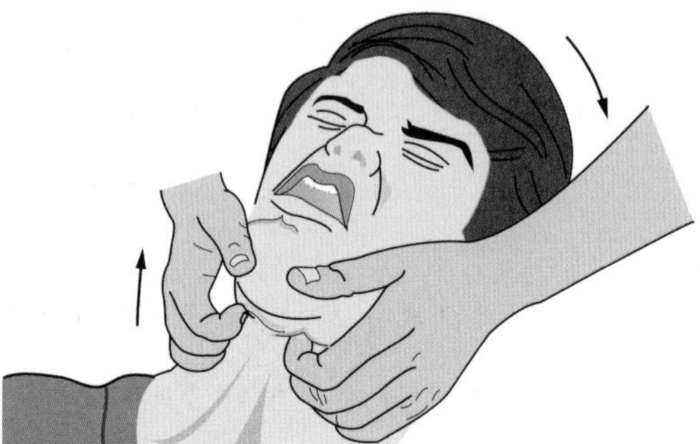

Figure 77. The head-tilt jaw-thrust technique.

Agonal breathing (occasional gasps, slow, laboured, or noisy breathing) is common in the early stages of cardiac arrest and should not be mistaken for a sign of life.

- If the patient has a pulse or other signs of life.
  - Urgent medical assessment is required. Depending on local protocols, this may be by the resuscitation team.
  - While awaiting the arrival of this team, assess the patient using the ABCDE approach.
  - Give the patient oxygen.
  - Attach monitoring.
  - Obtain venous access.
- If there is no pulse or other signs of life.
  - One person should start CPR as others call the resuscitation team and collect the resuscitation equipment. If only one member of staff is present, this will mean leaving the patient.
  - Give 30 chest compressions followed by 2 ventilations. Place your interlocked hands in the middle of the lower half of the sternum and depress the chest by 5–6 cm, aiming for a rate of 100–120 compressions per minute. The person providing the chest compressions should change every 2 minutes or earlier, with only minimal interruption to the chest compressions.
  - Maintain the airway and ventilate the lungs with the most appropriate equipment immediately at hand. A pocket mask, which may be supplemented by an oral airway, is usually readily available. If no equipment is immediately at hand, give mouth-to-mouth ventilation unless there are clinical reasons to avoid mouth-to-mouth contact.
  - Use an inspiratory time of 1 second and give enough volume to produce a chest rise as in normal breathing. Add supplemental oxygen as soon as possible.
  - Once the airway has been secured, continue chest compressions uninterrupted at a rate of 100–120 compressions per minute and ventilate the lungs at approximately 10 breaths per minute. Only stop compressions for defibrillation or pulse checks.

- Upon arrival of the defibrillator, apply self-adhesive defibrillation pads to the patient without interrupting chest compressions and analyse the rhythm.
- If using an automated external defibrillator (AED), switch on the machine and follow the visual prompts.
- For manual defibrillation, minimise the interruption to CPR to deliver a shock.
- Pause briefly to assess the heart rhythm. With a manual defibrillator, if the rhythm is VF or pulseless VT (VF/VT), charge the defibrillator and restart chest compressions.
- Once the defibrillator is charged, oxygen sources have been removed, and all the rescuers apart from the one doing the chest compressions are clear, pause the chest compressions, rapidly check that everyone is clear (tell the remaining rescuer to "*stand clear*"), and deliver the shock. Restart the chest compressions immediately. This sequence should be planned before stopping the chest compressions.
- Continue resuscitation until the resuscitation team arrives or until the patient shows signs of life. If using an AED, follow the voice prompts. If using a manual defibrillator, follow the algorithm for ALS (see *Station 88*).
- Prepare intravenous cannulae and drugs likely to be used by the resuscitation team (e.g. adrenaline).
- Identify one person to be responsible for handover to the resuscitation team leader and locate the patient's notes.

• If the patient is not breathing but has a pulse (respiratory arrest).
  - Ventilate the patient's lungs as described above, checking for a pulse after every 10 breaths (about every minute).
  - If there are any doubts about the presence of a pulse, start chest compressions until more experienced help arrives.
• If a patient has a monitored and witnessed cardiac arrest.
  - Confirm cardiac arrest and shout for help.
  - If the initial rhythm is VF/VT, give up to three quick successive (stacked) shocks. Start chest compressions immediately after the third shock and continue CPR for 2 minutes.
  - A pre-cordial thump in these settings works rarely and may succeed only if given within seconds of the onset of a shockable rhythm. It should not delay calling for help or accessing a defibrillator.

Adapted from Resuscitation Council (UK) 2010 Guidelines.

Advanced Life Support

Specifications: A mannequin in lieu of a patient.

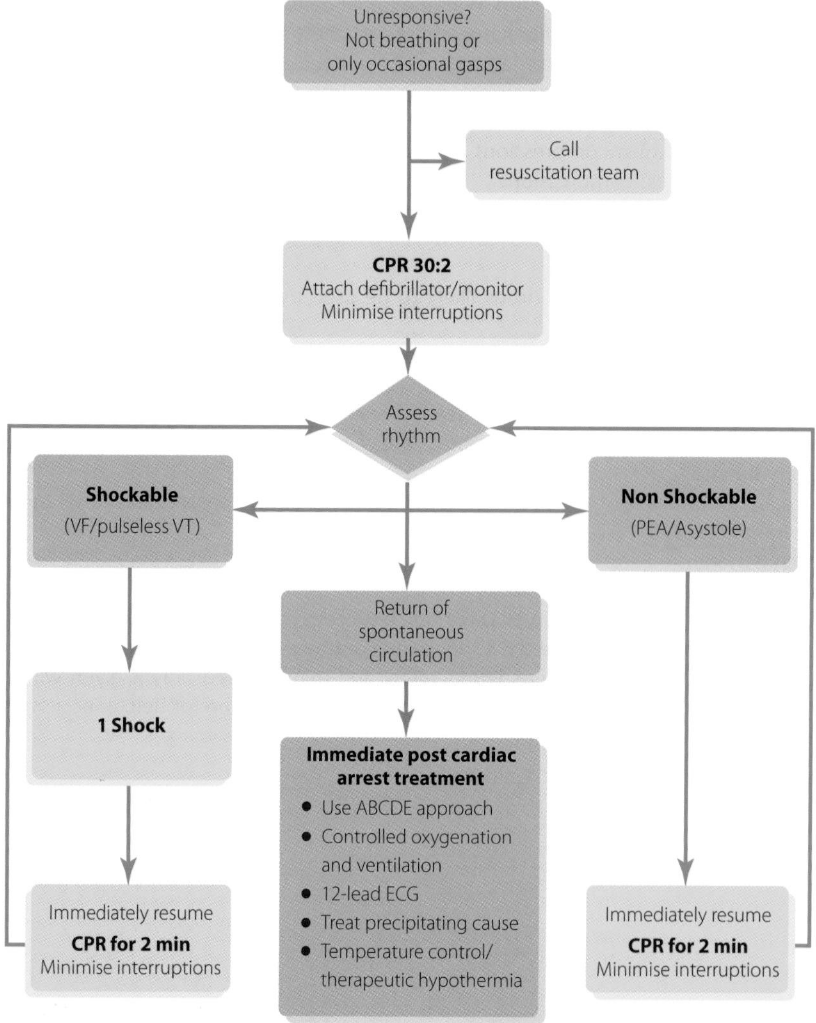

During CPR

- Ensure high-quality CPR: rate, depth, recoil
- Plan actions before interrupting CPR
- Give oxygen
- Consider advanced airway and capnography
- Continuous chest compressions when advanced airway in place
- Vascular access (intravenous, intraosseous)
- Give adrenaline every 3–5 min
- Correct reversible causes

Reversible Causes

- Hypoxia
- Hypovolaemia
- Hypo-/hyperkalaemia/metabolic
- Hypothermia

- Thrombosis (coronary or pulmonary)
- Tamponade, cardiac
- Toxins
- Tension pneumothorax

Figure 78. Advanced Life Support algorithm.

The patient has arrested and CPR is under way. The defibrillator/monitor has just been attached.

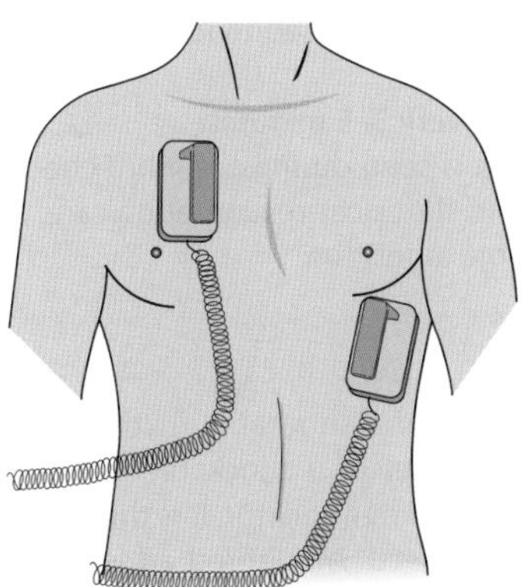

Figure 79. Positioning of the defibrillator paddles. One paddle goes under the right clavicle and the other goes in the V6 position in the mid-axillary line.

- Assess the rhythm.

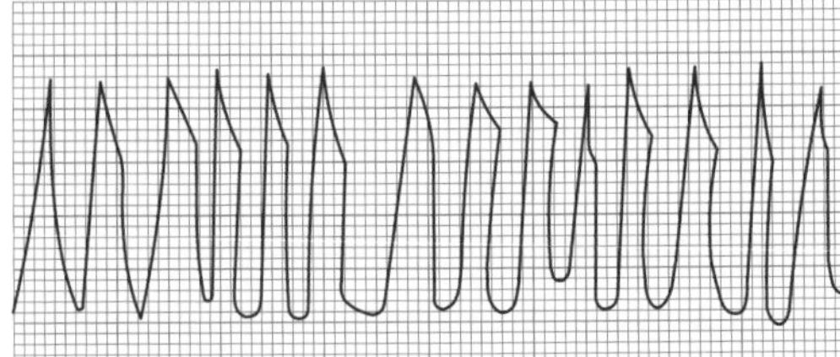

Ventricular tachycardia

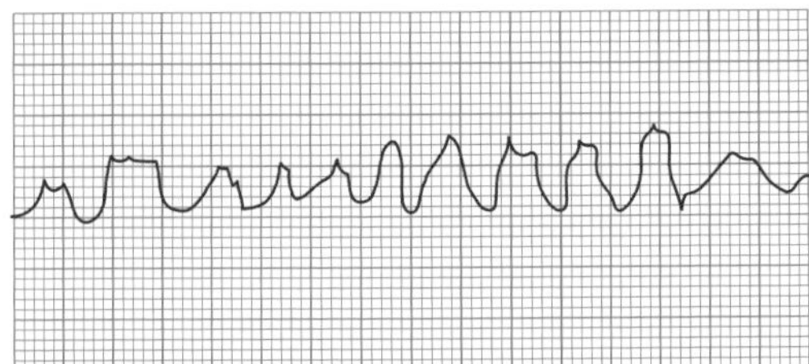

Ventricular fibrillation

Figure 80. ECG traces of ventricular fibrillation and ventricular tachycardia.

- Pause briefly to check the monitor, confirm VF/VT from the ECG, and resume the chest compressions immediately.
- Select the appropriate energy on the defibrillator (150–200 J biphasic for the first shock and 150–360 J biphasic for subsequent shocks) and press the charge button.
- Once the defibrillator is charged, oxygen sources have been removed, and all the rescuers apart from the one doing the chest compressions are clear, pause the chest compressions, rapidly check that everyone is clear (tell the remaining rescuer to *"stand clear"*), and deliver the shock. Restart the chest compressions immediately. This sequence should be planned before stopping the chest compressions.
- Continue CPR for 2 minutes at a ratio of 30:2.
- Pause briefly to check the monitor. If VF/VT persists, repeat the relevant steps above to deliver a second shock.
- If VF/VT still persists repeat the relevant steps above to deliver a third shock.

- Resume chest compressions immediately and perform CPR for a further 2 minutes, during which time give adrenaline 1 mg IV and amiodarone 300 mg IV.
- Keep on repeating this 2 minute CRP – rhythm/pulse check – defibrillation sequence for as long as VF/VT persists.
- Give further adrenaline 1 mg IV after alternate shocks, i.e. after every 3–5 minutes.
- If organised electrical activity compatible with a cardiac output is seen during a rhythm check (and not otherwise), check for central pulse. If a pulse is present, start post-resuscitation care. If a pulse is absent, continue CPR and switch to the non-shockable algorithm.

Precordial thump

A single precordial thump has a very low success rate for cardioversion of a shockable rhythm and is only likely to succeed if given within the first few seconds of the onset of a shockable rhythm. Delivery of a precordial thump must not delay calling for help or accessing a defibrillator. It is therefore appropriate therapy only when several clinicians are present at a witnessed, monitored arrest, and when a defibrillator is not immediately to hand. Using the ulnar edge of a tightly clenched fist, deliver a sharp impact to the lower half of the sternum from a height of about 20 cm, then retract the fist immediately to create an impulse-like stimulus. A precordial thump is most likely to be successful in converting VT to sinus rhythm.

Non-shockable rhythms (PEA and asystole)

Survival after cardiac arrest with PEA or asystole is unlikely unless a reversible cause can be found and treated successfully.

Sequence of actions for PEA (cardiac electrical activity in the absence of any palpable pulse).

- Start CPR 30:2.
- Give adrenaline 1 mg IV as soon as IV access is achieved.
- Continue CPR 30:2 until the airway is secured, then continue chest compressions without pausing during ventilation.
- Consider possible reversible causes of PEA and correct any that are identified.
- Recheck the patient after 2 minutes.
- If there is still no pulse and no change in the ECG appearance:
  - continue CPR
  - recheck the patient after 2 minutes and proceed accordingly
  - give further adrenaline 1 mg IV after every 3–5 minutes (alternate loops)
- If VF/VT, change to the shockable rhythm algorithm
- If a pulse is present, start post-resuscitation care.

Sequence of actions for asystole and slow PEA (rate < 60 per minute).

- Start CPR 30:2.
- Without stopping CPR, check that the leads are attached correctly.
- Give adrenaline 1 mg IV as soon as IV access is achieved.
- Give atropine 3 mg IV (once only).
- Continue CPR 30:2 until the airway is secured, then continue chest compressions without pausing during ventilation.
- Consider possible reversible causes of PEA and correct any that are identified.
- Recheck the patient after 2 minutes and proceed accordingly.
- If VF/VT, change to the shockable rhythm algorithm.
- Give further adrenaline 1 mg IV after every 3–5 minutes (alternate loops).

Adapted from Resuscitation Council (UK) 2010 Guidelines, which can be found at www.resus.org.uk/pages/als.pdf and which you are encouraged to read.

The primary and secondary surveys

In this station, you are going to be asked to assess a patient with a medical emergency or who has suffered severe injury (e.g. from a road traffic accident). What follows is a general outline of the areas that you are going to need to cover.

Primary survey

The quick look

- Inspect the patient.
- Introduce yourself to him. Is he responsive? Try to elicit a response by shouting out his name.

Airway and cervical spine

- Assess the airway for obstruction.
- If necessary, clear and secure the airway. If there is suspicion of a cervical spine injury, use the jaw-thrust technique.
- If there is a suspicion of cervical spine injury, immobilise the cervical spine in a stiff collar. Place sandbags on either side of the head and tape them across the forehead.

Breathing

- Assess breathing: look, listen, feel.
- Expose the chest.
- Note the rate and depth of respiration.
- Look for asymmetries of chest expansion.
- Look for chest injuries.
- Palpate for tracheal deviation. Palpate, percuss, and auscultate the chest. Try to exclude flail segments, pneumothorax, or haemothorax.
- Attach a pulse oximeter.
- If appropriate, ventilate using a bag, mask, and oropharyngeal airway or endotracheal tube.

Circulation and haemorrhage control

- Control any visible haemorrhage by direct pressure.
- Look for clinical signs of shock: assess the pulse, skin colour, capillary refill time, JVP, heart sounds, and blood pressure. Try to exclude cardiac tamponade.
- Attach an ECG monitor.
- Place two large-bore (grey) cannulas into large peripheral veins.
- Take a sample of blood for group and cross-match.
- Start fluid replacement.

Disability (neurological assessment)

- Assess neurological function on the AVPU scale:
  - A Alert
  - V Voice elicits a response
  - P Pain elicits a response
  - U Unresponsive
- Assess the pupils for size and reactivity.
- Check that all limb extremities can be moved.

Exposure and environmental control

- Remove the patient's remaining clothing and inspect both his front and back. Log-roll him so that his spine remains immobilised.
- Cover him in a blanket.

Secondary survey

Once the patient is stable:

- Take a short, AMPLE history:
  - **A**llergies
  - **M**edications and tetanus immunity
  - **P**revious medical history
  - **L**ast meal
  - **E**vents leading to the injury
- Carry out a head-to-toe physical examination.
- Monitor ECG, BP, oxygen saturation, and core temperature.
- Insert a urinary catheter and, if necessary, a naso-gastric tube.
- Order investigations: full blood count, urea and electrolytes, liver function tests, amylase, glucose, coagulation profile, arterial blood gases, toxicology screen, and X-rays of the lateral cervical spine, chest, and pelvis.
- Encourage questions from the patient and address his concerns.

Management of medical emergencies

Acute asthma

You are called to see a 28 year old man in A&E. The patient is in obvious respiratory distress, and is struggling to speak. The nurse tells you that the patient has a history of asthma. PEFR is 40% of expected, and oxygen saturation is 91%. What is your immediate course of action?

- Assess the severity of the attack by carrying out a brief physical examination, including ABCs.

  A severe attack is indicated by:
  - PEFR <50% of predicted or best
  - respiratory rate >25/min
  - pulse rate of >110 beats/min
  - inability to complete sentences

  A life-threatening attack is suggested by:
  - oxygen saturation <92%
  - silent chest, cyanosis, poor respiratory effort
  - bradycardia, arrhythmia, or hypotension
  - exhaustion, confusion, or coma
- If this is a severe attack, call for senior or specialist help and inform an anaesthetist and the ITU. Begin treatment immediately.
- Sit the patient up and give 100% oxygen through a non-rebreather mask with a reservoir bag.
- Give 5 mg salbutamol and 0.5 mg ipratropium bromide nebulised with oxygen.
- Give a corticosteroid such as hydrocortisone 100 mg IV, and consider adding prednisolone 30–60 mg (if the patient is not too distressed to take tablets).
- Once the patient is stable, carry out investigations including arterial blood gases (ABGs) and a chest X-ray. A life-threatening attack can be confirmed on ABGs by a $PaO_2 > 8$ kPa, a $PaCO_2 > 5$ kPa (due to poor respiratory effort), and a pH < 7.35 (due to CO_2 retention or lactic acidosis from tissue ischaemia). ABGs can also be used to monitor serum electrolytes, particularly K^+ which may be decreased. Chest X-ray is helpful in excluding differentials such as inhalation of a foreign body, pneumothorax, pulmonary oedema, and acute exacerbation of COPD.
- If initial measures fail, add magnesium sulphate 1.2–2 g IV over 20 minutes and give salbutamol nebulisers every 15 minutes.
- Continue monitoring the patient at regular intervals. If he is still not improving, consider aminophylline IV. Discuss with your seniors and with the ITU.

Acute pulmonary oedema

You are called to the ward to see a 55 year old lady with acute shortness of breath. She was admitted with severe diarrhoea and vomiting, and was therefore being aggressively rehydrated. An old ECG suggests left ventricular damage. On physical examination you find a raised JVP, gallop rhythm, and bilateral crackles. What is your immediate course of action?

- Sit the patient up.
- Give 100% oxygen through a non-rebreather mask with a reservoir bag. Care must be taken if the patient has COPD.
- Obtain IV access and attach an ECG monitor. Treat any arrhythmias as appropriate.
- Give GTN spray 2 puffs SL, unless the patient is hypotensive.
- Give diamorphine 2.5–5 mg IV slowly. Care must be taken if the patient has COPD.
- Give frusemide 40–80 mg IV slowly. Note that both diamorphine and frusemide are primarily acting as vasodilators in this context.

- Once the patient has stabilised, further investigations can be carried out such as arterial blood gases, chest X-ray, cardiac enzymes, and U&Es. Continue monitoring the patient at regular intervals.
- Start a nitrate infusion, e.g. isosorbide dinitrate 2–10 mg/h unless the patient is hypotensive. (If systolic BP is < 100 mmHg, treat as cardiogenic shock.)
- If the patient deteriorates, discuss with your seniors and with ITU. Consider increasing the nitrate infusion or giving more frusemide. Re-consider alternative diagnoses such as asthma, COPD, pneumonia, and pulmonary embolism.
- As this patient has left ventricular failure, an ACE-I is indicated once her condition has stabilised.

Acute myocardial infarction

You are tending to a 65 year old gentleman with known cardiovascular disease when he suddenly clutches his chest in severe pain. You look up at the cardiac monitor and see prominent ST elevation. What is your immediate course of action?

- Assess ABCs.
- Give 100% oxygen through a non-rebreather mask with a reservoir bag.
- If not already in place, set up continuous cardiac monitoring and obtain a 12-lead ECG.
- Gain IV access and take blood for baseline troponins, FBC, U&Es, glucose, and lipids.
- If possible, carry out a brief assessment of the patient, including brief history and focused physical examination.
- Give morphine 5–10 mg IV with an antiemetic. Two puffs of GTN SL can be given to provide further relief if the patient is not hypotensive.
- Give aspirin 300 mg PO.
- If the patient is diabetic or the blood glucose is >11 mmol/l, an insulin sliding scale may be indicated.
- For a STEMI, thrombolysis should ideally be given within 90 minutes, e.g. streptokinase 1.5 million units in 100 ml saline IVI over 1 hour. Alteplase may be indicated if the patient has previously received streptokinase. In equipped centres, primary percutaneous coronary angioplasty can be considered in lieu of thrombolysis.

The indications for thrombolysis are:

- ST elevation of >2 mm in 2 or more chest leads
- ST elevation of >1 mm in 2 or more limb leads
- New onset LBBB
- Posterior MI, as evidenced by dominant R waves and ST depression in leads V1–3

Ensure that there are no contraindications to thrombolysis such as internal bleeding or severe liver disease. If so, consider urgent angioplasty instead of thrombolysis.

- Following thrombolysis, give a beta blocker such as atenolol 5 mg IV and an ACE inhibitor such as lisinopril 2.5 mg (unless contraindicated).
- For a NSTEMI, give LMWH, a beta blocker such as atenolol 5 mg IV, and IV nitrates (unless contraindicated). Medium and high risk patients should be given an infusion of GPIIb/IIIa and urgent angiography. Low risk patients may be discharged following a stress test (exercise ECG/stress echo).
- Following an MI, and unless there are any contraindications, the patient should receive:
  - long term low-dose aspirin
  - clopidogrel (4 weeks for STEMI, 3 months for NSTEMI)
  - long term statin
  - long term beta blocker
  - long term ACE inhibitor

Massive pulmonary embolism

You are fast-bleeped to the ward, where a 48 year old lady who had surgery for ovarian carcinoma 12 days ago has collapsed on the toilet. She has developed acute dyspnoea with pleuritic chest pain. You assess ABCs and carry out a brief physical examination and find tachycardia, hypotension, and signs of right ventricular strain. What is your immediate course of action?

- Give 100% oxygen through a non-rebreather mask with a reservoir bag.
- Obtain IV access. Take blood for FBC, clotting screen, D-dimers, cardiac enzymes, U&Es, and creatinine. ABGs should also be taken and may reveal reduced PaO_2, reduced $PaCO_2$, and acidosis.
- Give morphine 10 mg IV with an anti-emetic.
- Start unfractionated heparin 10000 U IV bolus, then 18 U/kg/h IVI as guided by APTT. Low molecular weight heparin can be given as an alternative.
- If systolic BP is >90 mmHg, confirm the diagnosis by carrying out ECG, chest X-ray, and computed tomographic pulmonary angiogram (CTPA) which is the gold standard for diagnosing PE. Chest X-ray is most often normal, but is useful in excluding other chest disease such as pneumothorax and pneumonia. ECG may reveal sinus tachycardia or AF, right ventricular strain, RBBB, and, uncommonly, the S_I, Q_{III}, T_{III} pattern: deep S waves in lead I, Q waves in lead III, and inverted T waves in lead III.
- Start warfarin 10 mg OD PO. Stop heparin once INR is in the range 2–3.
- If systolic BP is <90 mmHg, give a rapid colloid infusion and call for senior help. The patient may require inotropic support and thrombolysis. Surgical embolectomy is an alternative if immediately available.

Status epilepticus

You are the duty A&E doctor when a fitting patient is brought in by ambulance. You establish that the fitting started more than 20 minutes ago. What is your immediate course of action?

- Assess ABCs
- Secure the airway.
- Place the patient in the recovery position.
- Give 100% oxygen through a non-rebreather mask with a reservoir bag to prevent cerebral hypoxia from seizure activity. Regular suctioning may also be required.
- Record and monitor blood pressure.
- Obtain IV access.
- Take bloods for ABGs, glucose, U&Es, calcium, magnesium, LFTs, FBC, toxicology screen, and anticonvulsant levels to try to determine the cause of the seizures, e.g. hypoglycaemia, metabolic disturbance, alcohol, drugs, inadequate anticonvulsant dose, cerebral lesion or infection, and, if the patient is pregnant, eclampsia. Pseudo-seizures are a possibility to bear in mind. Obtain some information about the patient, e.g. from an accompanying relative, if at all possible.
- If hypoglycaemia is suspected to be the cause, give 50 ml of 50% dextrose IV. If alcohol is suspected to be the cause, give thiamine 250 mg IV over 10 minutes.
- To stop the seizures, give a benzodiazepine such as lorazepam 4 mg IV slowly or diazepam 10 mg IV/PR. IV benzodiazepines should only be given if resuscitation facilities are available.
- If this measure is unsuccessful, the next step is a phenytoin IV infusion. With a blood pressure and ECG monitor attached, give 15–18 mg/kg, at less than 50 mg/min.
- If this is unsuccessful, call for senior help and for an anaesthetist. General anaesthesia in ITU may be required.

Diabetic ketoacidosis

A 17 year old boy with no previous medical history presents to A&E complaining of vomiting and abdominal pain. When you see him, he appears severely dehydrated and is breathing heavily. You can smell ketones on his breath. What is your immediate course of action?

- Assess ABCs.
- Obtain a rapid blood glucose and urine dipstick for urinary ketones.
- Establish IV access and take blood for laboratory glucose, osmolality, U&Es, HCO_3^-, amylase, FBC, and blood cultures. Obtain an arterial sample for blood gases.
- Give IV fluids. Be careful, as one of the commonest causes of death in DKA (diabetic ketoacidosis) is from cerebral oedema from over-rapid rehydration. One regimen is to give 1 l of normal saline over 30 min followed by 1 l over 1 hour, 1 l over 2 hour, 1 l over 4 hour, and 1 l over 6 hours. Change to 5% dextrose once blood glucose is 10–15 mmol/l.
- Start a sliding scale of insulin via an IVI pump. Add 50 U of Actrapid to 50 ml of saline in a syringe, and give insulin at an initial rate of 4–8 U/h (4–8 ml/h).
- Monitor vital signs, ECG, glucose, U&Es, and HCO_3^-. Aim for a fall in glucose of 5 mmol/h. Plasma K^+ falls as K^+ enters cells, so KCl should be added to IV fluids as appropriate.
- Investigate the cause of the episode and treat any precipitating factors such as infection.
- Other measures:
  - give unfractionated heparin 5000 units TDS SC for venous thromboembolism prophylaxis
  - consider a naso-gastric tube if the patient is nauseated, vomiting, or unconscious
  - consider a urinary catheter if there is persistent hypotension, cardiac failure, renal failure, or no urine output for 2 hours
  - consider a CVP line in the frail and elderly or if there is cardiac failure or renal failure

Acute poisoning

- Carry out ABCs and take action as appropriate. Nurse in semi-prone position if unconscious.
- If possible, take a focussed history from the patient or friends/relatives focussing in particular on:
  - the drugs ingested and their quantities
  - associated alcohol or drug use
  - symptoms, including vomiting
  - other aspects of the history, particularly past medical history, past psychiatric history, and drug history

Carry out a full physical examination. If no history is available, try to identify the ingested drug from your findings.

Table 26. Acute poisoning – identifying the ingested drug

Drug	Signs and symptoms
Paracetamol	Initially: none or nausea, vomiting, and RUQ pain Later: jaundice, hypoglycaemia, encephalopathy, renal failure
Salicylates	Vomiting, dehydration, increased respiratory rate, hyperventilation, sweating, warm extremities, bounding pulse, tinnitus, vertigo, deafness, metabolic disturbances, pulmonary oedema, renal failure, seizures, coma
Opiates	Pin-point pupils (sometimes absent if other drugs are involved), nausea, vomiting, drowsiness, respiratory depression, coma

- Obtain IV access and take blood for FBC, U&Es, creatinine, LFTs, INR/PT/clotting screen, blood glucose, paracetamol and salicylate levels, other specific drug levels (as appropriate, contact senior colleagues or the National Poisons Information Service if unsure). Other investigations that need to be carried out include urine/serum toxicology screen, ABGs, and an ECG.
- Monitor vital signs such as respiratory rate, oxygen saturation, pulse rate, blood pressure, and temperature. Consider attaching a cardiac monitor to monitor ECG and inserting a urinary catheter to monitor urinary output.

- If appropriate, consider
  - gastric emptying and lavage, NB: gastric lavage alone is rarely used
  - activated charcoal (50 g in 200 ml water) to reduce the absorption of, for example, paracetamol or salicylates from the gut

Paracetamol

- Specialist help from the gastroenterology team should be sought early if severe liver damage is likely. In adults, 150 mg/kg or more may be fatal.
- Transfer to a specialist unit if systolic BP < 80 mmHg, blood pH < 7.3, INR > 2, creatinine > 200, or there are signs of encephalopathy or increased intracranial pressure.
- Repeat paracetamol level, ideally at 4 hours post-ingestion.
- If < 8 hours post-ingestion and paracetamol level is above the normal treatment line, give N-acetylcysteine (NAC, Parvolex) IVI as per protocol. If the patient is malnourished (e.g. in anorexia or alcoholism), or on an enzyme-inducing drug, prefer the high-risk treatment line instead (Figure 70).
- If > 8 hours post-ingestion and the patient has taken a significant overdose, start *N*-acetylcysteine and stop if paracetamol level returns below the treatment line and INR/ALT is normal. Note that paracetamol level is unreliable after 15 hours or in the event of a staggered overdose; simply treat according to the initial amount ingested.

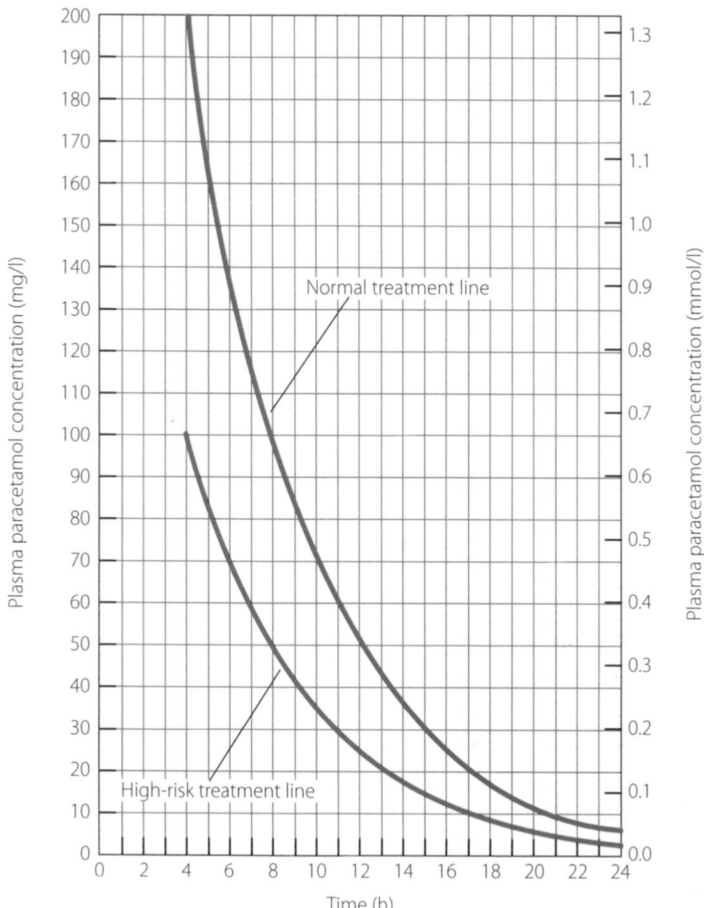

Figure 81. Paracetamol poisoning: normal and high-risk treatment lines.

- Continue monitoring vital signs at regular intervals and repeat U&Es, creatinine, LFTs, and INR/PT on the next day.

Salicylates

- IV fluid to correct any dehydration, with particular attention to K+ supplements.
- Give 1.26% sodium bicarbonate IVI to correct any metabolic acidosis.
- Repeat salicylate level at 2 hours post-ingestion: levels above 700 mg/l are potentially fatal: call for senior or specialist help.
- If plasma level > 700 mg/l or severe acidosis, renal failure, heart failure, or seizures, consider haemodialysis.
- Monitor salicylate levels, ABGs, blood glucose, U&Es, and urinary output.

Opiates

- Naloxone, e.g. 0.4–2 mg IV, titrated to response.
- As naloxone has a shorter half-life than opiates, it may need to be given often or as an intravenous infusion to prevent re-occurrence of signs and symptoms. If the patient is threatening to self-discharge, it can be given IM.
- Naloxone may precipitate severe withdrawal in high-dose opiate misusers, who may be very angry at you for ruining their 'trip'.

Once the patient is medically stable, he should be referred for a psychiatric assessment.

Bag-valve mask ventilation

Specifications: A mannequin in lieu of a patient.

- Open the airway using the head-tilt, chin-lift method. Remove any visible obstruction from the mouth.
- Identify the need for a Guedel airway (e.g. if the airway is obstructed or the patient is unconscious).
- Size the Guedel airway by measuring the distance from the incisors to the angle of the jaw. The most commonly used sizes are 2 for a small adult, 3 for a medium adult, and 4 for a large adult.
- Insert the Guedel airway so that its concave side faces away from the tongue. After inserting it almost to the back of the pharynx, rotate it 180 degrees and slide it in to its full extent.
- Choose an appropriately sized bag-valve mask.
- Attach the bag-valve mask to an oxygen supply. Adjust the flow rate to 15 l per minute.
- Hold the mask over the face with your dominant hand. Place your thumb over the nose and support the jaw with the middle and ring fingers (*Figure 82*). Ensuring a tight seal is difficult, so make sure you get sufficient practice.
- Maintain the head-tilt, chin-lift position.
- Use your free hand to compress the bag.
- Look for a rise in the chest.

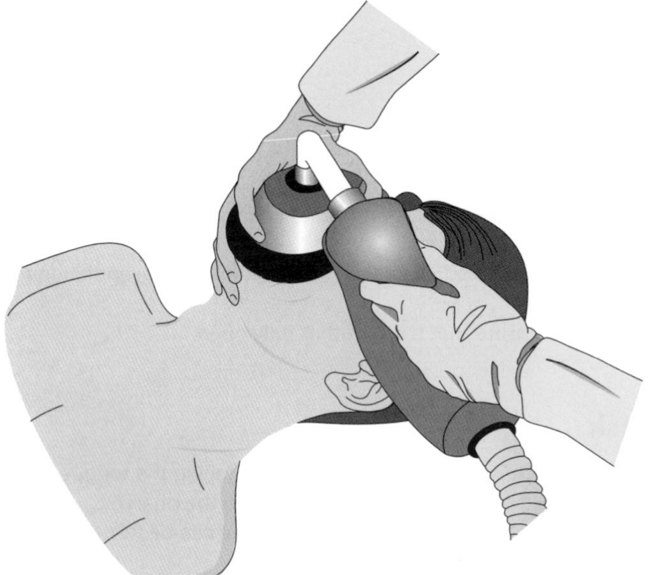

Figure 82. Bag-valve mask ventilation technique.

If a second person is available (e.g. the examiner), use both hands to hold the mask and get him to squeeze the bag.

- Ventilate at a rate of 10 compressions per minute until the patient starts breathing or until the patient can be intubated and put on a ventilator.

Laryngeal mask insertion

Specifications: A mannequin in lieu of a patient.

Table 27. Laryngeal mask sizes

Size 1	Infant
Size 2	Child
Size 3	Small adult
Size 4	Normal adult
Size 5	Large adult

The equipment

Gather in a tray:

- A pair of non-sterile gloves.
- Laryngeal mask of appropriate size (see *Table 27*).
- Lubricant.
- An air-filled syringe.
- A bandage.

Before inserting the laryngeal mask

- Don the gloves.
- Assemble the equipment.
- Check inflation and deflation of the laryngeal mask.
- Lubricate the laryngeal mask.
- Ensure that the patient has received adequate anaesthesia (the cough reflex should be suppressed).
- Ensure that the patient has been pre-oxygenated, or pre-oxygenate him by bag ventilation for 1 minute.
- Use the head-tilt, chin-lift technique to ensure that the mouth is fully open.
- Check the state of the dentition.

Inserting the laryngeal mask

- Insert the tip of the mask into the mouth, ensuring that the aperture is facing the tongue.
- Press the tip of the mask against the hard palate as you introduce it into the pharynx.
- Use your index finger to guide the tube into the pharynx until resistance can be felt.
- Check that the black line on the tube is facing the upper lip.

If you do not succeed in inserting the laryngeal mask within 30 seconds, you must pre-oxygenate the patient a second time before you try again.

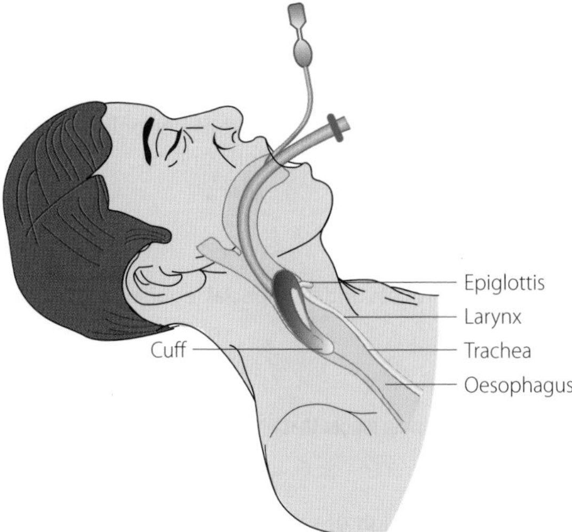

Figure 83. Laryngeal mask insertion.

After inserting the laryngeal mask

- Inflate the cuff, ensuring that you do not over-inflate it. A size 3 mask needs <20 ml of air, a size 4 <30 ml, and a size 5 <40 ml.
- Attach the breathing system and check that the patient is being satisfactorily ventilated.
- Secure the cuff in place by means of a length of bandage.

Pre-operative assessment

The surgical pre-assessment is about half the job of a surgical house officer, so is not unlikely to be examined in a final year OSCE. The aims of the pre-operative assessment are primarily to:

- Ascertain that the patient is fit for surgery and anaesthesia.
- Take appropriate action if he is not.
- Ensure that he fully understands the proposed procedure.
- Ensure that he fully understands the peri-operative process and any special requirements of the proposed procedure.
- Minimise any remaining fears or anxieties.

[Note] The responsibility for gaining informed consent from the patient is no longer that of the junior house officer, but that of the operating surgeon.

Specifications: In this station you may be asked to talk through or carry out a part or parts of the pre-operative assessment.

Before starting

- Introduce yourself to the patient.
- Explain that you are going to ask him some questions and carry out a physical examination to assess his fitness for surgery.
- Ensure that he is comfortable.

The assessment

History

- Medical history, in particular:
  - previous surgery and anaesthesia – ask specifically about history of anaesthetic complications, e.g. suxamethonium apnoea, malignant hyperpyrexia
  - previous hospital admissions
  - cardiovascular: hypertension, palpitations, angina, myocardial infarction, cardiac failure, orthopnoea, other 'heart problems', stroke or TIA
  - respiratory: dyspnoea, asthma, cough, tuberculosis
  - GI and renal: dysphagia, heartburn, liver disease, renal failure
  - other: diabetes, sickle cell anaemia, epilepsy, neuromuscular problems
- Drug history:
  - prescribed medication – ask specifically about recent changes in medication, insulin, and anticoagulants
  - over-the-counter and alternative medication
  - recreational drugs (especially cocaine, ecstasy, and narcotics)
- Allergies including to antiseptic, plaster, and latex.
- Smoking.
- Alcohol.

[Note] Most drugs should be taken as normal on the day of the surgery, although special advice is needed for insulin and anticoagulants.

- Family history of allergic reactions, anaesthetic complications, medical and surgical conditions.
- Social history, e.g. level of support in post-operative period.

Physical examination

- Record height and weight and calculate his body mass index as given by weight in kilograms/(height in metres)^2, e.g. 70 kg/(1.8 m)^2 = 21.6 (normal 20–25).
- Examine the cardiovascular, respiratory, gastrointestinal, and neurological systems.
- Assess neck mobility by asking the patient to flex and extend his neck.
- Assess jaw mobility by asking the patient to open and close his mouth.
- Inspect the state of the dentition.
- Carry out a Mallampati pharyngeal assessment. To do this you need to ask the patient to open his mouth as wide as possible and to extend his tongue (*Figure 84*).

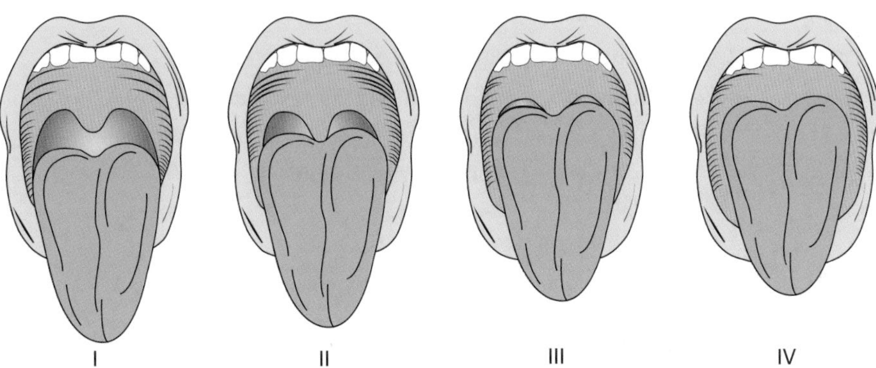

Figure 84. Mallampati pharyngeal assessment:
I – Pharyngeal pillars, soft palate, and uvula visible;
II – Soft palate and uvula visible;
III – Soft palate and the base of the uvula visible;
IV – Soft palate not visible
NB: Mallampati scores of III or IV are relative contraindications to surgery

- Determine the ASA physical status rating, a health index at the time of surgery (*Table 28*).

Table 28. The ASA physical status rating

1*	Healthy, no systemic disturbance
2*	Mild/moderate systemic disease. No activity limitation.
3*	Severe systemic disturbance. Some activity limitation.
4*	Life-threatening systemic disturbance. Severe activity limitation.
5*	Moribund with limited chance of survival.

* Add suffix *E* for emergency.

Pre-operative investigations

Table 29. Indications for pre-operative investigations	
Group and save/cross-match	Group and save for e.g. cholecystectomy, ERCP, mastectomy, amputation Cross-match for e.g. laparotomy (2 units), TURP (3 units), hip replacement (4 units), liver surgery (6 units), aneurysm repair (4 units if elective, 10 units if emergency)
FBC	Cardiorespiratory disease, anaemia, blood loss, chronic disease, blood disorders, on an oral anticoagulant, alcohol misuse, female patients, male patients > 40 years
Clotting screen	Liver disease, alcohol misuse, on an anticoagulant
Sickle cell screening	Patients from Africa, the Caribbean, and the Mediterranean
U&Es	Hypertension, heart failure, renal failure, liver disease, diabetes, dehydration, starvation, on diuretics, digoxin, steroids, or lithium, age > 60 and having major surgery
Glucose	Diabetes, obesity, on steroids
LFTs (including clotting screen)	Liver disease, alcohol misuse, malignancy, malnutrition
ECG	Arrhythmias, angina, myocardial infarction, heart murmurs, heart failure, cardiovascular risk factors, age > 50
CXR	Hypertension, cardiorespiratory disease or symptoms, malignancy, > 60 years old and having major surgery, recent immigrant
Cervical spine X-ray	Severe chronic rheumatoid arthritis, cervical spondylosis
Other	TFTs in thyroid disease Amylase in abdominal pain or hepatobiliary surgery Lung function tests in severe respiratory disease Drug levels, e.g. if on digoxin or lithium HIV

Peri-operative management

Explain about:

- Fasting, in most cases:
  - stop solids from 6 hours before the operation
  - stop milky drinks from 4 hours
  - stop clear fluids (and chewing gum) from 2 hours
- Pre-medication:
  - benzodiazepines can be given before the operation to help the patient feel sleepy or less anxious
- The anaesthetic procedure:
  - patient information about different anaesthetic procedures can be obtained from www.kch.nhs.uk/patients/general-information/leaflets/ – look for "You and Your Anaesthetic"
- Post-operative pain relief:
  - oral analgesia, e.g. paracetamol, cocodamol, NSAIDs such as diclofenac and ibuprofen, tramadol, opiates

- parenteral analgesia
- suppositories
- local anaesthetics and regional blocks
- patient-controlled analgesia
- patches

- Post-operative nausea and vomiting:
  - explain to the patient that he may feel sick after the operation and reassure him that this is quite normal and that he can be given an anti-sickness tablet or injection
- Going home and driving.

After the procedure

- Ask the patient if he has any remaining questions or concerns.
- Thank the patient.
- Order the appropriate investigations (*Table 29*) and remember to check up on the results!
- Talk to the anaesthetist if you have any concerns.

Syringe driver operation

There are two different sorts of syringe driver: the 50 ml syringe pump, frequently used for heparin, glyceryl trinitrate, and insulin infusions, and for epidural and patient-controlled analgesia; and the Graseby syringe driver, which installs a 10 ml or 20 ml syringe and is frequently used in palliative care. There are two varieties of the Graseby syringe driver: the blue Graseby MS 16A, which is designed to be programmed at an hourly rate, and the green Graseby MS 26, which is designed to be programmed at a 12, 24, or 48 hourly rate. In this station, you may be required to set up and operate a Graseby syringe driver for two drugs, e.g. diamorphine and cyclizine.

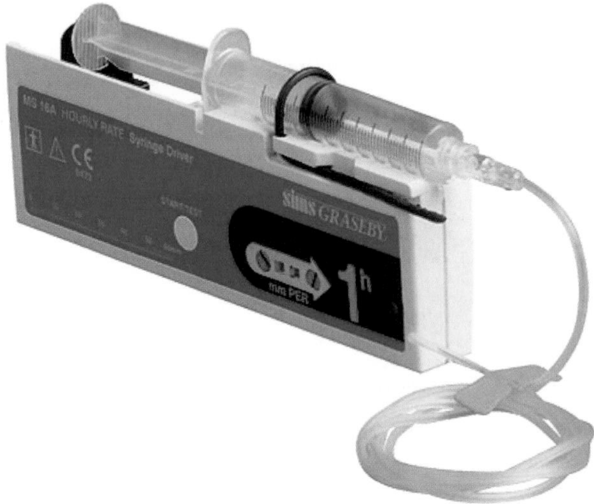

Figure 85. The blue Graseby MS 16A, designed to be programmed at an hourly rate.

Before starting

- Introduce yourself to the patient.
- Explain the need for a syringe driver and the procedure involved, and gain consent.
- Gather the appropriate equipment.

The equipment

- Non-sterile gloves.
- Graseby syringe driver (check the battery is in place and the device is functioning).
- Luer-lock syringe (10 ml or 20 ml).
- Subcutaneous giving set.
- Drug.
- Diluent (sterile water or normal saline).

The procedure

- Consult the prescription chart and check:
  - the identity of the patient
  - the prescription: drug(s), dose(s), diluent, route of administration, duration of the infusion, date and time of starting
  - drug allergies
- Check the name, dose, and expiry date of the drug(s) on the vial(s).
- Ask a colleague (registered nurse or doctor) to confirm the name, dose, and expiry date of the drug(s) on the vial(s).
- Don a pair of non-sterile gloves.
- Draw up the correct doses of the drugs into the Luer-lock syringe.
- Draw up the correct diluent to make up the requested volume (stated on the prescription chart) and shake the syringe with the needle capped.
- Connect the giving set to the syringe and run the infusion through it.
- Calculate the rate of infusion by measuring the length of liquid in the syringe in millimetres and dividing it by the number of hours (Graseby 16A) or days (Graseby MS 26) over which the infusion should be given.
- Label the syringe with:
  - the patient's name, date of birth, and hospital number
  - the date and time of preparation
  - drugs used and their doses
  - diluent used and its volume
  - rate of infusion
  - your name
- Place the syringe into the syringe driver and secure the device.
- Set the syringe driver to the rate required.
- Place the giving set subcutaneously and start the infusion.

After the procedure

- Sign the drug chart, and have your checking colleague countersign it.
- Ask the patient if he has any questions or concerns.
- Ensure that he is comfortable.

Patient-Controlled Analgesia (PCA) explanation

In PCA, the patient presses a button to activate an infusion pump and receive a pre-prescribed intravenous bolus of analgesic, most commonly morphine or another opioid such as diamorphine, pethidine, or fentanyl.

Advantages

- Prevents delays in analgesic administration and thereby minimises pain. In the post-operative period this may forestall a number of adverse events such as disability, pressure sores, DVT, PE, atelectasis, and constipation.
- Minimises the amount of analgesic used, as the patient only activates the pump if he is actually in pain. Other people, such as relatives, should be told not to activate the pump.
- Provides a reliable indication of the patient's pain, and its evolution over time.
- Reduces the chance of dangerous medication errors, as the pump is programmed according to a set prescription and 'locks out' if the patient tries to activate it too often. A typical dose regimen is a 0.5–2.0 mg bolus of morphine with a lock-out of 10–15 minutes.

Disadvantages

- Patients may not receive enough analgesia (see later). In particular, patients may wake up in pain, as they cannot press the button when they are asleep.
- Patients may be physically or mentally unable to press a button.
- The pumps are expensive and may malfunction, especially if the battery is not adequately charged.

Side-effects

Side-effects of morphine include:

- respiratory depression
- sedation
- nausea and vomiting
- constipation
- urinary retention
- pruritus

Some of these side-effects can be controlled by additional prescriptions of, for example, anti-emetics, laxatives, or antihistamines. If the patient is suffering from significant respiratory depression or sedation, the dose should be decreased and alternative analgesia considered. (Remember that respiratory depression or sedation can also be caused by important post-operative complications, so do not omit to exclude these.)

Monitoring

Patients should be reviewed at regular intervals for pain, analgesic usage, and side-effects; observations should be made of the patient's pain score, analgesic usage, pulse, blood pressure, respiratory rate, and oxygen saturation. If pain relief is inadequate, the dose regime should be altered. In some cases, a continuous 'background' infusion might be considered.

Epidural analgesia explanation

Epidural analgesia, or 'epidural', is a form of regional anaesthesia involving the injection of local anaesthetics and/or opioids through a catheter inserted into the epidural space. Epidurals can be indicated for analgesia in labour (often simply as a matter of patient choice), for surgical anaesthesia in certain operations, e.g. caesarean section, and as an adjunct to general anaesthesia in others, e.g. laparatomy, hysterectomy, hip replacement. They can also be indicated for post-operative analgesia, back pain, and palliative care.

Advantages

- Permits analgesia to be delivered as a continuous infusion and/or to be patient-controlled.
- Effective and safe, with a mortality of only about 1 in 100 000.
- In post-operative analgesia, reduces the risk of certain post-operative complications such as nausea and vomiting, chest infections, and constipation.

Disadvantages

- 5% failure rate.
- In labour, increases the risk of an assisted delivery.

Contraindications

Absolute

- Raised intracranial pressure.
- Coagulopathy/anticoagulation.
- Hypovolaemia.
- Skin infection at epidural site.
- Septicaemia.

Relative

- Un-cooperative patient.
- Anatomical abnormalities or previous spinal surgery.
- Certain neurological disorders.
- Certain heart-valve problems.

Procedure

Epidurals are normally performed by a trained anaesthetist with the patient either in the preferred sitting position or in the left lateral position. The planned entry site is identified and marked. After the skin is cleaned and local anaesthetic administered, a Tuohy needle is advanced until a loss of resistance is felt anterior to the *ligamentum flavum*. The cathether, a fine plastic tube, is then threaded through the needle and the needle is removed, leaving the catheter in place. As epidurals are usually carried out in the mid-lumbar region, there is very little risk of injuring the spinal cord.

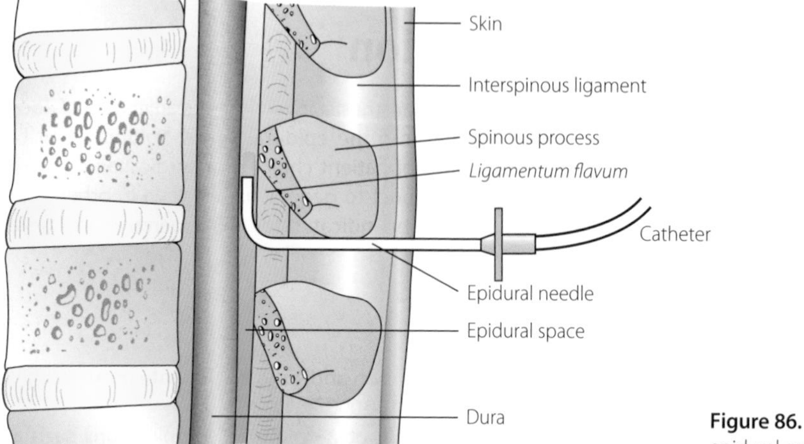

Figure 86. Anatomy of the epidural space.

Side-effects and complications

- Side-effects of opioids.
- In higher doses can result in loss of other modalities of sensation (such as touch and proprioception) and motor function.
- Hypotension, most often resulting from loss of sympathetic function.
- Urinary retention.
- Accidental dural puncture resulting in a leak and a severe headache that is exacerbated by raising the head above horizontal.
- Accidental infusion into the CSF resulting in a high block or, more rarely, a total spinal involving profound hypotension, respiratory paralysis, and unconsciousness.
- Epidural haematoma that can cause spinal compression.
- Abscess formation.

Monitoring

Patients receiving epidural analgesia should be monitored for pain intensity, drug-related side-effects, and signs of complications due to the epidural procedure.

Wound suturing

Specifications: A pad of 'skin' in lieu of a patient. This station most likely requires you to talk through the parts of the procedure and then to demonstrate your suturing technique. For this second part, there can be no substitute for practice, practice, and more practice!

Before starting

- Introduce yourself to the patient.
- Explain the procedure and ask for his consent to carry it out.
- Examine the wound, looking for debris, dirt, and tendon damage.
- Indicate that you would request an X-ray to exclude a foreign body.
- Assess distal motor, sensory, and vascular function.
- Position the patient appropriately and ensure that he is comfortable.

The equipment

Gather in a tray or on a trolley:

- a pair of sterile gloves
- a suture pack
- a suture of appropriate type (monofilament non-absorbable for superficial wounds, absorbable for deep wounds) and size (3/0 for scalp and trunk, 4/0 for limbs, 5/0 for hands, 6/0 for face)
- a 5 ml syringe, 21G and 25G needles, and a vial of local anaesthetic (e.g. 1% lignocaine)
- antiseptic solution
- a sharps bin

The procedure

- Wash your hands.
- Open the suture pack, thus creating a sterile field.
- Pour antiseptic solution into the receptacle.
- Open the suture, the syringe, and both needles onto the sterile field.
- Wash your hands using sterile technique.
- Don the non-sterile gloves.
- Attach a 21G needle to the syringe.
- Ask an assistant (the examiner) to open the vial of local anaesthetic and draw up 5 ml of local anaesthetic. For an average 70 kg adult, up to 20 ml of 1% lignocaine can be safely used, although 5–10 ml is usually sufficient. Epinephrine may be used with lignocaine to minimise bleeding. The maximum safe dose of lignocaine with or without epinephrine is 7 mg/kg and 3 mg/kg respectively. However, avoid injecting epinephrine when anaesthetising the extremities due to the risk of ischaemic tissue necrosis.
- Discard the needle into the sharps bin and attach the 25G needle to the syringe.
- Clean the wound (use forceps) with antiseptic-soaked cotton wool and drape the field. Dirty wounds may benefit from cleansing with povidone iodine, whereas normal saline can be used to cleanse and irrigate 'clean' wounds.
- Inject the local anaesthetic into the apices and edges of the wound. Make sure to pull back on the plunger before injecting.
- Discard the needle into the sharps bin.
- Indicate that you would give the anaesthetic 5–10 minutes to operate (or as long as it takes).

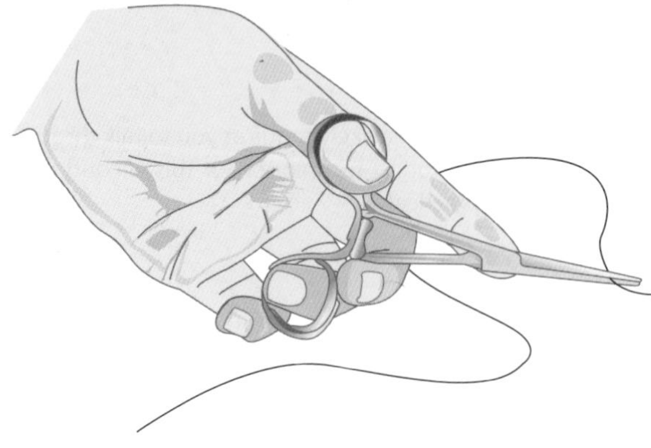

Figure 87. Use needle-holding forceps to hold the needle approximately two-thirds from the needle tip.

- Apply the sutures approximately 3 mm from the wound edge and 5–10 mm apart. Use needle-holding forceps to hold the needle and toothed forceps to pick up the skin margins. Knot the sutures around the needle-holding forceps.

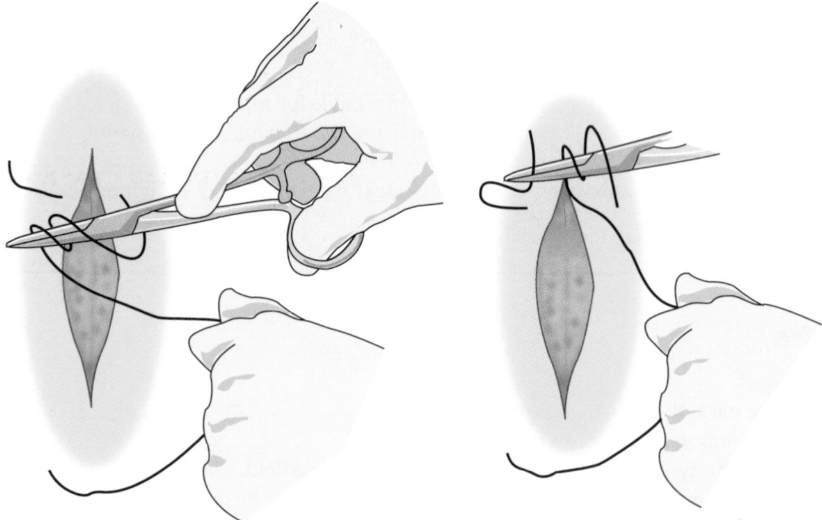

Figure 88. Suggested approach for suturing. Knot the sutures around the needle-holding forceps: loop the suture twice around the nose of the needle-holding forceps using your hand. Then take hold of the short end of the suture with the needle-holding forceps and carry it through the loops, gently pulling the knot tight. Two further single loops are then added in a similar fashion to secure the knot. Each loop is pulled in the opposite direction across the wound edge.

After the procedure

- Clean the wound and indicate that you would apply a dressing.
- Assess the need for a tetanus injection.
- Give appropriate instructions for wound care and indicate the date sutures should be removed (e.g. face 3–4 days, scalp 5 days, trunk 7 days, limbs 7–10 days, feet 10–14 days).
- Ask if the patient has any questions or concerns.
- Thank the patient.

Blood glucose measurement and interpretation

Specifications: In this station you are far more likely to be asked to talk through the procedure rather than carry it out on a patient or actor.

Before starting

- Introduce yourself to the patient.
- Explain the procedure and ask for his consent to carry it out.
- Establish when he last ate (fasting blood glucose is usually carried out in the morning before the patient has had anything to eat or drink).

The equipment

In a tray, gather:

- a pair of gloves
- an alcohol wipe
- a glucose monitor
- test strips
- a spring-loaded pricker
- a lancet
- cotton wool

The procedure

- Ask the patient to wash and dry his hands, or use an alcohol wipe to clean the finger that you are going to prick.
- Massage the finger from its base to its tip to increase its perfusion.
- Turn on the glucose monitor and ensure that it is calibrated.
- Check that the test strips have not expired.
- Insert a test strip into the glucose monitor.
- Load the lancet into the pricker and prick the side of the finger.

It is less painful to prick the side rather than the tip of a finger because there are comparatively fewer nerve endings there.

- Squeeze the finger to obtain a droplet of blood. If no or insufficient blood is obtained, prick the finger again. If this happens, be sympathetic to the patient's plight.
- Place the droplet of blood on the test strip, so as to cover the sensor entirely.
- Give the patient some cotton wool to stop any bleeding.
- Record the reading on the monitor. Units are in millimoles per litre.

After the procedure

- Tell that patient their blood glucose and explain its significance and any further action that needs to be taken, e.g. fasting blood glucose, glucose tolerance test, laboratory measurement. Note that the diagnosis of diabetes in a symptomatic patient should never be made on the basis of a single abnormal blood glucose measurement.
- Ask the patient if he has any questions or concerns.
- Thank the patient.

Table 30. Blood glucose measurement: interpretation of result (normal results vary from lab to lab)

	Units are in millimoles per litre
Normal	
fasting glucose	< 6.0
non-fasting glucose*	< 7.8
Impaired glucose tolerance	
fasting glucose	6–7
non-fasting glucose	7.8–11.1
Diabetes mellitus	
fasting glucose	≥ 7.0
non-fasting glucose	≥ 11.1

* 2-h post 75 g glucose.

Examiner's questions

Complications of type II diabetes

Hyperosmolar non-ketotic coma (HONK), retinopathy and cataracts, nephropathy progressing to renal failure, cardiovascular disease predisposing to increased risk of myocardial infarction and stroke, peripheral vascular disease, peripheral and autonomic neuropathy (most frequently distal symmetric sensorimotor polyneuropathy in a glove-and-stocking distribution and oculomotor mononeuropathy), infections, foot ulcers progressing to diabetic foot disease, impotence, miscarriage, stillbirth.

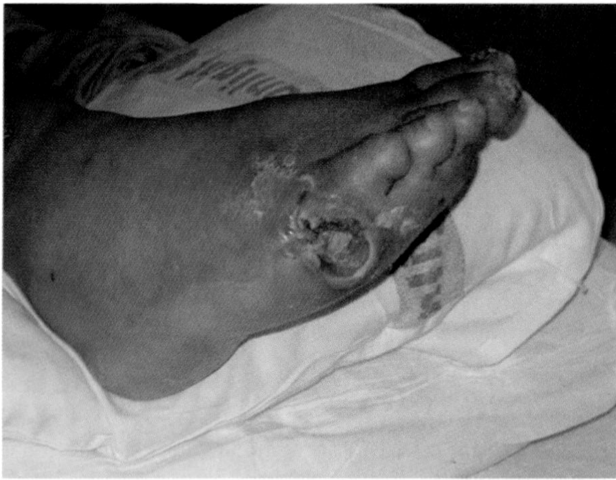

Figure 89. Diabetic foot.

Reproduced with permission from www.londonvascularclinic.com.

Urine sample testing and interpretation

Before starting

- Introduce yourself to the patient.
- Take a very brief history from him.
- Explain that you are going to test his urine and explain why.
- Ensure that the urine specimen is fresh and that it has been appropriately collected (genitalia have been cleaned, bottle has not come into contact with body, only mid-stream urine has been collected).

The equipment

- Urine dipstick and urine dipstick bottle.
- A pair of gloves.
- A pen and paper (or the patient's case notes).

The procedure

- Put on the gloves.
- Inspect the colour and appearance of the urine.
- Stir the urine bottle to ensure that the urine is mixed.
- Check the expiry date on the urine dipstick jar.
- Briefly immerse the urine dipstick into the urine specimen.
- Tap off any excess urine from the dipstick.
- Hold the strip horizontally.
- After 2 minutes, read each colour pad using the colour chart on the dipstick bottle.
- Report and record the results.
- Discard the used urine dipstick and the gloves.
- Wash your hands.

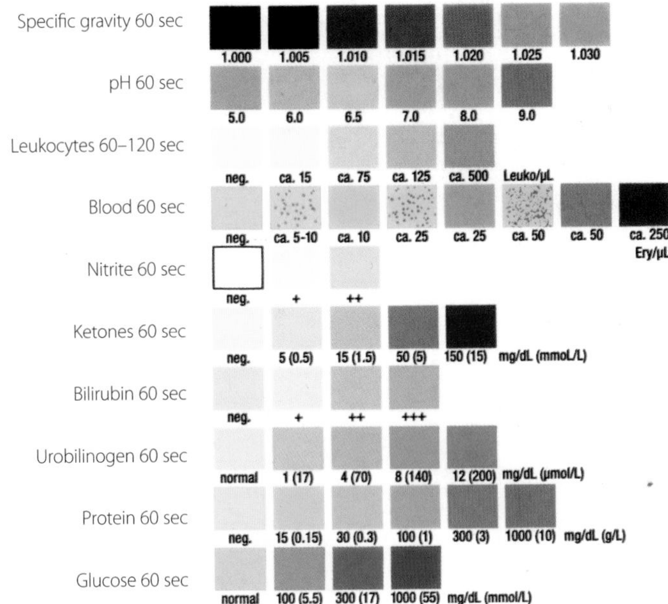

Figure 90. The colour chart on the urine dipstick bottle.

After testing the urine

- Explain the results to the patient.
- Document the results in the patient's notes.
- If abnormal, suggest obtaining a second sample of urine or sending the urine for laboratory analysis.
- Thank the patient.

Table 31. Urine dipstick: interpretation of results

Leukocytes	Urinary tract infection
Nitrites	Bacteriuria, contaminated sample
Protein	Kidney damage or disease, standing upright for prolonged periods, exercise, fever, pregnancy, rarer causes, e.g. leukaemia, multiple myeloma, pre-eclampsia
Blood	Kidney damage or disease, urinary calculi, urinary tract infection, contaminated sample, exercise, dehydration, myoglobinuria
Ketones	Diabetic ketoacidosis, starvation, alcohol intoxication
Glucose	Diabetes mellitus, pregnancy

Blood test interpretation

1. Reference ranges are based on a Gaussian or normal distribution, and usually include about 95% of the population. This means that a result only slightly outside the reference range is not necessarily 'abnormal'.
2. Reference ranges do vary from one laboratory to another – don't let this confuse you!

Full blood count

	Normal range
Hb	13–18 g/dl (males); 11.5–16 g/dl (females)
RCC	4.5–6.5 × 10^{12}/l (males); 3.9–5.6 × 10^{12}/l (females)
PCV	0.4–0.54 (males); 0.37–0.47 (females)
MCV	76–96 fl
MCHC	30–36 g/dl
WCC	4.0–11.0 × 10^9/l
neutrophils	2.0–7.5 × 10^9/l (40–75% WCC)
lymphocytes	1.3–3.5 × 10^9/l (20–45%)
eosinophils	0.04–0.44 × 10^9/l (1–6%)
basophils	0–0.10 × 10^9/l (0–1%)
monocytes	0.2–0.8 × 10^9/l (2–10%)
Platelets	150–400 × 10^9/l

- Haemoglobin (Hb) and red cell count (RCC) are increased in dehydration, chronic hypoxia, or polycythaemia. The term 'anaemia' describes a Hb of < 13 g/dl in males and < 11.5 g/dl in females. Anaemia has many causes, including iron deficiency, folate or vitamin B12 deficiency, chronic illness, blood loss, and blood cell destruction.
- Packed cell volume (PCV) or 'haematocrit' is the fraction of total blood volume occupied by red cells; it decreases in anaemia and increases in dehydration, chronic hypoxia, and polycythaemia.
- Mean corpuscular volume (MCV) is the average volume of a red blood cell, and is thus equivalent to PCV/RCC; it decreases in iron deficiency, chronic disease, thalassaemia, and sideroblastic anaemia and increases in folate or vitamin B12 deficiency, alcoholism, liver disease, hypothyroidism, pregnancy, reticulocytosis (e.g. in haemolysis), and other haematological diseases.
- Mean corpuscular haemoglobin concentration (MCHC) is the average concentration of haemoglobin in red cells, and decreases in iron deficiency, chronic disease, and chronic blood loss.
- A raised white cell count (WCC) or leukocytosis may indicate infection, inflammation, major tissue damage, or certain lymphoproliferative disorders. The *differential* white cell count is useful in determining the probable cause of a leukocytosis. For example, a raised neutrophil count or neutrophilia may indicate acute bacterial infection, acute inflammation, or major tissue damage, and a raised eosinophil count or eosinophilia may indicate an allergic reaction or parasitic infection.
- A raised platelet count or thrombocytosis may result from haemorrhage, chronic inflammatory conditions, hyposplenism, and certain myeloproliferative disorders, e.g. chronic myelogenous leukaemia. A low platelet count or thrombocytopaenia may result from decreased platelet production (e.g. folate or vitamin B12 deficiency, infection, cancer treatment), increased platelet destruction (e.g. immune thrombocytopaenic purpura, disseminated intravascular coagulation, systemic lupus erythematosus), or certain drugs.

Iron studies (haematinics)

	Normal range
Serum iron	14–31 μmol/l (males); 11–30 μmol/l (females)
Ferritin	12–200 μg/l
TIBC	54–75 μg/l
Folate	2.1 μg/l
Vitamin B12	0.13–0.68 nmol/l

- Ferritin is the main protein that stores iron, and so serum ferritin reflects the body's iron stores.
- Total iron binding capacity (TIBC) reflects the amount of transferrin, a protein that transfers iron from the gut, in the serum.
- Iron deficiency and chronic disease may both lead to a decrease in serum iron, and therefore to a microcytic anaemia. In investigating the cause of a microcytic anaemia, serum iron must be looked at in conjuction with serum ferritin and TIBC. In iron deficiency anaemia, serum ferritin is decreased and TIBC is increased. In contrast, in anaemia of chronic disease, serum ferritin is often increased and TIBC often decreased. Note that, in some cases, anaemic of chronic disease can also present with a normal MCV. Other causes of a normocytic anaemia include acute blood loss and renal failure.
- By contrast, folate and vitamin B12 deficiency result in a macrocytic anaemia. Folate levels decrease if dietary intake of folate is inadequate or if demand for folate is increased (e.g. pregnancy, increased cell turnover) and in alcoholism, malabsorption, pernicious anaemia, and treatment with certain drugs such as phenytoin and sodium valproate. Vitamin B12 levels decrease if dietary intake of vitamin B12 is inadequate, and in malabsorption and pernicious anaemia.

Coagulation tests

	Normal range
PT	10–14 s
APTT	35–45 s
TT	10–15 s
INR	0.9–1.2
D-dimers	<0.5 mg/l

- A lack of factors I, II, V, VII, and X or fibrinogen leads to an increase in prothrombin time (PT). PT thus tests the extrinsic system and is prolonged by warfarin treatment, vitamin K deficiency, liver disease, and DIC.
- A lack of factors I, II, V, VIII, IX, XI, or XII leads to an increase in activated partial thromboplastin time (APTT). APTT thus tests the intrinsic system and is prolonged by heparin treatment, haemophilia, liver disease, and DIC.
- Thrombin time (TT) is prolonged by a deficiency of factor I (fibrinogen), heparin treatment, and DIC.
- INR is the ratio of PT to mean PT in a normal population, and should thus be around 1. Target INR for DVT and PE prophylaxis is 2–3 (3.5 if recurrent), but 3–4 for prosthetic metallic heart valves.
- D-dimers are a fibrin degradation product, and are raised in DVT, PE, and DIC, but also in inflammatory states.

ESR

	Normal range
ESR	< 20 mm/h Or, for males, (age in years)/2, and for females (age in years + 10)/2

- A raised erythrocyte sedimentation rate (ESR) is a non-specific finding that often results from inflammation, but sometimes also from injury or malignancy. Serial ESR measurements can be used to monitor disease severity and treatment response in inflammatory disorders such as rheumatoid arthritis and temporal arteritis.

Thyroid function tests

	Normal range
TSH	0.5–5.7 mU/l
Thyroxine (T4)	70–140 nmol/l
Free T4	9–22 pmol/l
Tri-iodothyronine (T3)	1.2–3 nmol/l
TBG	7–17 mg/l

- Typical findings in hyperthyroidism are decreased TSH (thyroid-stimulating hormone) and increased (or normal) T4, free T4, and T3.
- Typical findings in hypothyroidism are increased TSH and decreased (or normal) T4 and free T4.
- Increased TSH and increased T4 suggest a TSH-secreting tumour.
- Decreased TSH, T4, and T3 suggest pituitary disease or 'sick euthyroidism', which can be seen in any systemic illness.
- T4 and T3 are increased if TBG (thyroxine-binding globulin) is increased (e.g. in pregnancy or oestrogen therapy) and vice versa.

Liver function tests

	Normal range
Bilirubin	3–17 μmol/l
ALT	5–35 U/l
AST	5–35 U/l
ALP	30–150 U/l
GGT	11–51 U/l (males); 7–33 U/l (females)
Albumin	35–50 g/l

- The amount of bilirubin in the blood reflects the balance between that produced by red cell destruction and that removed by the liver. A raised bilirubin level results either from diseases causing increased red blood cell destruction, diseases causing hepatocellular damage, or diseases causing biliary obstruction and thereby restricting the excretion of bilirubin. The latter is suggested by a high ratio of conjugated bilirubin to unconjugated bilirubin.
- Raised ALT and AST suggest hepatocellular damage. ALT (alanine aminotransferase) is a relatively specific marker of hepatocellular damage, and is most raised in the acute phase. Although ALT is also present in cardiac muscle, the rises seen in myocardial infarction are comparatively small. AST is a less specific marker of hepatocellular damage than ALT and may also be raised in myocardial infarction, skeletal muscle damage, haemolysis, shock, pregnancy, and exercise.

- Raised ALP and GGT suggest biliary obstruction. ALP (alkaline phosphatise) is raised in biliary obstruction, hepatocellular damage, some bone diseases, and pregnancy. GGT (gamma-glutamyl transferase) is raised in alcohol consumption, and also in biliary obstruction and hepatocellular damage.
- Albumin is a genuine test of liver function and falls in chronic liver disease. Other causes for a fall in albumin include malnutrition, malabsorption, nephrotic syndrome, burns, pregnancy, and overhydration, e.g. with IV fluids. A rise in albumin is usually the consequence of dehydration.

Urea and electrolytes

	Normal range
Sodium	135–145 mmol/l
Potassium	3.5–5.0 mmol/l
Calcium (total)	2.12–2.65 mmol/l
Bicarbonate	24–28 mmol/l
Urea	2.5–6.7 mmol/l
Creatinine	70–150 µmol/l

Hyponatraemia

- Hyponatraemia is commonly caused by the syndrome of inappropriate secretion of antidiuretic hormone (SIADH), which itself has a large number of causes including malignancy, pulmonary disorders, central nervous system disorders, and drugs. Other common causes of hyponatraemia are inappropriate fluid therapy, diuretic treatment, diarrhoea and vomiting, and cardiac and renal failure. For the causes of hyponatraemia, see *Figure 91*. Note that high serum glucose, urea, proteins, or lipids can increase serum volume and result in a pseudohyponatraemia.

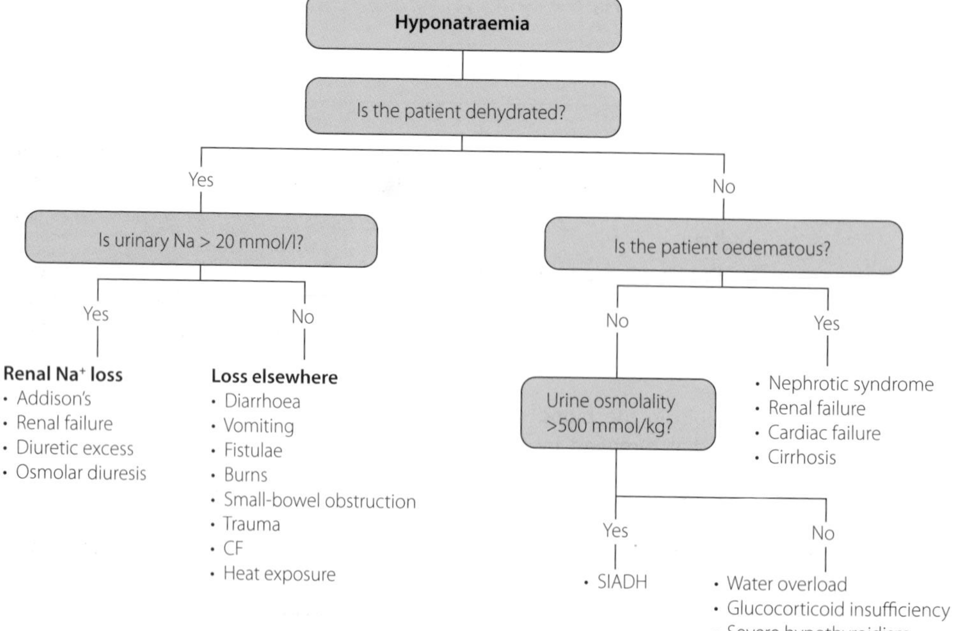

Figure 91. Causes of hyponatraemia.

- Hyponatraemia may be asymptomatic or may produce nausea, vomiting, headache, confusion, convulsions, and coma.
- Treat the cause. It is important to determine the volume status of the patient. If the patient is hypovolaemic, a normal saline infusion may be indicated. Particularly in chronic hyponatraemia, correction should be cautious and gradual (a maximum of 15 mmol/day) so as to avoid the complication of central pontine myelinosis. If the patient is hypervolaemic, fluid restriction (with or without frusemide) may be indicated. Hypertonic saline should only be used in emergency situations.

Hypernatraemia

- Causes include:
  - insufficient water intake
  - inappropriate fluid therapy
  - fluid loss, e.g. through diarrhoea, vomiting, and burns
  - diuretic treatment
  - osmotic diuresis, e.g. in hyperglycaemia
  - diabetes insipidus
  - mineralocorticoid excess as in Conn's syndrome or Cushing's syndrome
- Symptoms include thirst, confusion, convulsions, and coma.
- Treat through oral rehydration or a 5% dextrose infusion, e.g. 4 litres over 24 hours. Note that over-rapid correction of hypernatraemia can lead to cerebral oedema and convulsions, brain damage, and death.

Hypokalaemia

- Causes include:
  - gastrointestinal losses as in vomiting, diarrhoea, laxative use, villous adenoma
  - renal losses as in thiazide or loop diuretic treatment (most common cause), mineralocorticoid excess (e.g. Conn's syndrome, Cushing's syndrome), and renal tubular acidosis
  - shift into cells as in insulin treatment, metabolic alkalosis, high catecholamines (e.g. due to pain)
  - poor intake as in prolonged fasting, eating disorders
  - re-feeding syndrome
  - hypomagnesaemia
- In mild cases, hypokalaemia is often asymptomic. In severe cases, the clinical picture is dominated by muscle weakness which can progress to flaccid paralysis and, rarely, respiratory failure. ECG changes may include T wave flattening, ST segment depression, appearance of U waves, and tachyarrhythmias.
- Treatment involves addressing the cause and supplementing potassium, either orally or as an intravenous infusion, depending on severity. Note that too concentrated an infusion is painful and damages peripheral veins, and too fast an infusion predisposes to ventricular tachyarrhythmias.

Hyperkalaemia

- Causes include:
  - artefact due to haemolysis of the blood sample (repeat the measurement)
  - excessive intake, most likely in the form of potassium supplements
  - impaired excretion as in renal insufficiency, Addison's disease (reduced mineralocorticoids), treatment with potassium-sparing diuretics and NSAIDs
  - shift out of cells as in diabetic ketoacidosis and other metabolic acidoses
  - excessive release from cells, as in burns, rhabdomyolysis, tumour lysis, massive blood transfusion

- Although hyperkalaemia is usually asymptomatic, it can lead to cardiac arrhythmia and sudden death. For this reason, an ECG should be carried out as soon as hyperkalaemia is suggested. ECG findings include tall, tented T waves, broadened QRS complex, prolonged PR interval, P wave flattening, and a sine wave appearance.
- In mild hyperkalaemia, potassium intake should be restricted. In severe hyperkalaemia, or if there are ECG changes, IV calcium gluconate should be administered to stabilise the myocardium. IV insulin with glucose, the potassium-binding resin calcium resonium, and dialysis can then be used to reduce potassium.

Calcium

- Calcium (total) needs to be adjusted for albumin by adding 0.1 mmol/l for every 4 g/l that albumin is below 40 g/l, and subtracting 0.1 mmol/l for every 4 g/l that albumin is above 40 g/l.
- Hypocalcaemia may be caused by hypomagnesaemia, hyperphosphataemia, hypoparathyroidism, pseudohypoparathyroidism (failure of cells to respond to parathyroid hormone), vitamin D deficiency, and chronic renal failure. Symptoms include depression, perioral paraesthesiae, carpo-pedal spasm (hence Trousseau's sign), neuromuscular excitability (hence Chvostek's sign), tetany, laryngospasm, and cardiac arrhythmias. Treatment involves treating the cause and, depending on severity, oral or IV calcium replacement.
- 90% of cases of hypercalcaemia are accounted for by either malignancy or hyperparathyroidism. Symptoms include fatigue, confusion, depression, anorexia, nausea and vomiting, constipation, abdominal pain, polyuria, renal calculi, and cardiac arrest. Management involves treating the hypercalcaemia and its underlying cause. Treating the hypercalcaemia involves fluids (normal saline), frusemide, and bisphonates, e.g. pamidronate.

For acid–base disturbances, see *Station 101*.

Urea and creatinine

- Urea is increased in renal disease, renal hypoperfusion (e.g. in severe dehydration), and urinary tract obstruction. It is also increased by a high-protein diet, bleeding into the GI tract, tissue damage, and certain drugs. It is decreased in overhydration, advanced liver disease, malnutrition, and eating disorders.
- Serum creatinine provides a crude estimate of glomerular filtration. It is increased in renal disease, renal hypoperfusion, urinary tract obstruction, and rhabdomyolysis. It is decreased in advanced liver disease, malnutrition, eating disorders, and muscle loss. A better estimate of glomerular filtration is creatinine clearance.

Arterial blood gas sampling and interpretation

Specifications: An anatomical arm in lieu of a patient.

Before starting

- Introduce yourself to the patient.
- Explain the procedure and ensure that the patient consents to it.
- Check the case notes for anticoagulant treatment or platelet or clotting abnormalities.
- Note the patient's oxygen requirements and body temperature.
- Gather the required equipment in a tray.

The equipment

- Non-sterile gloves.
- Alcohol wipes.
- Lignocaine 1%.
- 2 ml syringe and cap for syringe.
- Heparin 1000 U/ml (or a heparinised 2 ml syringe).
- 23G (blue) needle (×2).
- Gauze.
- Sharps bin.

The procedure

- Wash and dry your hands or cleanse them with alcohol gel.
- Position the patient's arm so that the wrist is extended.
- Palpate the radial artery over the head of the radius and locate the site of maximum pulsation.
- Don the gloves.
- Cleanse the site with an alcohol wipe.
- Drape the area.
- Inject lignocaine intradermally around the chosen area, taking care not to puncture the vessel or mask its pulsation. (This step can be omitted depending on patient preference.)
- If you do not have a heparinised syringe, attach a 23G needle to the 2 ml syringe and draw up a little heparin into the syringe.
- Discard the needle into a sharps bin.
- Attach a second 23G needle to the syringe.
- Fix the chosen area between the index and middle fingers of your non-dominant hand.
- Warn the patient to expect a 'sharp scratch' or some other gross euphemism.
- Insert the needle at 30 degrees to the skin.
- Advance the needle a few millimetres in line with the direction of the artery until you obtain a flashback of bright red arterial blood into the syringe. Gentle aspiration from the syringe may in some cases be required.
- Allow the syringe to fill with 2 ml of arterial blood.
- Pick up a gauze with your non-dominant hand.
- Withdraw the needle and press firmly over the puncture site with the gauze. State that you would do this for 5 minutes, checking regularly for the formation of a haematoma.
- Discard the needle into a sharps bin.
- Expel any air bubbles from the syringe and cap it.
- State that you would immediately take the blood to a blood gas machine for analysis. At this point the examiner may hand you a print out from the machine.

After the procedure

- Ensure that the patient is comfortable.
- Interpret the print out, if any (see *Table 32*).
- Feedback to the patient/examiner.
- Ask the patient if he has any questions or concerns.
- Clear up.

Arterial blood gas interpretation (suggested approach for an OSCE station)

1. Assess PaO_2 (9.3–13.3 kPa, higher readings may indicate that the patient is receiving oxygen).
2. Assess pH

   ≤ 7.35 is acidosis.

   ≥ 7.45 is alkalosis.
3. Assess $PaCO_2$
   - If > 6.0 kPa there is either respiratory acidosis or respiratory compensation for metabolic alkalosis.
   - If < 4.7 kPa there is either respiratory alkalosis or respiratory compensation for metabolic acidosis.
4. Assess standardised HCO_3
   - If < 22 there is metabolic acidosis or renal compensation for respiratory alkalosis.
   - If > 28 there is a metabolic alkalosis or renal compensation for respiratory acidosis.
5. Combine information from 2, 3, and 4 above to determine the primary disturbance and whether there is any renal or respiratory compensation occurring (see *Table 32*).

Example

pH = 7.30

$PaO_2 = 6.8$

$PaCO_2 = 7.45$

$HCO_3 = 26.0$ mmol/l

This is uncompensated respiratory acidosis due to abruptly impaired ventilation, e.g. asthma attack.

Table 32. Arterial blood gas interpretation

	pH	$PaCO_2$	HCO_3
Respiratory acidosis	↓	↑	→, ↑*
Respiratory alkalosis	↑	↓	→, ↓*
Metabolic acidosis	↓	→, ↓**	↓
Metabolic alkalosis	↑	→, ↑**	↑
Mixed acidosis	↓	↑	↓
Mixed alkalosis	↑	↓	↑

* Renal compensation occurring.

** Respiratory compensation occurring.

Examiner's questions regarding disorders of acid–base balance	
Respiratory acidosis	• Results from alveolar hypoventilation. • Common causes include airway obstruction, respiratory disease, impaired lung motion, neuromuscular disease, central nervous system depression, and obesity (Pickwickian syndrome). • Symptoms are often those of the underlying cause, and in severe cases 'CO_2 narcosis' may supervene. Respiratory acidosis does not have a marked effect on serum electrolytes. • Management involves oxygen therapy, but particular care must be taken in patients with COPD. Where possible, treat the cause.
Respiratory alkalosis	• Results from alveolar hyperventilation. • Common causes include anxiety, pyrexia, CNS causes such as stroke and subarachnoid haemorrhage, liver failure, drugs such as salicylates and nicotine, high altitude, and mechanical ventilation. • There may be signs and symptoms of hypocalcaemia (including positive Trousseau and Chvostek signs) without a fall in total serum calcium levels (due to increased binding of calcium). • Management involves treating the cause.
Metabolic acidosis	• Results from increased production of hydrogen ions, or the inability to form bicarbonate in the kidney. • Causes are various: some increase the anion gap and others do not. The anion gap (normal range 10–18 mmol/l) is a measure of organic acids and is given by $([Na^+]) - ([Cl^-] + [HCO_3^-])$ • Causes that increase the anion gap include renal failure, massive rhabdomyolysis, diabetic ketoacidosis, lactic acidosis, and intoxication with ethanol or methanol. • Causes that do not increase the anion gap include chronic diarrhoea and renal tubular acidosis. • Symptoms are various and non-specific. In extreme cases there may be cardiac arrhythmias, and coma and seizures. • Depending on severity, management may involve IV bicarbonate or dialysis.
Metabolic alkalosis	• Results from decreased hydrogen ion concentration or increased bicarbonate concentration. • Principal causes include vomiting, diuretic treatment, hypokalaemia (due to intracellular shift of hydrogen ions), hyperaldosteronism, base ingestion, and over-compensation of respiratory acidosis. • Symptoms include symptoms of hypocalcaemia (due to increased binding of calcium), symptoms of hypokalaemia (due to intracellular shift of potassium), hypoventilation, arrhythmias, and seizures. • Metabolic alkalosis involving the loss of chloride ions is termed chloride responsive, because it typically corrects with IV administration of normal saline, whereas chloride-unresponsive metabolic alkalosis does not and typically involves severe hypokalaemia or mineralocorticoid excess. • Treat the cause. Correct hypovolaemia and hypokalaemia. In severe cases, consider dialysis.

ECG recording and interpretation

Before starting

- Introduce yourself to the patient.
- Explain the procedure to him, specifying that it is not painful, and ask him for his consent to carry it out.
- Position him so that he is lying on a couch.
- Ask him to expose his upper body and ankles.

The equipment	
• A 12-lead ECG machine.	• Electrode sticky pads.

The procedure

- Indicate that you may need to shave the patient's chest to apply the electrode pads.
- Attach the electrode pads as per the leads.
- Attach the limb leads, one on each limb. The longest leads attach to the legs, above the ankles, and the mid-length leads attach to the upper arms.

Table 33. Colour codes for ECG limb and chest leads

Limb leads		Chest leads	
Red	Right arm	Red	V1
Yellow	Left arm	Yellow	V2
Green	Left leg	Green	V3
Black	Right leg	Brown	V4
		Black	V5
		Violet	V6

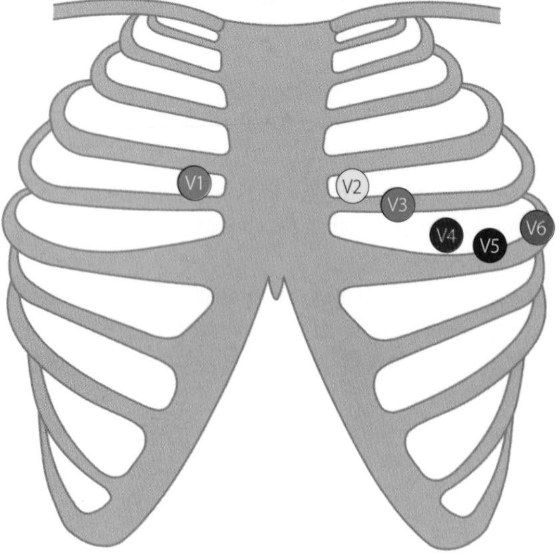

Figure 92. Lead placement.

- Place the chest leads (the shortest leads) such that (see *Figure 92*):
  - V1 is in the fourth intercostal space at the right sternal margin
  - V2 is in the fourth intercostal space at the left sternal margin
  - V3 is midway between V2 and V4
  - V4 is in the fifth intercostal space in the left mid-clavicular line
  - V5 is at the same horizontal level as V4, but in the anterior axillary line
  - V6 is at the same horizontal level as V4 and V5, but in the mid-axillary line
- Turn the ECG machine on and check calibration (1 mV = 1 cm in height) and paper speed (25 mm/s).
- Ensure that the patient is relaxed and comfortable and press on 'Analyse ECG' or a similar button.

See *Figure 93* for an example of a normal ECG trace.

After recording the ECG

- Analyse the ECG for any life-threatening abnormalities.
- Remove the leads.
- Discard the electrode pads.
- Ensure that the patient is comfortable.
- Thank the patient.

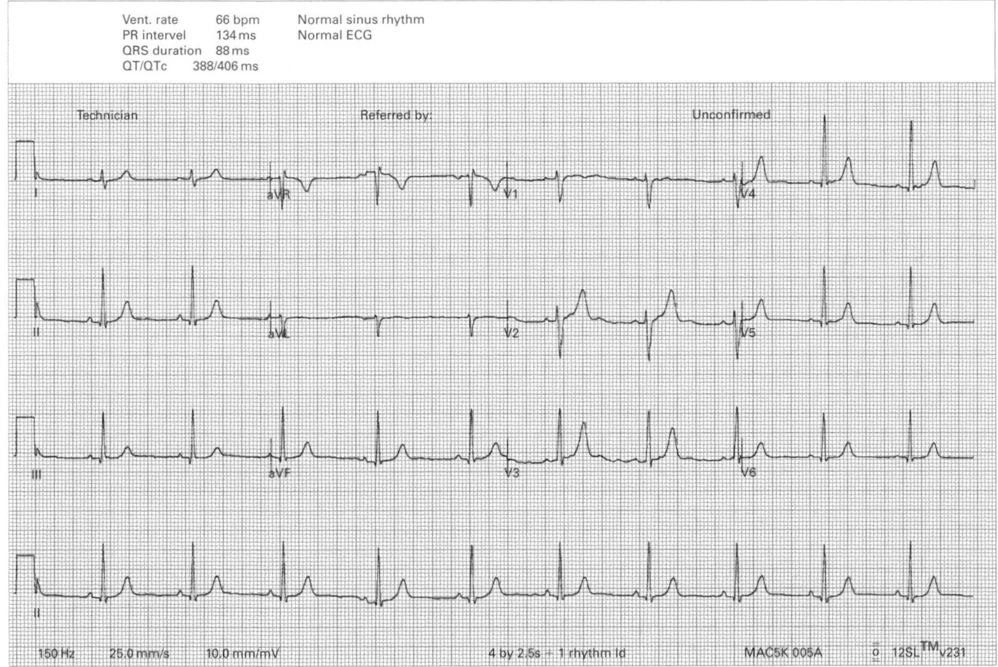

Figure 93. Normal ECG.

ECG interpretation in 10 steps (suggested approach for an OSCE station)

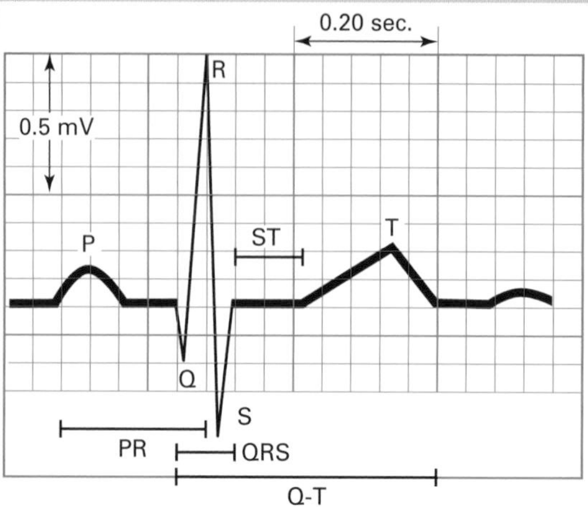

Figure 94. The basic ECG complex.

1. Check labelling (name, date, calibration, paper speed, etc.) and eyeball the ECG.
2. Rate: divide 300 by the number of large squares between consecutive R waves.
3. Rhythm: ensure that each P wave is followed by a QRS complex. Use a pen and card to determine whether the rhythm is regular or irregular.
4. Axis:
   - normal axis: the QRS complexes are predominantly positive in both leads I and II
   - left axis deviation: the QRS complex is predominantly positive in lead I but is predominantly negative in lead II
   - right axis deviation: the QRS complexes are predominantly negative in both leads I and II
5. P waves: normal is less than 2.5 mm in height and 0.11 s in width in lead II.
6. PR interval: normal is 0.12–0.20 s or 3–5 small squares in duration.
7. QRS complex:
   - normal is < 0.12 s or 3 small squares in duration
   - the sum of the S wave in V2 and an R wave in V5 or V6 should not be greater than 35 mm
   - Q waves should not be deeper than one small square or 25% of the following R wave
8. ST segment: the ST segment should not be elevated or depressed.
9. T waves: T waves should not be tall, flattened, or inverted. T wave inversion in leads I, II, and V4–6 is always abnormal.
10. QT interval: normal is less than 400 ms or 2 large squares or half the R–R interval.

ECG interpretation in 10 easy steps – in more detail

1. Check **labelling** (name, date, indication, calibration 1 cm/mV, paper speed 25 mm/s).
2. **Rate:** either divide 300 by the number of large squares between consecutive R waves (1 large square = 0.2 s, 1 small square = 0.04 s) *or* count the number of R waves in the rhythm strip and multiply by 6 (as the rhythm strip is 10 s long).
   Sinus bradycardia (<~50 bpm and regular): athletes, hypothermia, hypothyroidism, intracranial hypertension, obstructive jaundice, SA node disease or ischaemia, beta blockade.
   Sinus tachycardia (>~90 bpm and regular): exercise, pain, fever, hypovolaemia, anaemia, pregnancy, thyroxicosis, vasodilators, vagolytics such as atropine.
3. **Rhythm:** ensure that each P wave is followed by a QRS complex. Use a pen and card to determine whether rhythm is regular or irregular. *Sinus arrhythmia* describes an increase in heart rate upon inspiration.
4. **Axis**
   a. *Normal axis*: the QRS complexes are predominantly positive in both leads I and II.
   b. *Left axis deviation*: the QRS complex is predominantly positive in lead I but is predominantly negative in leads II and III. Left axis deviation may indicate left anterior fascicular block and a number of other conditions, but not usually left ventricular hypertrophy.
   c. *Right axis deviation*: the QRS complexes are predominantly negative in both leads I and II. Right axis deviation may indicate right ventricular hypertrophy due to pulmonary conditions or congenital heart disease.

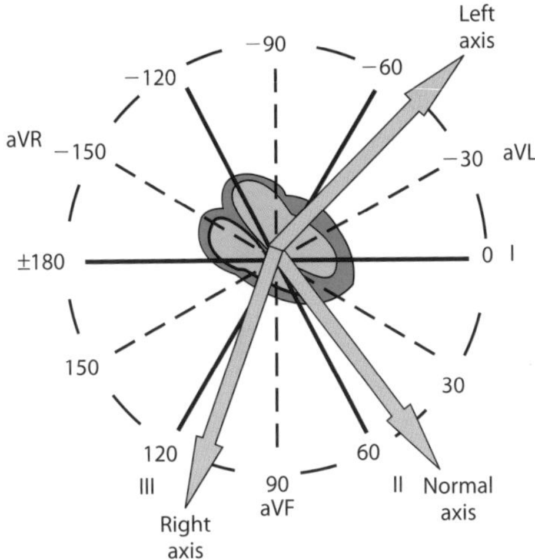

Explanation: normally the depolarising wave spreads towards leads I, II, and III and is therefore associated with a predominantly upward QRS deflection in all these leads, but greatest in lead II.

- In right axis deviation, the axis swings to the right so that the QRS deflection in lead I becomes negative and the deflection in lead III becomes most positive.
- In left axis deviation, the axis swings to the left, so that the deflection in lead III becomes negative. Left axis deviation is not significant until the deflection is also negative in lead II.

5. **P waves**: normal is less than 2.5 mm in height and 0.11 s in width *in lead II*. An inverted P wave in V1 is likely to indicate an incorrect recording. A tall P wave (P pulmonale) is due to right atrial enlargement and is seen most commonly in lung disease but also in tricuspid valve stenosis. A broad, bifid P wave (P mitrale) is due to left atrial enlargement and is seen most commonly in mitral stenosis.

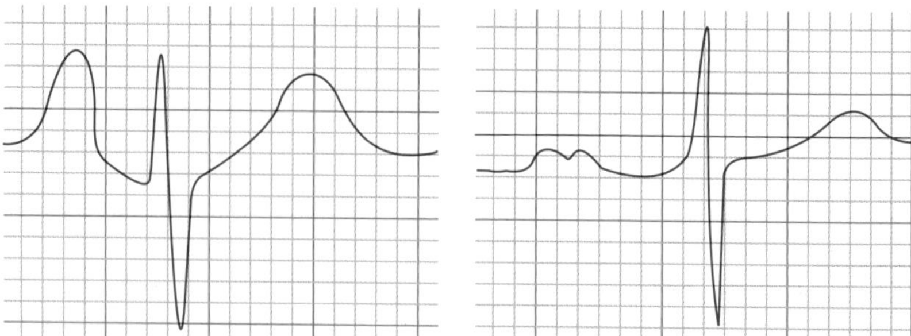

6. **PR interval**: normal is 0.12–0.20 s (3–5 small squares) in duration. Prolonged in heart block, shortened in conditions involving an abnormality on the fibrous insulating ring such that signals get past the AV node more quickly, e.g. Wolff–Parkinson–White syndrome.

   AV node blocks

   - First degree block: atrial conduction is delayed such that the PR interval is consistently prolonged. This may be a sign of coronary artery disease, acute rheumatic carditis, digitalis toxicity, or electrolye disturbances.
   - Second degree block: excitation completely fails to pass through the AV node. The causes of second degree heart block are the same as for first degree heartblock.
     - *Mobitz type I (Wenckebach phenomenon)*: there is progressive lengthening of the PR interval and then regular failure of conduction of an atrial beat, followed by a conducted beat with a short PR interval and then a repetition of this cycle.
     - *Mobitz type II*: most beats are conducted with a constant PR interval but occasionally there is an atrial contraction without a subsequent ventricular contraction. May herald complete heart block.

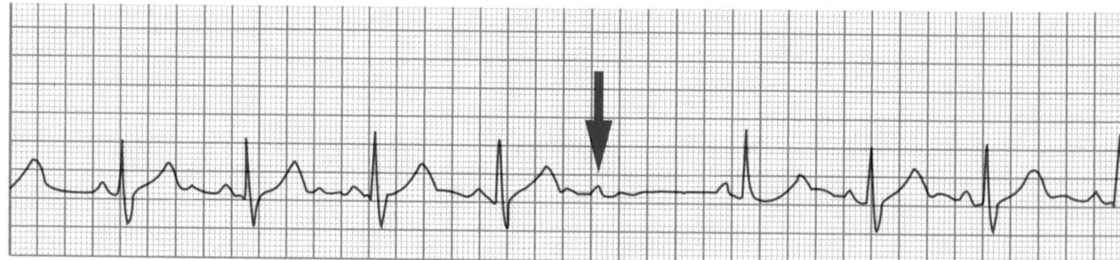

     - *2:1 (or 3:1) conduction*: there are alternate conducted and non-conducted atrial beats, giving twice (or three times) as many P waves as QRS complexes. May herald complete heart block in patients with MI.

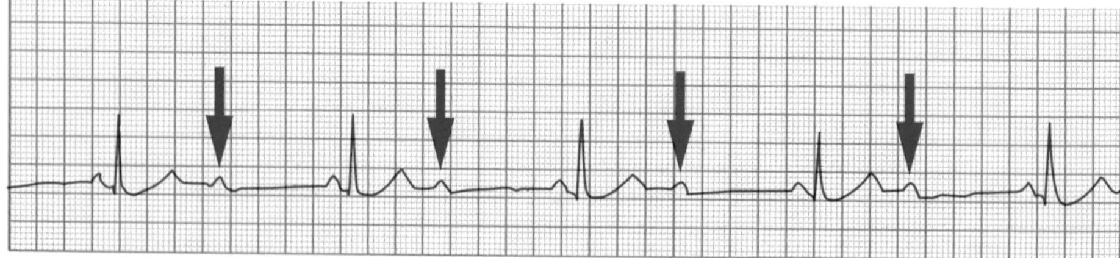

   - Third degree (complete) block: atrial contraction is normal but no beats are conducted to the ventricles. A ventricular escape rhythm takes hold, such that there is no relation between P and QRS. May occur after an MI (usually transient) or due to fibrosis around the bundle of His.

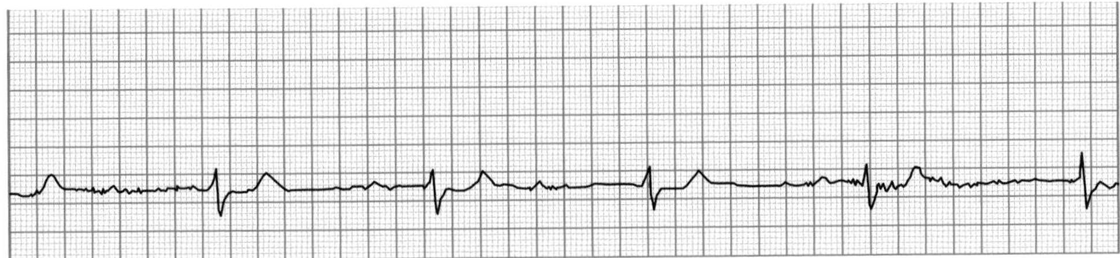

[Note] Heart block that is Mobitz type II or above requires pacing and is symptomatic (hypotension, dizziness, collapse). The choice between a temporary or permanent pacemaker depends on whether the underlying cause is transient or permanent.

SA node blocks can also occur but they are uncommon and usually asymptomatic (due to the establishment of a ventricular escape rhythm). SA node block is not to be confused with SA node *suppression*, which occurs when an arrhythmia prevents the SA node from generating an impulse.

7. **QRS complex**:
   a. Normal is <0.12 s or 3 small squares in duration. A broad QRS results either from depolarisation by a focus in the ventricular muscle or from a bundle branch block (BBB).
      i. Right BBB: can be normal, or may be caused by IHD, PE, or ASD.
      ii. Left BBB: LBBB invariably reflects underlying heart disease, but its presence precludes further interpretation of the ECG.

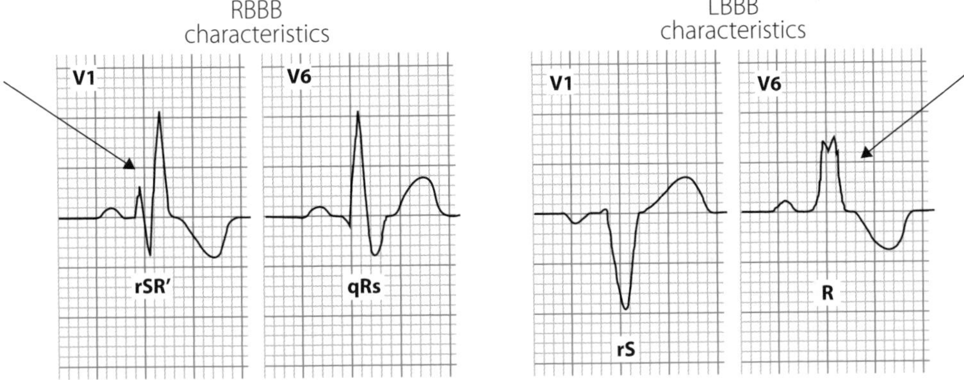

   b. The sum of the S wave in V2 and an R wave in V5 or V6 should not be greater than 35 mm. If it is, this indicates ventricular hypertrophy.
   c. Q waves should not be deeper than one small square or 25% of the following R wave. If they are, this indicates an old MI.

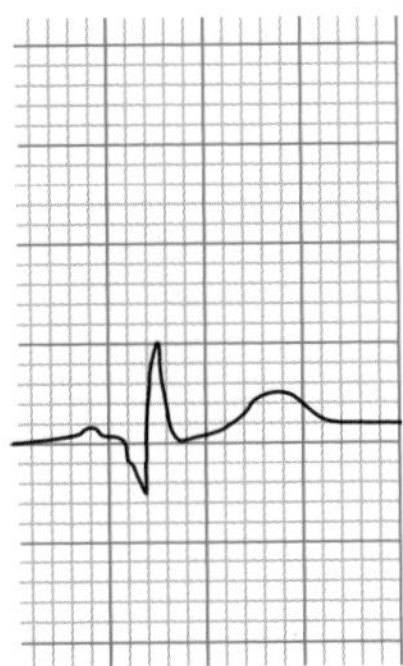

8. **ST segment**: the ST segment should not be elevated or depressed. Elevation of >1 mm indicates full thickness infarction of the myocardium.

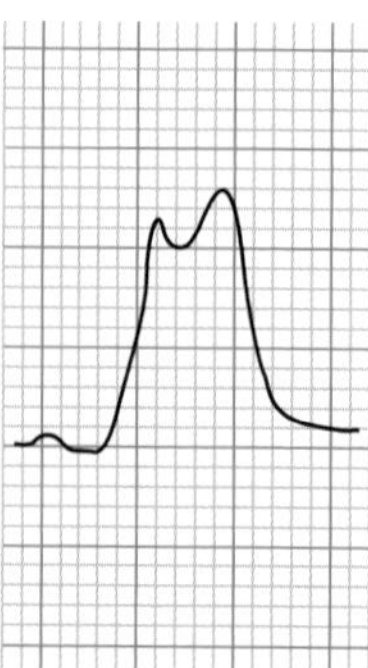

Depression of >0.5 mm indicates ischaemia, e.g. angina. In the presence of raised cardiac enzymes (e.g. troponin I) ST depression is indicative of MI (termed non-ST elevation MI). Saddle elevation in all the leads indicates pericarditis.

9. **T waves**: T waves should not be tall, flattened, or inverted. Tall, tented T waves indicate hyperkalaemia, flattened T waves indicate hypokalaemia. T wave inversion in leads I, II, and V4–6 is always abnormal, and indicates subendocardial (partial thickness) infarction, i.e. non-ST elevation MI, angina, or digoxin administration.
10. **QT interval**: normal is less than 400 ms (2 large squares) or half the R–R interval. Prolongation is usually secondary to drugs, e.g. antipsychotics, toxins, and electrolyte disturbances, and predisposes to potentially dangerous ventricular arrhythmias.

Abnormal rhythms

Supraventricular tachyarrhythmias (SVTs)

In SVTs the depolarisation spreads to the ventricles in the normal way via the His bundle so the QRS complex is normal and the same whether depolarisation was triggered by the SA node, the atrial muscle, or the junctional region.

Atrial extrasystoles

This example of atrial extrasystoles can be described as non-compensated atrial quadrigeminy: 'quadrigeminy' because there is one extrasystole after every three normal beats; 'non-compensated' because there is no compensatory pause after the extrasystole. Atrial extrasystoles are common in healthy people with normal hearts, and also occur in certain conditions such as cardiac failure and mitral valve disease.

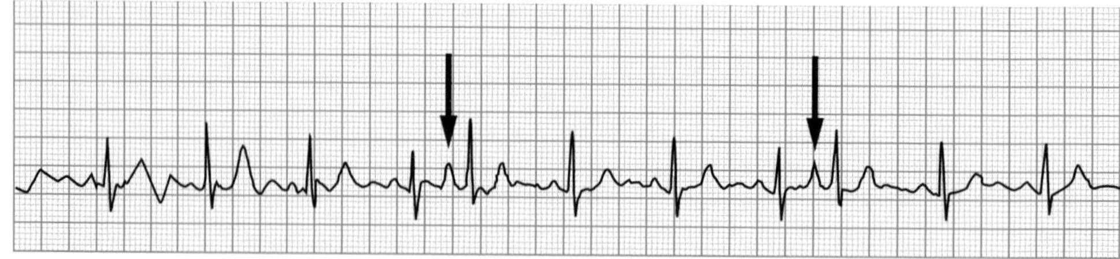

Atrial tachycardia

In atrial tachycardia, there is a heart rate of about 150 with P waves superimposed on preceding T waves. Atrial tachycardia typically arises from an ectopic source in the atrial muscle and is often paroxysmal in nature. Although it is sometimes seen in patients with diseased hearts, it is nearly always benign.

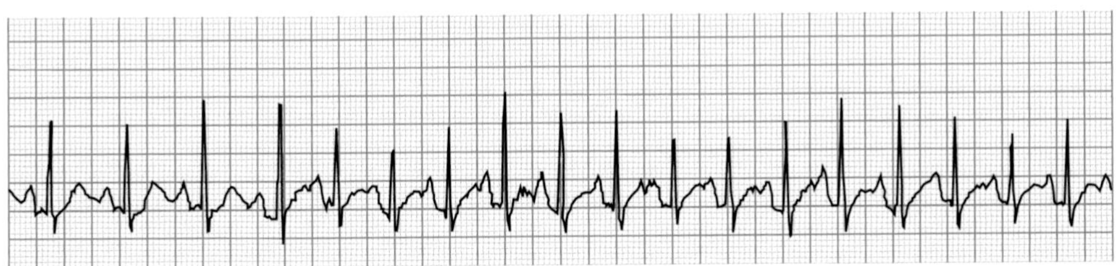

Atrial flutter

In atrial flutter, the atrial rate is commonly 300 bpm and there is usually a 2:1 block, resulting in a ventricular rate of **150 bpm**. Can occur spontaneously in people with normal hearts, but most often occurs in people with cardiovascular disease. Frequently degenerates into AF.

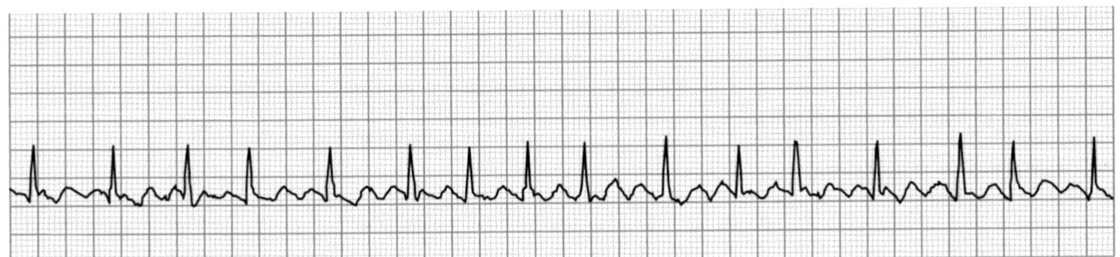

Atrial flutter with *variable* (2:1 and 3:1) block. Fast P waves produce a 'saw-tooth' appearance.

Atrial fibrillation (AF)

AF is associated with any disease affecting the heart. There is an 'irregularly irregular' ventricular rate with no true P waves but baseline irregularities representing atrial activation.

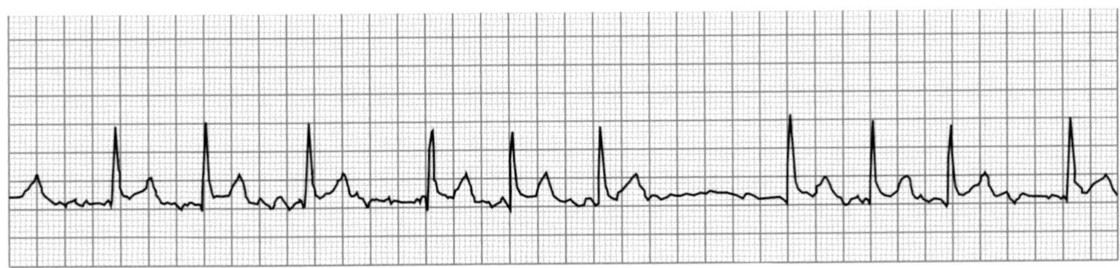

AV nodal re-entrant tachycardia (AV 'junctional' tachycardia)

A re-entrant circuit is set up in the atria, causing the ventricles to depolarise at fast rates of up to 200 bpm. P waves are often absent, hidden in the QRS.

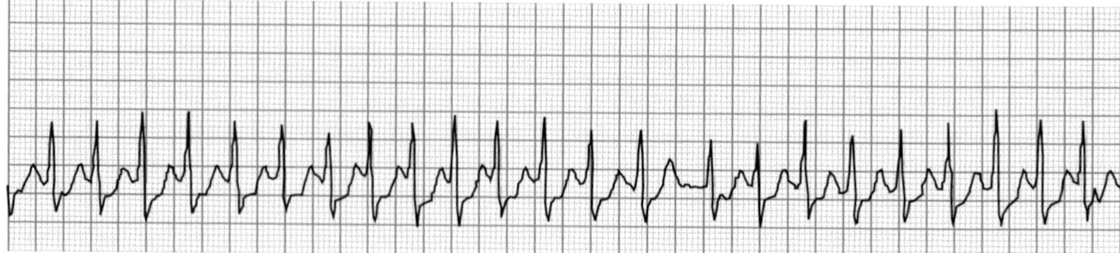

AV re-entrant tachycardia, via an accessory pathway e.g. Wolff–Parkinson–White syndrome

In WPW syndrome, some of the atrial depolarisation passes quickly to the ventricle before it gets through the AV node. The early depolarisation of the ventricle leads to a shortened PR interval and a slurred start to the QRS wave (delta wave).

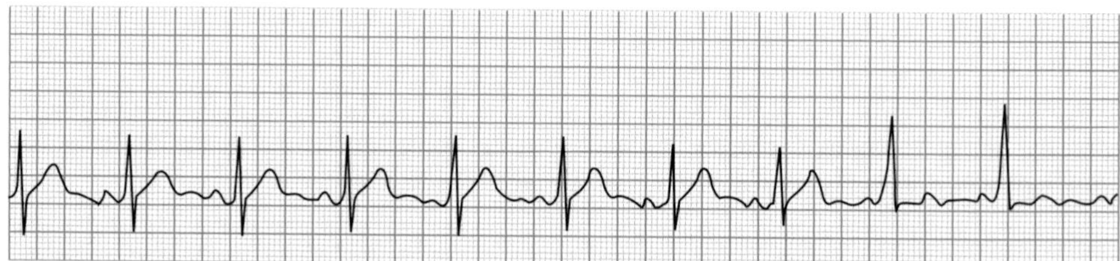

Ventricular tachyarrhythmias

Ventricular extrasystole (VE)

Ventricular extrasystoles arise from an ectopic focus leading to a broad and atypical QRS complex that is unrelated to a preceding P wave. If a VE occurs early in the T wave of a preceding beat it can induce ventricular fibrillation.

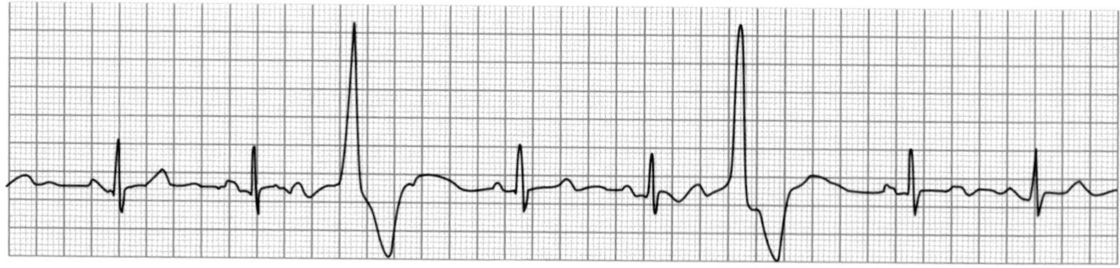

Ventricular trigeminy.

Parasystole refers to a lack of coupling between VEs and the sinus rhythm. This may result in a number of fusion beats, in which a VE merges into the sinus beat.

Ventricular tachycardia (VT)

Two ventricular extrasystoles are termed a couplet but three or more are termed VT. Sustained VT can degenerate into ventricular fibrillation and death. Note the obvious dissociation between atria and ventricles.

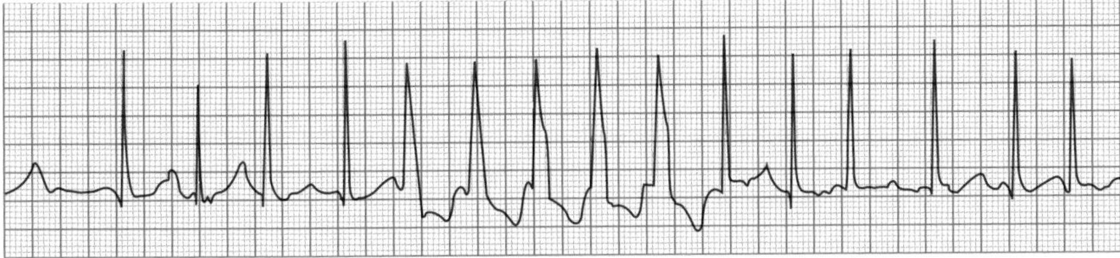

* Accelerated idioventricular rhythm can look like VT, but the rate is <120 and the condition is benign. For this reason, VT should not be diagnosed unless the heart rate is >120.

** VT can be very difficult to differentiate from SVT with a BBB (as the BBB produces a broad QRS complex).

Ventricular fibrillation (VF)

Ventricular fibrillation is a chaotic ventricular rhythm which rapidly results in death.

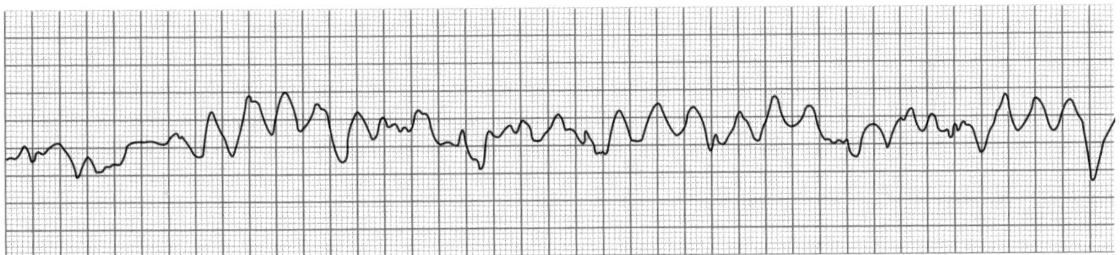

Ventricular flutter

Ventricular flutter is a relatively uncommon and short-lived sine-wave like rhythm that usually degenerates into VF.

Bradycardias

Most abnormal rhythms are tachycardias, but they can also be bradycardias. The heart rate is normally controlled the SA node. However, if the SA node fails to depolarise, the heart rate is taken over by a focus in the atrial muscle or in the region around the AV node (the junctional region) both of which have spontaneous depolarisation frequencies of about 50 per min. If these also fail, or if the His bundle is blocked, the heart rate is taken over by a ventricular rhythm of about 30 per min. These slow, protective rhythms are collectively referred to as 'escape rhythms'. It is important to recognise them as such, because trying to suppress them can have dire consequences. The trace below shows a junctional escape rhythm:

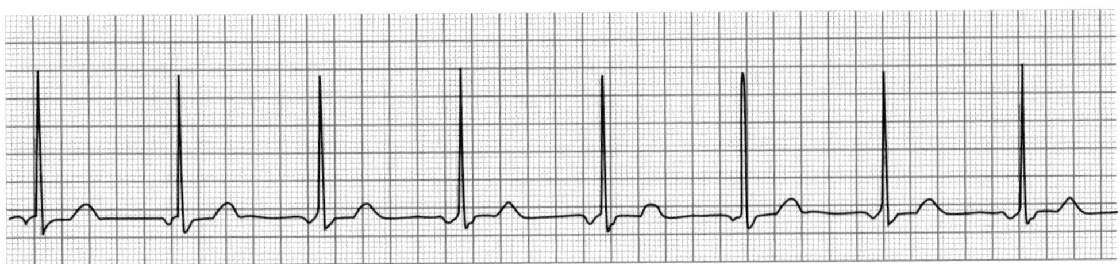

ECG patterns

Myocardial infarction (MI)

In the 'hyperacute' phase, there are tall R waves and ST elevation which is sloped upwards and which often merges into tall, broad T waves. In established MI, there are prominent Q waves, elevated ST segments, and inverted 'arrowhead' T waves.

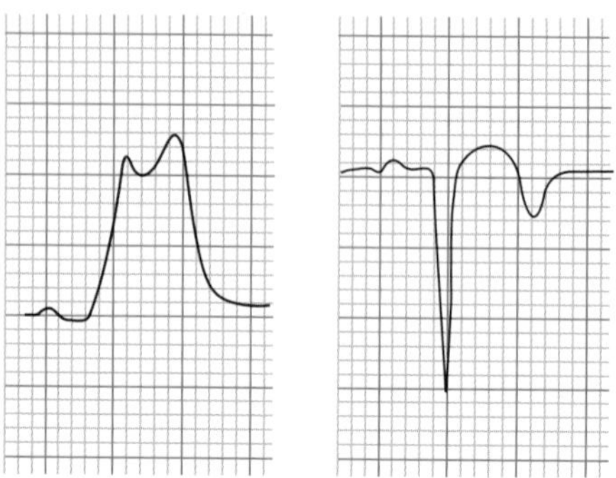

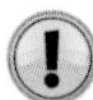

In posterior MI, posterior wall changes are mirrored in the leads opposite the lesion, i.e. V1 and V2, leading to a tall R, ST depression, and upright 'arrowhead' T waves. Note that there may be no ECG changes in MI, so don't rely solely on the ECG!

Angina

ST segment depression of 1 mm or greater (Sheffield criteria) or ST elevation in Prinzmetal's angina.

Myocarditis

Tachycardia, atrial and ventricular extrasystoles, first degree and LAHB (left anterior hemi-block) heart blocks, ST changes.

Pericarditis

Sinus tachycardia, widespread 'saddle' elevation of the ST segment, T wave abnormalities.

Pericardial effusion

Diminished amplitude of ECG deflections and possibly also T wave inversion and electrical alternans (alternating QRS amplitude = tall one beat, short the next, and so on).

Pulmonary thromboembolism

Sinus tachycardia. Other ECG abnormalities are uncommon and the classical $S_IQ_{III}T_{III}$ syndrome only occurs in under 10% (prominent S in lead I, Q and inverted T in lead III). There may also be right atrial enlargement, atrial tachyarrhythmias, right ventricular hypertrophy or ischaemia, and RBBB.

Hyperkalaemia

Initially, tall tented T waves, then disappearance of P waves and, finally, broadened and distorted QRS complexes leading to ventricular arrhythmia or cardiac standstill.

Hypokalaemia

Flattened T waves and more prominent U waves which may be falsely interpreted as QT prolongation. There may also be first or second degree AV heart block.

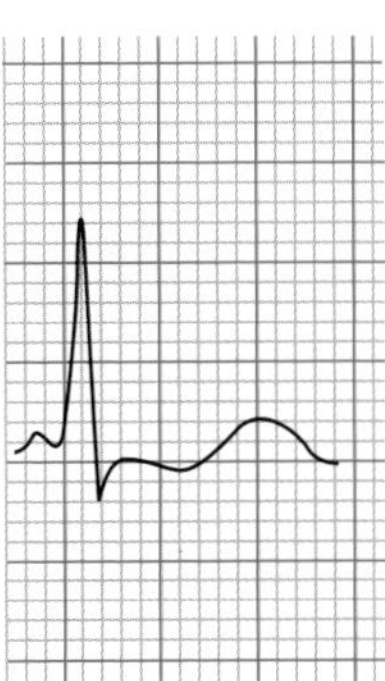

Hypothermia

Sinus bradycardia, prominent 'J' wave, QRS and QT prolongation, leading to blocks, ventricular extrasystoles and, finally, VF.

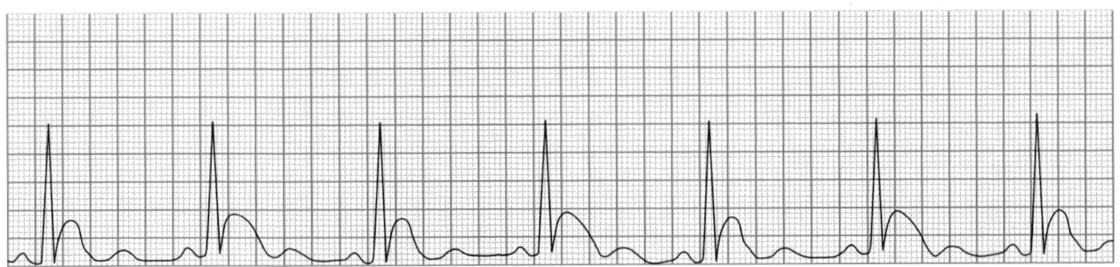

Try to familiarise yourself with different patterns of ECG, e.g. left ventricular hypertrophy, ischaemic heart disease, acute myocardial infarct, atrial fibrillation, heart block, pulmonary embolus. Study ECG libraries such as the one that can be found at www.ecglibrary.com/ecghome.html.

Chest X-ray interpretation

A systematic approach to interpreting X-rays not only fills out the time and impresses the examiner, but also minimises your chances of missing any abnormalities. Before saying anything, it is an excellent idea to spend one minute looking at the X-ray, rubbing your chin and organising your thoughts.

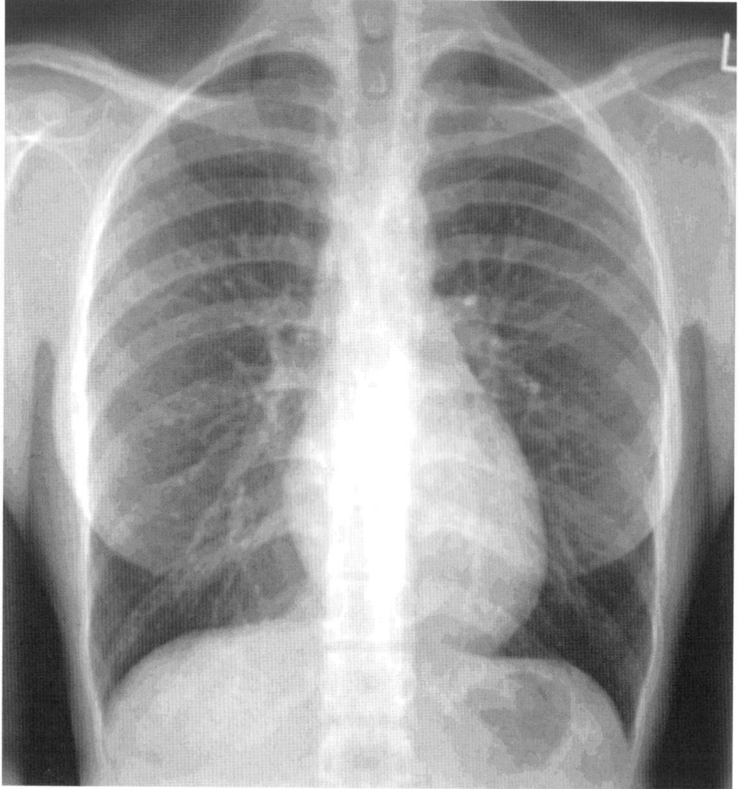

Figure 95. Normal chest X-ray.

1. The X-ray

- Name and age of the patient.
- Date of the X-ray.
- PA, AP, or lateral?
- Erect or supine?
- Rotation – if there is no rotation, the distances from the vertebral spines to the medial ends of the clavicles should be equal.
- Penetration – if penetration is normal, the upper half of the thoracic spine should be discernible.

Erect or supine?

An X-ray can be confirmed as having been taken in the erect position if the gastric air bubble is found lying under the left hemidiaphragm.

AP films are almost invariably taken supine, and this has major implications for interpretation. A supine film differs from an erect film in that:

- there is an enlarged heart size
- the diaphragm is higher, resulting in an apparent decrease in lung volume
- pleural fluid levels lie vertically, resulting in an opacification of the lung field
- any prominence of upper zone vessels does not suggest left heart failure

2. Interventions

Make a note of any chest drains, ECG pads, etc., that may be visible on the X-ray.

3. The skeleton

Inspect the ribs, the shoulder girdles, and the spine.

4. The soft tissues

Inspect the breasts, the chest wall, and the soft tissues of the neck. Look for any distortion, and for any opacities and translucencies.

5. The lungs and hila

The lungs: check the lung volumes, then carefully inspect the lung fields for any opacity or radiolucency.

The hila: inspect the hila, the densities created by the pulmonary arteries and the superior pulmonary veins of either lung for any abnormal opacities. Check their positions: the left hilum should be 2–3 cm higher than its right counterpart.

6. The pleura

Systematically check *all* lung margins, looking for pleural opacity, pleural displacement, and loss of clarity of the pleural edge (the so-called *silhouette sign*).

7. The diaphragm

Inspect the diaphragm and the area underneath it. The right hemidiaphragm should be at least 3 cm higher than the left.

8. The mediastinum and heart

First look for any mediastinal shift. Then calculate the cardiothoracic ratio (CTR) by dividing the maximal diameter of the heart by the maximal diameter of the chest. In a PA film the CTR should be 0.5 or less. Inspect the trachea and right and left main bronchi. Then inspect the aortic arch, the pulmonary artery, and the heart. Are there any abnormal opacities (masses) or radiolucencies (pneumomediastinum)?

9. Summarise your findings

Conditions most likely to appear in a chest X-ray interpretation station
Pneumonia (see *Figure 96*) • Air space filling with pus is the hallmark of bacterial pneumonias; viral pneumonias tend to cause a more interstitial pattern and predominantly hazy ground glass opacification. Pneumonia may be accompanied by a pleural effusion.
Pleural effusion (see *Figure 97*) • Depending on the size of the effusion: blunting of the costophrenic angle; obscuring of the outline of the hemidiaphragm; opacification of the inferior hemithorax associated with a meniscus shape of the fluid at its upper, lateral margin; opacification of the entire hemithorax; displacement of the mediastinum to the contralateral side.
Pulmonary oedema • In cardiogenic pulmonary oedema, the pattern may include cephalization of the pulmonary vessels, Kerley B lines or septal lines, peribronchial cuffing, perihilar haziness and blurring of the normally sharp hilar vessels, 'bat's wing' haziness, cardiomegaly, pleural effusion.
COPD (see *Figure 98*) • Hyperinflated lungs with flattened hemi-diaphragms, hyperlucent lungs, bullae.
Interstitial pulmonary fibrosis • Bilateral reticular or reticulo-nodular pattern, loss of lung volume, honeycomb lung in late stages.
Pneumothorax (see *Figure 99*) • Radiolucent area beyond collapsed lung with absence of pulmonary vessel markings beyond the white line of the pleura; in tension pneumothorax, displacement of the mediastinum to the contralateral side, flattening of the hemi-diaphragm, soft tissue emphysema.
Tuberculosis • Multifocal consolidation or nodularity with spread to regional lymph nodes and subsequent scarring with calcification of the lung parenchyma and lymph nodes; cavitation, if seen, tends to occur later in the course of the disease. Pleural effusion and pneumothorax might also be seen.
Lung cancer
Rib fractures

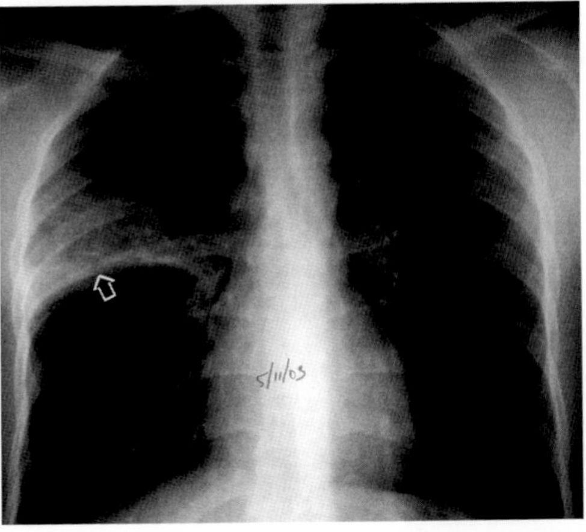

Figure 96. Frontal chest X-ray of adult male with pneumonia (marked with arrow).

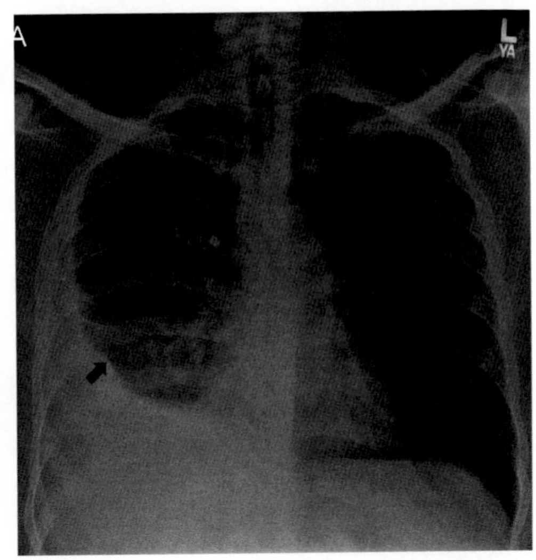

Figure 97. Frontal chest X-ray of adult with a right-sided pleural effusion (marked with arrow).

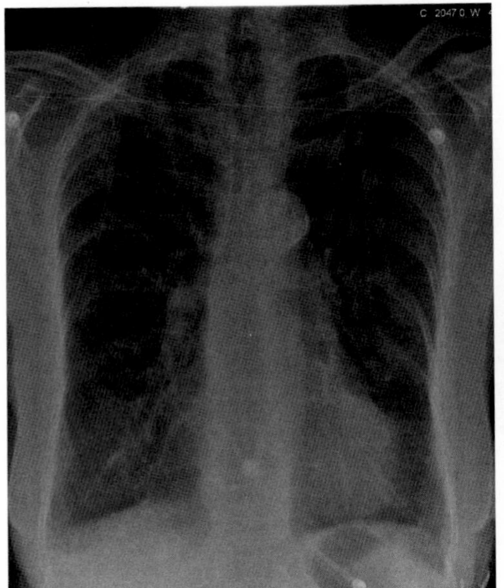

Figure 98. Frontal chest X-ray of a long term smoker with COPD.

Figures 96–99 all reproduced from *Interpreting Chest X-Rays* by Stephen Ellis.

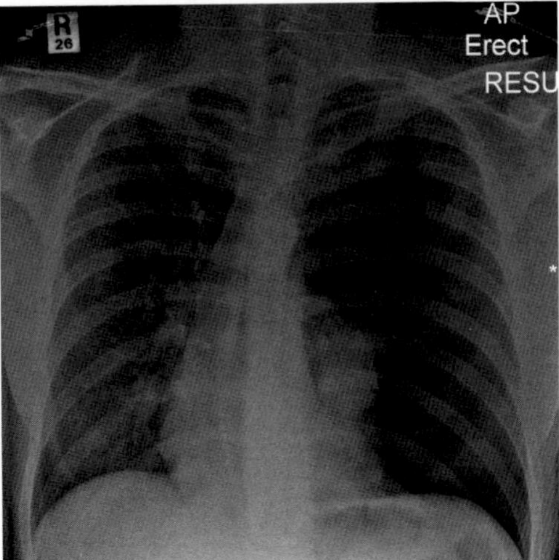

Figure 99. Anterior–posterior chest X-ray of adult with a left pneumothorax which has completely collapsed the left lung.

Abdominal X-ray interpretation

A systematic approach to interpreting X-rays not only fills out time and impresses the examiner, but also minimises your chances of missing any abnormalities. Before saying anything, it is an excellent idea to spend one minute looking at the X-ray and organising your thoughts.

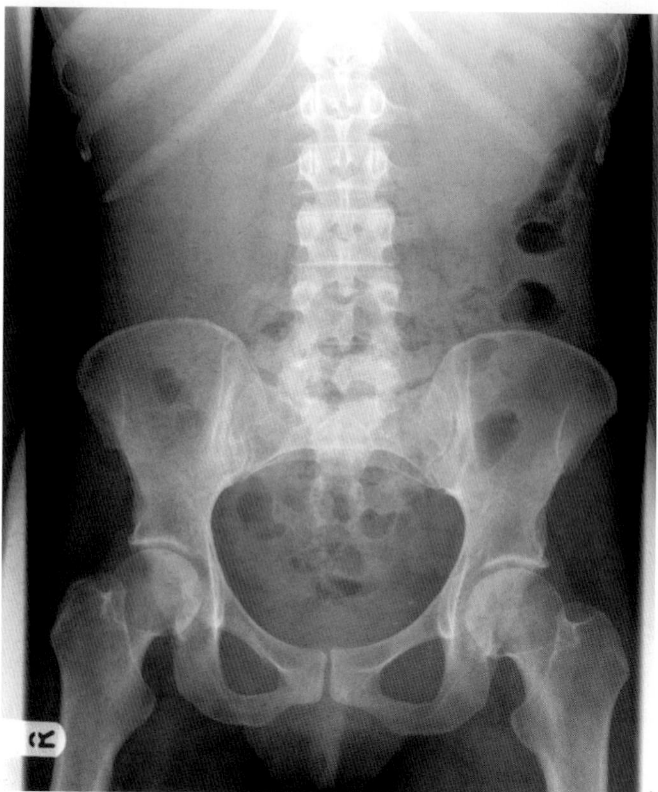

Figure 100. Normal adult supine PA abdominal X-ray.

1. The X-ray

- Name, age, and sex of the patient.
- Date of the X-ray.
- Confirm size of area covered.
- PA or AP? (They are usually PA.)
- Supine (usual), erect, or lateral decubitus? (Look at gastric air bubble and fluid levels.)
- Penetration (lumbar vertebrae should be visible).

2. Interventions or artefacts

- Make a note of any clearly visible interventions or artefacts (*Table 34*).

Table 34. Abdominal X-ray: interventions and artefacts	
Interventions	Surgical clips, retained surgical instruments or swabs, nasogastric tube, CVP line, intrauterine contraceptive device, renal or biliary stents, endoluminal aortic stent, inferior vena caval filter
Artefacts/other	Pyjama bottoms, coins in pockets, body piercings, bullets, drugs ('bodypackers'), even, unfortunately, small animals

3. Skeleton

Inspect the:

- lower rib cage
- lumbar vertebrae
- sacrum and sacroiliac joints
- pelvis
- hip joints and femora

4. Organs

Inspect the:

- liver
- spleen: usually not visualised
- kidneys: about three vertebrae in size, the left kidney is higher than the right
- bladder: not visualised if empty
- prostate: only visualised if calcified
- stomach
- small bowel
- large bowel

Large bowel usually frames a central area containing small bowel loops, not all of which are likely to be visible on an X-ray. If need be, large bowel and small bowel can be distinguished by their different mucosal markings: large bowel has haustra that cross only part of the bowel wall whereas small bowel has valvulae that cross its full width.

5. Gas, fluid levels, and faecal matter

- Gas: depending on its amount and distribution, intraluminal gas may be normal, but intramural or extraluminal gas should be considered abnormal. The small bowel should not be greater than 3 cm in diameter, the colon 5 cm in diameter, and the caecum 9 cm in diameter. Look for gas under the diaphragm (pneumoperitoneum), even though this is best visualised on an erect chest X-ray.
- Fluid levels: a fluid level in the stomach and caecum is a normal finding, but multiple fluid levels in the colon should be considered abnormal.
- Faecal matter: the amount and distribution of faecal matter can be revealing of underlying pathology.

6. Abnormal calcification

- Calculi (kidneys, ureters, bladder, gall bladder, and biliary tree).
- Pancreas.
- Kidneys.
- Abdominal aorta and arteries.
- Costal cartilages, although note that calcification of the costal cartilages is a benign finding in the older age population.

7. Summarise your findings

Conditions most likely to appear in an abdominal X-ray interpretation station
Faecal impaction or overload • Faecal matter, which is solid, liquid, and gas, has a grey and mottled appearance.
Obstruction (mass, stricture, volvulus, intussusception) • In large bowel obstruction, there is a cut-off point with proximal gas–faecal dilatation of the large bowel (diameter >5 cm, caecum >9 cm) and few but long fluid levels; the small intestine is not normally involved. In contrast, in small bowel obstruction there is gas–fluid dilatation of the small bowel (diameter >5 cm) and many but short fluid levels at different heights ('step-ladder' appearance); the large intestine is not involved. Volvulus may yield a grossly distended inverted U-shaped colonic loop, loss of haustra, and the 'coffee-bean' sign from a doubled-up loop of distended, oedematous sigmoid colon. Intussusception may yield the target sign, a pair of concentric circular radiolucent lines, or the crescent sign, a crescent shaped lucency with a soft tissue mass.
Paralytic ileus • In contrast to mechanical obstruction, paralytic ileus manifests as distension along the full length of both the large and small bowel.
Perforation • On an erect chest X-ray, there may be sub-diaphragmatic gas especially visible on the right side. On an abdominal X-ray, there may be a circular gas lucency in the central abdomen (the 'football' sign), and the bowel may take on a 3D appearance due to air on both the luminal and peritoneal side of the bowel wall (the Rigler sign).
Biliary, renal, or bladder calculi • Gallstones may be seen as laminated, faceted, and often multiple radio-opacities in the right upper quadrant, although only in 10-20% of cases. • Renal calculi may be seen in 80–90% of cases as small, round radio-opacities along the urinary tract; they often obstruct at the level of the pelviureteric brim or vesicoureteric junction. The urinary tract is visualised by looking along the transverse processes of the vertebrae, across the sacroiliac joint to the level of the ischial spine. • Bladder calculi may be seen as often large and multiple radio-opacities in the pelvic region.
Appendicolith • Small, round, calcified radio-opacity in the region of the right Iliac fossa.
Artefacts (see *Table 34*)

Learn their signs, especially the barn-door ones such as apple-core and bird's beak.

Ordering investigations

Request forms for laboratory investigations (biochemistry, haematology, blood grouping and transfusion, microbiology, cellular pathology, immunology) and radiological investigations differ considerably from one hospital trust to another, so try to familiarise yourself with your local ones. Once you have seen the forms, they are actually pretty self-explanatory. Note that in some hospitals, investigations are ordered on a computer screen and paper forms are only used as a back-up.

On most forms you typically need to provide details about the:

Patient

- Last and first names
- Sex (usually 'M' or 'F', but sometimes 'U' for 'unknown')
- Date of birth
- Hospital number and NHS number

Use the patient's full name, e.g. 'Dorothy', not 'Dot or 'Dottie'. It is usually possible to omit the patient's hospital number and NHS number, but this is not best practice.

Request

- The ward or department that the report needs to go to ('Location for report'). Sometimes you are also able to specify a ward or department for a second copy of the report to go to ('Copy report').
- The speciality on behalf of which you are ordering the investigation, e.g. A&E, surgery.
- The name of the patient's consultant. If this is unclear, you can normally write the name of the consultant on take or on call.
- The patient's category (e.g. NHS, private, trial).
- The requesting doctor's name and signature.
- The requesting doctor's bleep or telephone number.

Specimen

- The type of specimen, e.g. blood, urine, sputum, other.
- Date and time of collection.
- The (anatomical) site of collection.

Clinical details

- The patient's clinical details, e.g.
  - chest pain, SOB, ECG changes, ? MI
  - pyrexia of unknown origin, ? cause
  - acute psychosis, due to start antipsychotic medication
- If the investigations are urgent, you can write 'Urgent please'. If the investigations are really urgent, take the sample and request form to the laboratory and speak to the technician in person.

On radiology request forms, you generally need to provide more specific clinical details, and specify what questions the examination should answer. You also need to specify the patient's transport (e.g. walking, chair, stretcher, bed) and other (e.g. oxygen, drip, escort) needs, and fill in a short risk assessment that is often in the form of a tick box list of questions (e.g. pregnancy, breast-feeding, allergies – yes/no).

Investigations requested

This obviously depends on the clinical situation. Commonly ordered laboratory and radiological investigations include FBC, haematinics, group and save, U&Es, LFTs, TFTs, glucose, lipids, CRP, ESR, amylase, D-dimers, blood cultures, MC&S, CXR, and AXR.

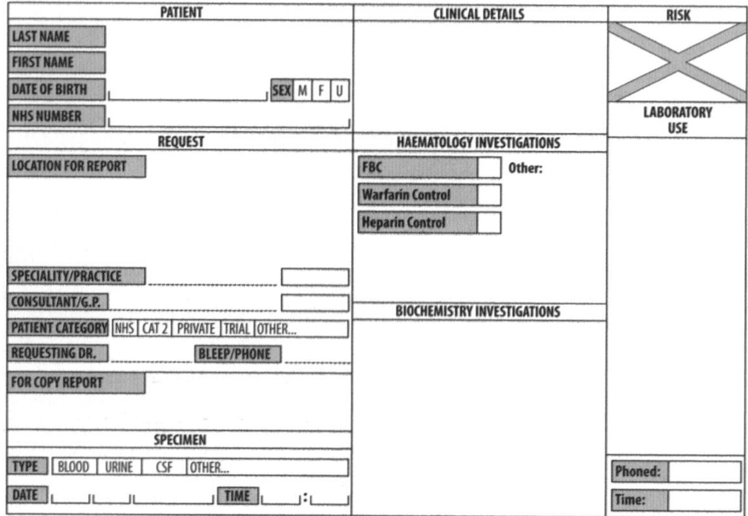

PATIENT
LAST NAME
FIRST NAME
DATE OF BIRTH SEX M F U
NHS NUMBER

CLINICAL DETAILS

RISK

LABORATORY USE

REQUEST
LOCATION FOR REPORT
SPECIALITY/PRACTICE
CONSULTANT/G.P.
PATIENT CATEGORY NHS CAT 2 PRIVATE TRIAL OTHER...
REQUESTING DR. BLEEP/PHONE
FOR COPY REPORT

HAEMATOLOGY INVESTIGATIONS
FBC Other:
Warfarin Control
Heparin Control

BIOCHEMISTRY INVESTIGATIONS

SPECIMEN
TYPE BLOOD URINE CSF OTHER...
DATE TIME :

Phoned:
Time:

Figure 101. A typical request form for laboratory investigations. Note that, in this hospital, biochemistry and haematology investigations are requested on the same form.

After completing the request form

Before you take the specimen, confirm the patient's name and date of birth. For blood specimens, most hospitals use a purple specimen tube for haematology, a pink tube for group and save and cross-matching, a yellow tube for biochemistry (e.g. U&Es, LFTs, TFTs, CRP, lipids), a grey tube for glucose, a black tube for ESR, and a light blue tube for coagulation screen. Label the specimen tubes using a black ball-point pen, ensuring that the information on the label matches that on the request form. Place the labelled specimen tube into the bag on the reverse of the request form, remove the protective strip, and fold the flap onto the bag so as to seal it. Note that blood cultures require two 'blood bottles' with specific media for aerobic and anaerobic organisms.

VACUTAINER TUBE GUIDE – Draw tubes in the order given		
Haemoguard Stopper	**Tube Content**	**Determinations**
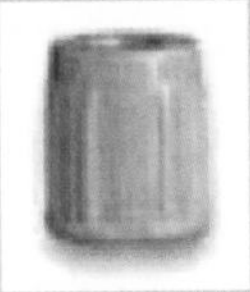	SODIUM CITRATE 1:9	Coagulation Screen, Prothrombin Time (INR), APTT, Thrombophilia Screen, Lupus Anticoagulant Screen
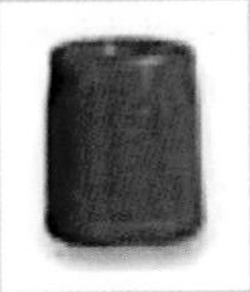	PLAIN (No Additive)	Anti-Cardiolipin antibodies
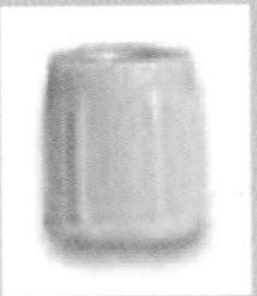	SST	All Biochemistry Tests not mentioned elsewhere (1 Tube), Microbiology (1 Tube)
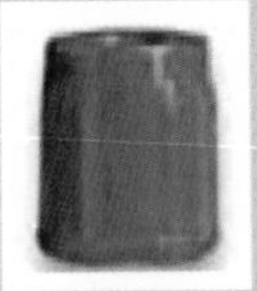	HEPARIN	Chromosome Studies, Lead, Amino Acids, Troponin
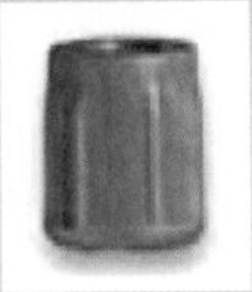	EDTA	FBC, Reticulocytes, Sickle Screen, Haemoglobinopathy Screen, G6PD, GF Test, Viscosity, Malarial Parasites, RBC Folate, ZPP, Marker Studies, Lead, Mercury Complement, Glycosylated Haemoglobin
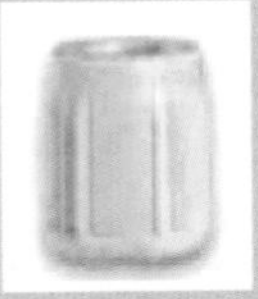	EDTA (cross match)	Blood Group, Save Serum, Crossmatch, Antibody Screening, Cord Blood Samples
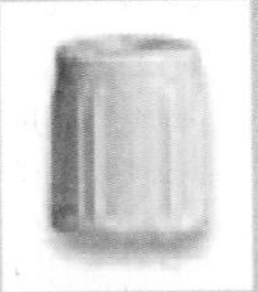	FLUORIDE/ OXALATE	Glucose, Ethanol (Alcohol), Lactate
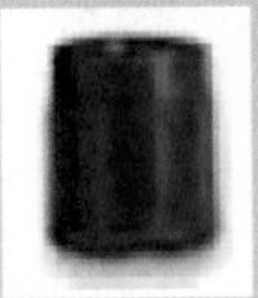	SODIUM HEPARIN	Copper, Selenium, Zinc

Figure 102. Specimen tube guide. Note that the colours used may differ from one hospital trust to another.

Drug and controlled drug prescription

Before prescribing a drug

- Look at the patient's medical notes. In particular, is there any hepatic or renal impairment/ failure?
- Find out if he is on any other drugs, and consider possible interactions.
- Ask him if he has any allergies and document these in the medical notes.
- Explain to him the reason for recommending the drug, its likely beneficial effects, and its common or dangerous side-effects.

Prescribing a drug

- Write legibly and in black ink.
- Avoid all abbreviations other than those that are in common usage (see *Table 35*).
- Use generic names (unless a particular drug preparation is required).

Table 35. Latin abbreviations commonly used in prescribing drugs

Abbreviation	Latin	English
OD	*omni die*	once a day
BD	*bis in die*	twice a day
TDS	*ter die sumendus*	three times a day
QDS	*quarter die sumendus*	four times a day
QQH	*quarta quaque horae*	every four hours
AC	*ante cibum*	before food
PC	*post cibum*	after food
OM	*omni mane*	every morning
ON	*omni nocte*	every night
PRN	*pro re nata*	as required
Stat.	*statim*	at once

Include:

- the date
- the full name, address, and date of birth of the patient
- the age of the patient if he is a child under the age of 12
- the generic name and formulation of the drug – prefer generic names unless a particular preparation is required
- the dose and frequency – avoid decimal points, e.g. 500 mg and not 0.5 g, and superfluous zeros, e.g. 4 mg and not 4.0 mg; if prescribing in micrograms, spell out 'micrograms' in full
- the minimum dose interval for PRN or 'as required' drugs only, e.g. cyclizine 5 mg 8 hourly
- the quantity to be supplied
- the signature of a registered medical practitioner – any alterations or mistakes should also be signed (or at least initialled)

Prescribing a controlled drug

In your own handwriting, include:

- the date
- the full name, address, and date of birth of the patient
- the generic name of the drug
- the formulation and strength of the preparation
- the required dose of the drug, frequency, and number of days it is to be taken
- the total amount of the preparation, or the total number of dose units in both words *and* figures
- your signature and address

> December 12, 2007.
>
> Mr John Adam Smith
> 42 West Register Street
> London XXXX XXX
>
> Date of birth: 01/09/1972
>
> Methadone 10mg tablets
> 10mg TDS for 7 days
> 210mg, two hundred and ten milligrams in total.
>
> Signed: Dr Peter Brown
> The Best Hospital
> London XXXX XXX
>
> SPECIMEN

Prescribing on a hospital drug chart

- Hospital drug charts vary slightly from one hospital to another, so be familiar with your local ones. Most drug charts have four main sections, for regular drugs, PRN drugs, 'once-only' drugs, and fluids.
- Always write in black ink and in block capitals.
- Write at least the patient's name, date of birth, and any allergies/adverse reactions on every page of the drug chart.
- If prescribing a set course of medication, e.g. a 7-day course of antibiotics, cross off subsequent days so as to 'gate' the prescription.
- Sign and date every prescription. *If re-writing a drug chart, the date is not the date today, but the date on which the drug was first prescribed.*
- Record any changes you have made in the patient's case notes.
- Fluids and drugs such as oxygen, insulin and anticoagulants are sometimes prescribed on separate documents, and it is important not to miss them out if they have become separated from the drug chart.

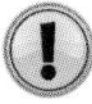

Avoid prescribing drugs you are unfamiliar with, high risk drugs such as anticoagulants and sedatives, and parenteral drugs without first consulting the British National Formulary *and senior colleagues.*

Example for a regular drug

PRESCRIPTION		Patient's Own Medicine	Date → / Time ↓		1/7/08	2/7/08	3/7/08	4/7/08	5/7/08	6/7/08	7/7/08	8/7/08						
Medicine (Approved Name) LANZOPRAZOLE		For use	6															
			(8)		AB	AB	AB	AB	AB	AB								
Dose 30 mg	Route ORAL	Quantity	12															
Notes	Start Date 1/7/08	Date	14															
Prescriber – sign + print A Doctor A DOCTOR		Pharmacy	18															
			22															

Example for a PRN drug

PRESCRIPTION		Patient's Own Medicine	AS REQUIRED THERAPY							
Medicine (Approved Name) PARACETAMOL		For use	Date							
			Time							
Dose + Frequency 1 g 4–6 hourly Max 4 g/24 hrs	Route PO/BR	Quantity	Dose/Route							
			Initials							
Notes FOR PAIN	Start Date 1/7/08	Date	Date							
			Time							
Prescriber – sign + print A Doctor A DOCTOR		Pharmacy	Dose/Route							
			Initials							

Example for a once-only drug

ONCE ONLY

Date	Time	Medicine (Approved Name)	Dose	Route	Prescriber – Sign + Print	Time Given	Given By
1/7/08	0800	CEFUROXIME	1.5 g	IV	A Doctor A DOCTOR	0800	AB
1/7/08	0800	METRONIDAZOLE	500 mg	IV	A Doctor A DOCTOR	0800	AB

Example for fluids

INFUSION THERAPY

Date	Infusion solution	Additives and dose	Volume	Rate	Route	Sign	Time Given	Given By
1/07/08	Normal saline	None	1 l	8°	IV	A Doctor	0800	AB
1/07/08	Normal saline	None	1 l	8°	IV	A Doctor		
1/07/08	5% Dextrose	20 mmol KCl	1 l	8°	IV	A Doctor		

After prescribing a drug

- If you haven't done so already, give the patient instructions for administration of the drug.
- Ask the patient is he has any questions or concerns.

Table 36. Some commonly prescribed drugs and their adult dosages

Name	Dose	Frequency	Route(s)
Analgesics			
Paracetamol	1 g	4–6 h, max 4 g / 24 h	PO/PR
Diclofenac	50 mg	TDS	PO/PR
Ibuprofen	400 mg	QDS	PO
Cocodamol 8/500 or 30/500	2 tabs	QDS	PO
Codeine phosphate	30–60 mg	4 h, max 240 mg / 24 h	PO/IM
Tramadol	50–100 mg	4 h	PO/IM/IV
Morphine	5–10 mg	4 h	PO/IM/SC
Antibiotics			
Trimethoprim	200 mg	BD	PO
Penicillin V	250–500 mg	QDS	PO
Penicillin G	300–600 mg	QDS	IV
Amoxycillin	250–500 mg	TDS	PO
Co-amoxiclav 250/125 or 500/125	1 tab	TDS	PO
Flucloxacillin	25–500 mg	QDS	PO
Cefuroxime	250–500 mg	BD	PO
Cefuroxime	750 mg–1.5 g	TDS	IV/IM
Ciprofloxacin	250–750 mg	BD	PO
Clarithromycin	250–500 mg	BD	PO
Erythromycin	250–500 mg	QDS	PO
Metronidazole	400 mg	TDS	PO

continued

Table 36. Some commonly prescribed drugs and their adult dosages – *continued*

Name	Dose	Frequency	Route(s)
Anticoagulants			
Tinzaparin DVT prophylaxis	3500 U	OD	SC
Tinzaparin DVT/PE treatment	175 U/kg	OD	SC
Dalteparin DVT prophylaxis	2500–5000 U	OD	SC
Dalteparin DVT/PE treatment	200 U/kg	OD	SC
Warfarin	As per hospital protocol and INR monitoring		
Antiemetics			
Cyclizine	50 mg	TDS	PO/IM/IV
Metoclopramide	10 mg	TDS	PO/IM/IV
Antihistamines			
Desloratadine	5 mg	OD	PO
Cetirizine	5–10 mg	OD	PO
Hypnotics			
Temazepam	10–20 mg	ON	PO
Zopiclone	3.75–7.5 mg	ON	PO
Proton pump inhibitors and antacids			
Lansoprazole	15–30 mg	OD	PO
Omeprazole	20–40 mg	OD	PO
Gaviscon®	10–20 ml	TDS	PO
Triple therapy (7 days)			
Lanzoprazole	30 mg	BD	PO
Amoxicillin	1 g	BD	PO
Clarithromycin	500 mg	BD	PO
Laxatives			
Lactulose	15 mls	BD	PO
Senna	2 tabs	ON	PO
Glycerin suppository	1–2	PRN	PR
Phosphate enema	1	PRN	PR
Movicol	1–3 sachets/day	Divided doses	PO
Other drugs			
Aspirin prophylaxis	75 mg	OD	PO
Simvastatin	10–40 mg	ON	PO
Bendrofluazide	2.5 mg	OD	PO
Lisinopril	2.5–20 mg	OD	PO

Station 107

Oxygen prescription

Table 37. Guide to oxygen masks

Type of mask	Oxygen concentration	Indications
Low flow masks Deliver a variable concentration of oxygen		
Nasal cannula	24–44% depending on the flow rate*	Patients with mild hypoxia who are otherwise stable; long-term domiciliary treatment
Simple face mask	Up to 60% at 6–10 l/min	Acutely breathless patients
Partial rebreather mask	60–80% at 10 l/min	As above
Non-rebreather mask	Up to 95% at 15 l/min	As above
High flow (Venturi) masks Deliver a fixed concentration of oxygen	24–60% in steps depending on the valve used (see *Table 38*)	'Carbon dioxide retainers' in whom oxygen control is a requirement**

* For every litre of flow delivered up to 6 litres, the oxygen concentration increases by about 4%, e.g. at 4 l/min, oxygen concentration is 36%.

**Note that the commonest cause of a high $PaCO_2$ is not carbon dioxide retention but ventilatory failure, in which the patient requires a high concentration of oxygen.

Table 38. Venturi mask valves

Valve colour	Flow rate (l/min)	Oxygen delivered (%)
Blue	2	24
White	4	28
Yellow	6	35
Red	8	40
Green	12	60

Before starting

- Introduce yourself to the patient.
- Explain the need for oxygen and ensure that the patient consents to being treated.
- Quickly observe the equipment around you. There should be a selection of oxygen masks and Venturi valves.

The procedure

- Determine the patient's oxygen saturation using a pulse oximeter, and comment upon it.
- Tell the examiner that you would like to take an arterial blood gas sample. At this point, the examiner is likely to provide you with an arterial blood gas reading.

- Interpret the arterial blood gas reading (see *Station 101*).
- Select the appropriate piece of equipment and assemble it by connecting one end of the tubing to the piece of equipment and the other end to the oxygen source.
- Adjust the oxygen flow rate as appropriate.
- Apply the equipment to the patient, ensuring a tight yet comfortable fit.
- Tell the examiner that you would like to take a second arterial blood gas sample after a certain period of time. If the examiner provides you with a second arterial blood gas reading, interpret it and make the appropriate changes (if any).

After the procedure

- Record the instructions and sign the prescription chart.
- Ask the patient if he has any questions or concerns.
- Thank the patient.

Station 108

Death confirmation

Golden lads and girls all must,
As chimney-sweepers, come to dust.

Cymbeline: Act II, Scene 2.
Shakespeare

Specifications: A mannequin in lieu of a cadaver (!)

- Take a history from a nurse (or indicate that you would do so) and consider the need for resuscitation.
- Ask for the patient's notes.
- Confirm the patient's identity: check his name tag.
- Observe the patient's general appearance and note the absence of respiratory movements.
- Ascertain that the patient does not rouse to verbal or tactile stimuli, such as pressure on a nail-bed.
- Confirm that the pupils are fixed and dilated.
- Use an ophthalmoscope to examine the fundi for segmentation of the retinal columns ('rail-roading' or 'palisading').
- Feel for the carotid pulses *on both sides*.
- Feel for the radial pulses.
- Feel for the femoral pulses.
- Auscultate over the precordium. Indicate that you would listen for one minute. Note whether the patient has a pacemaker or not (you can always look at a recent chest X-ray if you are not sure).
- Auscultate over the lungs. Indicate that you would listen for 3 minutes.
- Wash your hands.

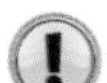

If any of your findings are non-corroboratory, you must consider the need for resuscitation.

- Make an entry in the patient's notes. Remember to include the time and date of death, and your examination findings.
- Indicate that you would:
  - consider the need for a post-mortem (see *Station 109: Death certificate completion*)
  - complete a death certificate (see *Station 109*)
  - inform the patient's GP and next of kin of the patient's death

Station 109

Death certificate completion

Legally, you can only fill in the death certificate if you have seen the patient in his last 14 days. Once the certificate is completed, it should be taken to the Registrar of Births and Deaths, usually by the patient's next of kin.

Before starting

You should understand the patient's history and the circumstances surrounding his death. You should have seen the patient's cadaver to confirm his death (or had the cadaver seen by a medically qualified colleague), noted if he had a pacemaker or radioactive implant, phoned his GP, and considered the need for a post-mortem examination (see *Table 39*).

Filling in the death certificate

In black ink, and as clearly and precisely as possible:

- Fill in the patient's:
  - name
  - date of death
  - age
  - place of death
- Fill in the date on which you last saw the patient alive.
- Circle one of the following statements:
  1. the certified cause of death takes account of information obtained from post-mortem
  2. information from post-mortem may be available later
  3. post-mortem not being held
  4. I have reported this death to the Coroner for further action
- Circle one of the following statements:
  a) seen after death by me
  b) seen after death by another medical practitioner but not by me
  c) not seen after death by a medical practitioner
- Fill in the cause of death: the disease that led directly to the patient's death is entered in Section I (a). The diseases that led to the disease entered in Section I (a) are entered in Sections I (b) and I (c).
- Fill in other significant diseases contributing to the death but not related to the disease having caused it in Section II.
- Tick the box if the death is related to employment.
- Sign the death certificate, fill in the date of issue, and print your name and medical qualification(s).
- Fill in the name of the consultant responsible for the overall care of the patient.
- Fill in the Counterfoil: record the patient's details and circumstances of death.
- Fill in the Note to Informant, and give it to the next of kin.

Table 39. Some reasons for referral to the coroner
The cause of death is uncertain.
The cause of death is due to industrial disease.
The cause of death is suspicious.
The cause of death is accidental.
The cause of death is violent.
The death is related to surgery or anaesthesia.
A doctor has not attended in the 14 days prior to the patient's death.

COUNTERFOIL

For use of Medical Practitioner, who should complete in all cases.

Name of deceased ....

Date of death ....

Age ....

Place of death ....

Last seen alive by me ....

Post-mortem/* Coroner 1 2 3 4

Whether seen after death* a b c

Cause of death:—

I (a) ....

(b) ....

(c) ....

II ....

Employment? ☐ *Please tick where applicable*

B. Further information offered?

....

Signature ....

Date ....

**Ring appropriate digit(s) and letter.*

BIRTHS AND DEATHS REGISTRATION ACT 1953

(Form prescribed by the Registration of Births and Deaths Regulations 1987)

MEDICAL CERTIFICATE OF CAUSE OF DEATH

For use only by a Registered Medical Practitioner WHO HAS BEEN IN ATTENDANCE during the deceased's last illness, and to be delivered by him forthwith to the Registrar of Births and Deaths.

Registrar to enter No. of Death Entry

Name of deceased ....

Date of death as stated to me .... day of .... Age as stated to me ....

Place of death ....

Last seen alive by me .... day of ....

1 The certified cause of death takes account of information obtained from post-mortem.
2 Information from post-mortem may be available later.
3 Post-mortem not being held.
4 I have reported this death to the Coroner for further action. *[See overleaf]*

Please ring appropriate digit(s) and letter

a Seen after death by me.
b Seen after death by another medical practitioner but not by me.
c Not seen after death by a medical practitioner.

CAUSE OF DEATH

The condition thought to be the 'Underlying Cause of Death' should appear in the lowest completed line of Part I.

I (a) Disease or condition directly leading to death† ....

(b) Other disease or condition, if any, leading to I(a) ....

(c) Other disease or condition, if any, leading to I(b) ....

II Other significant conditions CONTRIBUTING TO THE DEATH but not related to the disease or condition causing it. ....

SAMPLE

These particulars not to be entered in death register

Approximate interval between onset and death

The death might have been due to or contributed to by the employment followed at some time by the deceased. ☐ Please tick where applicable

†This does not mean the mode of dying, such as heart failure, asphyxia, asthenia, etc: it means the disease, injury, or complication which caused death.

I hereby certify that I was in medical attendance during the above named deceased's last illness, and that the particulars and cause of death above written are true to the best of my knowledge and belief.

Signature .... Qualifications as registered by General Medical Council ....

Residence .... Date ....

For deaths in hospital: Please give the name of the consultant responsible for the above-named as a patient ....

(Form prescribed by the Registration of Births and Deaths Regulations 1987)

NOTICE TO INFORMANT

I hereby give notice that I have this day signed a medical certificate of cause of death of

....

Signature ....

Date ....

This notice is to be delivered by the informant to the registrar of births and deaths for the sub-district in which the death occurred.

The certifying medical practitioner must give this notice to the person who is qualified and liable to act as informant for the registration of death (see list overleaf). Where the informant intends giving information for the registration outside of the area where the death occurred, this notice may be handed to the informant's agent.

DUTIES OF INFORMANT

Failure to deliver this notice to the registrar renders the informant liable to prosecution. The death cannot be registered until the medical certificate has reached the registrar.

When the death is registered the informant must be prepared to give to the registrar the following particulars relating to the deceased:

1. The date and place of death.
2. The full name and surname (and the maiden surname if the deceased was a woman who had married).
3. The date and place of birth.
4. The occupation (and if the deceased was a married woman or a widow the name and occupation of her husband).
5. The usual address.
6. Whether the deceased was in receipt of a pension or allowance from public funds.
7. If the deceased was married, the date of birth of the surviving widow or widower.

THE DECEASED'S MEDICAL CARD SHOULD BE DELIVERED TO THE REGISTRAR

PERSONS QUALIFIED AND LIABLE TO ACT AS INFORMANTS

The following persons are designated by the Births and Deaths Registration Act 1953 as qualified to give information concerning a death; in order of preference they are:

DEATHS IN HOUSES AND PUBLIC INSTITUTIONS

(1) A relative of the deceased, present at the death.

(2) A relative of the deceased, in attendance during the last illness.

(3) A relative of the deceased, residing or being in the sub-district where the death occurred.

(4) A person present at the death.

(5) The occupier* if he knew of the happening of the death.

(6) Any inmate if he knew of the happening of the death.

(7) The person causing the disposal of the body.

DEATHS NOT IN HOUSES OR DEAD BODIES FOUND

(1) Any relative of the deceased having knowledge of any of the particulars required to be registered.

(2) Any person present at the death.

(3) Any person who found the body.

(4) Any person in charge of the body.

(5) The person causing the disposal of the body.

*"Occupier" in relation to a public institution includes the governor, keeper, master, matron, superintendent, or other chief resident officer.

Complete where applicable

A	B
I have reported this death to the Coroner for further action. Initials of certifying medical practitioner.	I may be in a position later to give, on application by the Registrar General, additional information as to the cause of death for the purpose of more precise statistical classification. Initials of certifying medical practitioner. ....

The death should be referred to the coroner if:

- the cause of death is unknown
- the deceased was not seen by the certifying doctor *either* after death *or* within the 14 days before death
- the death was violent or unnatural or was suspicious
- the death may be due to an accident (whenever it occurred)
- the death may be due to self-neglect or neglect by others
- the death may be due to an industrial disease or related to the deceased's employment
- the death may be due to an abortion
- the death occurred during an operation or before recovery from the effects of an anaesthetic
- the death may be a suicide
- the death occurred during or shortly after detention in police or prison custody

LIST OF SOME OF THE CATEGORIES OF DEATH WHICH MAY BE OF INDUSTRIAL ORIGIN

MALIGNANT DISEASES	Causes include
(a) Skin	– radiation and sunlight – pitch or tar – mineral oils
(b) Nasal	– wood or leather work – nickel
(c) Lung	– asbestos – chromates – nickel – radiation
(d) Pleura and peritoneum	– asbestos
(e) Urinary tract	– benzidine – dyestuff manufacture – rubber manufacture
(f) Liver	– PVC manufacture
(g) Bone	– radiation
(h) Lymphatics and haematopoietic	– radiation – benzene
POISONING	
(a) Metals	e.g. arsenic, cadmium, lead
(b) Chemicals	e.g. chlorine, benzene
(c) Solvents	e.g. trichlorethylene

INFECTIOUS DISEASES	Causes include
(a) Anthrax	– imported bone, bonemeal hide or fur
(b) Brucellosis	– farming or veterinary
(c) Tuberculosis	– contact at work
(d) Leptospirosis	– farming, sewer or under-ground workers
(e) Tetanus	– farming or gardening
(f) Rabies	– animal handling
(g) Viral hepatitis	– contact at work
CHRONIC LUNG DISEASES	
(a) Occupational asthma	– sensitising agent at work
(b) Allergic alveolitis	– farming
(c) Pneumoconiosis	– mining and quarrying – potteries – asbestos
(d) Chronic bronchitis and emphysema	– underground coal mining

NOTE:—The Practitioner, on signing the certificate, should complete, sign and date the Notice to the Informant, which should be detached and handed to the informant. Where the informant intends giving information for the registration outside of the area where the death occurred, the notice may be handed to the informant's agent. The Practitioner should then, without delay, deliver the certificate itself to the Registrar of Births and Deaths for the sub-district in which the death occurred. Envelopes for enclosing the certificates are supplied by the Registrar.

Figure 103. Copy of death certificate.

Explaining skills

These skills can be used to explain a common condition, to explain an investigation, or to explain a procedure or treatment. They can also be used in your private life, although it may then be unwise to draw a diagram or hand out a leaflet.

What to do

- Introduce yourself.
- Summarise the patient's presenting symptoms.
- Tell the patient what you are going to explain.
- Determine how much the patient already knows.
- Determine how much the patient would like to know.
- Elicit the patient's main concerns.
- Deliver the information.
  - for a medical disorder: aetiology, epidemiology, clinical features, investigations/treatment, prognosis
  - for a pharmacological treatment: name, mechanism of action, procedure involved (dose, route of administration, frequency, precautions), principal benefits, principal side-effects, principal contraindications, alternatives including no treatment
  - for an investigative procedure: purpose, description of the procedure, principal risks, alternatives including no investigation, preparation required, after the procedure, results
  - for a surgical procedure: purpose, description of the procedure, principal risks, alternatives including no surgery, preparation required, anaesthetic procedure, post-operative care (e.g. recovery room, oxygen, blood pressure monitoring, etc.), analgesia
- Summarise and check understanding.
- Encourage and address questions.

How to do it

- Be empathetic.
- Explore the patient's feelings.
- Give the most important information first.
- Be specific.
- Regularly check understanding.
- Pitch the explanation at the patient's level. Use simple language and short sentences. If using a medical or technical term, explain it in layman's terms.
- Use diagrams, if appropriate.
- Hand out a leaflet.
- Be honest. If you are unsure about something, say you will find out later and get back to the patient.

What not to do

- Hurry.
- Reassure too soon.
- Be patronising.
- Give too much information.
- Use medical jargon.
- Confabulate (make things up).

"Really, now you ask me," said Alice, very much confused, "I don't think –"
"Then you shouldn't talk," said the Hatter.

Alice's Adventures in Wonderland: A Mad Tea-Party
Lewis Carroll

Some of the medical disorders, pharmacological treatments, investigative procedures, and surgical procedures that you may be asked to explain in an OSCE are listed below.
Information can be obtained from websites such as:
www.patient.co.uk
www.besttreatments.co.uk
www.kch.nhs.uk/patients/general-information/leaflets/

Medical disorders

- Asthma
- Diabetes
- Hypertension
- Angina
- Dementia
- Miscarriage
- Osteoarthritis/rheumatoid arthritis

Pharmacological treatments

- Statins
- Antibiotics
- Asthma inhalers
- Corticosteroids
- Insulin
- Antihypertensives
- Antidepressants
- Analgesics
- Glyceryl trinitrate
- Contraceptive pill (emergency pill, combined pill, progestogen-only preparations)
- Pessaries and suppositories
- Skin preparations, e.g. emollient, steroid cream, sunscreen

Investigative procedures

- Chest or abdominal X-ray
- CT scan
- MRI scan
- Ultrasound scan
- Echocardiography
- Flexible bronchoscopy
- Ventilation/perfusion scan
- Spirometry
- Oesophagogastroduodenoscopy (OGD)

- Barium swallow/meal/follow-through
- Barium enema
- Flexible sigmoidoscopy
- Colonoscopy
- Cystoscopy

Surgical procedures

- Angioplasty
- Laparoscopic cholecystectomy
- Endoscopic retrograde cholangiopancreatography (ERCP)
- Inguinal hernia repair
- Transurethral resection of the prostate (TURP)
- Hip/knee replacement
- Varicose vein stripping

Obtaining consent

Common questions

The purpose of gaining consent

Consent is needed on every occasion a doctor wishes to initiate an investigation or treatment or any other intervention, except in emergencies or where the law dictates otherwise (such as where compulsory treatment is authorised under the Mental Health Act).

How long is consent valid for?

Consent should be seen as a continuing process rather than a one-off decision. When there has been a significant period of time between the patient agreeing to a procedure and its start, consent should be reaffirmed.

Refusal of treatment

Competent adult patients are entitled to refuse treatment even when doing so may result in permanent physical injury or death. For example, a competent Jehovah's Witness can refuse a blood transfusion even if he will surely die as a result. An adult patient is competent if he can:

- Understand what the intervention is.
- Understand why the intervention is being proposed.
- Understand the alternatives to the intervention, including no intervention.
- Understand the principal benefits and risks of the intervention and of its alternatives.
- Understand the consequences of the intervention and of its alternatives.
- Retain the information for long enough to weigh it in the balance and reach a reasoned decision, whatever that decision may be. In some cases, the patient may not have the cognitive ability or emotional maturity to reach a reasoned decision, or may be unduly affected by mental illness.

Obtaining consent

When seeking to obtain consent, it is important not to be seen to be rattling through a list of 'must dos', but trying to elicit the patient's ideas, concerns, and expectations, and tailoring your explanations accordingly.

- The type of information that should be provided to obtain consent includes:
  - what the intervention is (use diagrams if this is helpful)
  - why the intervention is being proposed
  - alternatives to the intervention, including no intervention
  - the principal benefits and risks of the intervention and of its alternatives
  - the consequences of the intervention and of its alternatives
- Ask the patient to summarise the above information, and be certain that he is competent to give consent.
- Remind the patient that he does not have to make an immediate decision and that he can change his decision at any time.

Breaking bad news

What to do

- Introduce yourself.
- Look to comfort and privacy.
- Determine what the patient already knows.
- Determine what the patient would like to know.
- Warn the patient that bad news is coming.
- Break the bad news.
- Identify the patient's main concerns.
- Summarise and check understanding.
- Offer realistic hope.
- Arrange follow-up.
- Try to ensure there is someone with the patient when he leaves.

How to do it

- Be sensitive.
- Be empathetic.
- Maintain eye contact.
- Give information in small chunks.
- Repeat and clarify.
- Regularly check understanding.
- Give the patient time to respond. Do not be afraid of silence or of tears.
- Explore the patient's emotions.
- Use physical contact if this feels natural to you.
- Be honest. If you are unsure about something, say you will find out later and get back to the patient.

What not to do

- Hurry.
- Give all the information in one go, or give too much information.
- Use euphemisms or medical jargon.
- Lie or be economical with the truth.
- Be blunt. Words are like loaded pistols, as Jean-Paul Sartre once said.
- Prognosticate (*she's got six months, maybe seven*).

The angry patient or relative

I was angry with my friend:
I told my wrath, my wrath did end.
I was angry with my foe:
I told it not, my wrath did grow.

William Blake

The 'angry person' station can be rather unnerving, if only because medical students – and especially medical students in the earlier years of their training – are relatively sheltered from such persons.

The aim of the game is to diffuse the person's anger, *not* to ignore, placate or rationalise it. You should therefore try to be as empathetic and non-confrontational as possible.

What to do

- Introduce yourself.
- Acknowledge the person's anger.
- Try to find out the reason for his anger, e.g. frustration, fear, guilt.
- Validate his feelings.
- Let him vent his anger, or any feelings that led to his anger, e.g. frustration, fear, guilt.
- Offer to do something or for him to do something.

How to do it

- Sit at the same level as the person, not too close but not too far either.
- Make eye contact.
- Speak calmly and do not raise your voice.
- Avoid dismissive or threatening body language.
- Encourage the person to speak. Ask open rather than closed questions, and use verbal and non-verbal cues to show that you are listening.
- Empathise as much as you can.

What not to do

- Glare at the person.
- Confront him.
- Interrupt him.
- Patronise him.
- Get too close to or touch him.
- Block his exit route.
- Put the blame on others/seek to exonerate yourself.
- Make unreasonable promises.
- If the person is a patient's relative, be mindful of potential confidentiality issues.

The anxious or upset patient or relative

What to do

- Look to comfort and privacy.
- Introduce yourself and try to establish rapport.
- Acknowledge the person's emotional state, e.g. *"You seem to be very upset."*
- Explore his feelings, e.g. *"What's making you so upset?"*
- Validate his feelings, e.g. *"I think that most people would feel that way in your situation."*
- Provide honest and accurate information about the situation.
- Offer to do something or for him to do something.
- Summarise and conclude.

How to do it

- Encourage him to speak, e.g. by asking open rather than closed questions and by prompting him on, e.g. *"Can you tell me more about that?"*
- Show that you are listening, e.g. by making appropriate eye contact, adjusting your body posture, and using appropriate verbal and non-verbal cues.
- Be empathetic.
- Use silence at appropriate times. If the person sheds tears, give him the time and space to do so and hand him a tissue.
- Use physical contact if this feels natural to you.
- Remain poised: speak calmly, use simple sentences, and pace the information that you give.
- Repeat and clarify the information that you give, and check understanding.
- Encourage questions.

What not to do

- Ask only closed questions.
- Interrupt or rush him.
- Do all the talking.
- Dismiss or trivialise his feelings.
- Reassure too soon.
- Offer inappropriate reassurance or false hope, e.g.
  - *"There's absolutely nothing to be afraid of, everything will be just fine."*
  - *"Sure she's dead, but you'll get over her much sooner than you think."*
  - *"I'm sure your father's in a better place now."*
- If the person is a patient's relative, be mindful of potential confidentiality issues.

Cross-cultural communication

You do not need to have a Masters in anthropology from the School of Oriental and African Studies to score highly in this station. All you need to do is use some basic communication strategies, as detailed here. It is also important that you are seen to respect the patient's beliefs and/or values.

- Introduce yourself to the patient, and ensure that he is comfortable.
- Ask the patient's name, age, and occupation.
- Determine the patient's reason for attending.
- Elicit the patient's:
  - **I**deas
  - **C**oncerns
  - **E**xpectations

  (**ICE**)
- Establish:
  - the patient's cultural or religious group
  - the implications that this has on his reason for attending
  - the patient's individual beliefs and values
- Check that you have understood the patient's problems.
- Explore possible solutions, and agree a mutually satisfactory course of action.
- Summarise the consultation.
- Check the patient's understanding.
- Thank the patient.

Discharge planning and negotiation

Setting the scene

- Introduce yourself to the patient.
- Summarise the situation to him.
- Explore the impact that the illness/hospitalisation has had on him.
- Explore his current mood and disposition.

Going home and after

- Explain that you are considering for the patient to go home.
- Elicit and address any concerns that he may have about going home. Reassure him that transport can be organised, if need be.
- Explore his home situation and support system.
- In people who are elderly or disabled, assess Activities of Daily Living (ADL): grooming, bathing, dressing, feeding, bladder, bowels, toilet use, transfer, mobility, stairs.
- Consider any extra help that can be offered to the patient, for example, social services, home help, *meals on wheels*, health visitor, district nurse, specialist nurses, palliative care team, dietician, occupational therapist, speech (language) therapist, physiotherapist, psychologist, continence advisor, self-help group, day centre.
- Discuss medication and compliance. Check that the patient doesn't have any concerns about taking his discharge medication and reassure him that the pharmacy can supply a Dossett box, if need be.
- Address risk factors. Suggest lifestyle changes that the patient may benefit from, such as stopping smoking, eating a balanced diet, taking regular exercise, etc.
- Offer the patient a follow-up appointment either at his GP surgery or in the Out-Patient Department.

Before finishing

- Summarise what has been said.
- Check the patient's understanding of what has been said.
- Ask the patient if he has any further questions or concerns.
- Thank the patient.

Clinical Skills for OSCEs DVD

John Goodfellow and Neel Burton

There is much about clinical skills that cannot be conveyed through the written word and that students find difficult to visualise in their mind's eye. This DVD aims to expose you to a range of different clinicians, all performing near the level of the gold standard, and to a range of different patients. For each clinical skill, you should be able to get a feel not only for the steps involved, but also for their orchestration, and for the type of doctor–patient interaction that they call upon.

Of course, the DVD cannot feature each and every clinical skill, and priority has been given to those clinical skills that are used most regularly by most junior doctors, and that are most commonly examined in the course of undergraduate training.

Film 1. Venepuncture/phlebotomy
Film 2. Cannulation and setting up a drip
Film 3. Scrubbing up for theatre
Film 4. Chest pain history
Film 5. Cardiovascular examination
Film 6. Peripheral vascular system examination
Film 7. Breathlessness history
Film 8. Respiratory system examination
Film 9. Abdominal pain history
Film 10. Abdominal examination
Film 11. Nasogastric intubation
Film 12. Urological history
Film 13. Male catheterisation
Film 14. Female catheterisation
Film 15. History of headaches
Film 16. History of 'funny turns'
Film 17. Cranial nerve examination
Film 18. Depression history
Film 19. Suicide risk assessment
Film 20. Alcohol history
Film 21. Hearing and the ear examination
Film 22. Vision and the eye examination
Film 23. Lump in the neck examination
Film 24. HIV risk assessment
Film 25. Hand and wrist examination
Film 26. Hip examination
Film 27. Adult basic life support
Film 28. Syringe driver operation
Film 29. Wound suturing

The DVD also includes 100 mock marking schemes for you to practise with in pairs or in small groups.